EMOTION AND CONSCIOUSNESS

Emotion *and*
CONSCIOUSNESS

Edited by

Lisa Feldman Barrett

Paula M. Niedenthal

Piotr Winkielman

THE GUILFORD PRESS
New York   London

© 2005 The Guilford Press
A Division of Guilford Publications, Inc.
72 Spring Street, New York, NY 10012
www.guilford.com

Printed in the United States of America

This book is printed on acid-free paper.

Last digit is print number: 9   8   7   6   5   4   3   2   1

Library of Congress Cataloging-in-Publication Data

Emotion and consciousness / edited by Lisa Feldman Barrett, Paula M.
   Niedenthal & Piotr Winkielman.
        p. cm.
   Includes bibliographical references and index.
   ISBN 1-59385-188-X (cloth)
   1. Consciousness.   2. Emotions.   3. Emotions and cognition.
   I. Barrett, Lisa Feldman.   II. Niedenthal, Paula M.
   III. Winkielman, Piotr.
   BF311.E4855 2005
   152.4—dc22

                                                    2005001276

About the Editors

Lisa Feldman Barrett, PhD, completed her doctoral training at the University of Waterloo, Canada, and is now a professor of psychology at Boston College. Her major research focus addresses questions about the experience of emotion from social-psychological, psychophysiological, cognitive science, and neuroscience perspectives. Dr. Barrett's research has been funded by the National Science Foundation, and she currently holds an Independent Research Scientist Award from the National Institute of Mental Health. She is currently a fellow of the American Psychological Society and a consulting editor for *Emotion,* the *Journal of Personality and Social Psychology, Personality and Social Psychology Bulletin,* and *Personality and Social Psychology Review,* and edited, with Peter Salovey, *The Wisdom in Feeling: Psychological Processes in Emotional Intelligence* (2002, Guilford Press).

Paula M. Niedenthal, PhD, received her doctorate in social psychology from the University of Michigan and was an assistant professor at Johns Hopkins University until she moved to Indiana University in 1993. She was promoted to full professor there in 1998 but, while on sabbatical in Aix-en-Provence, decided to relocate to France. Dr. Niedenthal is now Director of Research in the National Centre for Scientific Research (CNRS) and is a member of the Laboratory in Social and Cognitive Psychology at Blaise Pascal University, Clermont-Ferrand, France. Author of more than 65 academic articles and chapters and several books, she has recently been associate editor of the journals *Cognition and Emotion* and *Personality and Social Psychology Bulletin.* Dr. Niedenthal is a fellow of the Society for Personality and Social Psychology and is currently at work on a textbook on the study of emotion in social psychology with colleagues Silvia Krauth-Gruber and François Ric, both at René Descartes University, Paris.

Piotr Winkielman, PhD, completed his doctorate at the University of
Michigan and received postdoctoral training in social neuroscience at The
Ohio State University, after attending the University of Warsaw in Poland
and the University of Bielefeld in Germany for his undergraduate studies.
He is now an associate professor of psychology at the University of
California–San Diego. Dr. Winkielman's current research focuses on the
relation between emotion, cognition, body, and consciousness using
psychological and psychophysiological approaches. His research has been
supported by the National Science Foundation and National Alliance for
Autism Research and he has served on the editorial boards of the *Journal
of Personality and Social Psychology* and *Personality and Social Psychology
Bulletin.*

Contributors

Ralph Adolphs, PhD, Department of Neurology, Division of Cognitive Neuroscience and Behavioral Neurology, University of Iowa College of Medicine, Iowa City, Iowa, and Department of Psychology and Neuroscience,California Institute of Technology, Pasadena, California

Anthony P. Atkinson, PhD, Department of Psychology, University of Durham Science Site, Durham, United Kingdom

Jo-Anne Bachorowski, PhD, Department of Psychology, Vanderbilt University, Nashville, Tennessee

Lisa Feldman Barrett, PhD, Department of Psychology, Boston College, Chestnut Hill, Massachusetts

Lawrence W. Barsalou, PhD, Department of Psychology, Emory University, Atlanta, Georgia

Kent C. Berridge, PhD, Department of Psychology, University of Michigan, Ann Arbor, Michigan

Mark E. Bouton, PhD, Department of Psychology, University of Vermont, Burlington, Vermont

Todd S. Braver, PhD, Department of Psychology, Washington University, St. Louis, Missouri

David B. Centerbar, PhD, Department of Psychology, University of Virginia, Charlottesville, Virginia

Louis C. Charland, PhD, Department of Philosophy, Department of Psychiatry, and Faculty of Health Sciences, University of Western Ontario, London, Ontario, Canada

Gerald L. Clore, PhD, Department of Psychology, University of Virginia, Charlottesville, Virginia

Beatrice de Gelder, PhD, Faculty of Social and Behavioral Sciences, Tilburg University, Tilburg, The Netherlands

Jeremy R. Gray, PhD, Department of Psychology, Yale University, New Haven, Connecticut

Silvia Krauth-Gruber, PhD, Social Psychology Laboratory, René Descartes University, Paris, France

Daniel Lundqvist, PhD, Psychology Section, Department of Clinical Neuroscience, Karolinska Institute, Stockholm, Sweden

Steven B. Most, PhD, Department of Psychology, Yale University, New Haven, Connecticut

Roland Neumann, PhD, Department of Psychology, Würzburg University, Würzburg, Germany

Paula M. Niedenthal, PhD, Laboratory of Social and Cognitive Psychology, Blaise Pascal University, Clermont-Ferrand, France

Arne Öhman, PhD, Psychology Section, Department of Clinical Neuroscience, Karolinska Institute, Stockholm, Sweden

Michael J. Owren, PhD, Department of Psychology, Cornell University, Ithaca, New York

Elizabeth A. Phelps, PhD, Department of Psychology, New York University, New York, New York

Jesse J. Prinz, PhD, Department of Philosophy, University of North Carolina, Chapel Hill, North Carolina

Drew Rendall, PhD, Department of Psychology and Neuroscience, University of Lethbridge, Lethbridge, Alberta, Canada

François Ric, PhD, Social Psychology Laboratory, René Descartes University, Paris, France

Michael D. Robinson, PhD, Department of Psychology, North Dakota State University, Fargo, North Dakota

Alexandre Schaefer, PhD, Department of Psychology, Yale University, New Haven, Connecticut

Klaus R. Scherer, PhD, Department of Psychology, University of Geneva, Geneva, Switzerland

Eliot R. Smith, PhD, Department of Psychology, Indiana University, Bloomington, Indiana

Justin Storbeck, MA, Department of Psychology, University of Virginia, Charlottesville, Virginia

Julia L. Wilbarger, PhD, Department of Psychology, University of Wisconsin–Madison, Madison, Wisconsin

Piotr Winkielman, PhD, Department of Psychology, University of California–San Diego, San Diego, California

Contents

PART III. UNCONSCIOUS EMOTIONAL BEHAVIOR

PART IV. THE EXPERIENCE OF EMOTION

PART V. PERSPECTIVES ON
THE CONSCIOUS–UNCONSCIOUS DEBATE

CHAPTER 1

Introduction

Lisa Feldman Barrett
Paula M. Niedenthal
Piotr Winkielman

The idea that emotion reflects a combination of conscious and unconscious processes dates back to the beginning of Western philosophy, when Plato and Aristotle noticed that some emotions, such as anger, can arise via careful deliberation (e.g., about injustice), via an impulsive reaction (e.g., to pain), or via a combination of both. Scientific interest in the role of consciousness in emotion was perhaps first stimulated by William James, who asserted that emotion is a *conscious* perception of bodily changes, which themselves can have *unconscious* origins. This interest in the interplay between conscious and unconscious contributions to emotional responding has reemerged in recent years, as scientists have placed the study of emotion at the center of scientific inquiry about the human condition, and as the study of consciousness has, again, become scientifically respectable. Fields with broadly differing epistemological frameworks (e.g., cultural anthropology, philosophy, psychology, cognitive science, and various forms of neuroscience) all study something called "emotion." And, as emotion research in these fields progresses at many levels of analysis, questions about the relationship between emotion and consciousness remain at the center of the investigations (even if only to highlight that consciousness is *not* the defining feature of an emotional state). Questions about the interplay of emotion and consciousness have expanded from examining the place of conscious feelings in emotional responding to include related issues, such as (1) how unconscious analysis of the incoming stimulus might produce emotional responses, (2) how conscious processes regulate emotional responding (and vice versa), (3) the role of consciousness in the integration of emotion and cognition, (4) the role of bodily responses in conscious and unconscious aspects of emotion, (5) how unconscious processes produce a conscious feeling of emotion, and so on.

Unfortunately, it is commonplace for researchers who work on these diverse questions to proceed independently of one another, and to focus on one question in the absence of addressing the others. Often, theoretical models of this and that phenomenon do not have sufficient contact with one another to allow for development of large-scale theory building about emotion. Further, the existing models often fail to keep pace with the flood of experimental findings that have been generated. In addition to these problems of communication, progress in understanding the nature of emotion is hampered by disagreements about how the two critical terms, *emotion* and *consciousness*, should be defined. It often seems as if researchers who approach the study of emotion from different perspectives and who define these terms differently, inhabit different planets that orbit one another but rarely, if ever, make contact.

The present volume came about as an attempt to address these issues and bring needed coherence to the scientific study of emotion and consciousness. This interdisciplinary book brings together researchers who are working on different components of emotion processing and presents the major themes guiding their research. These major themes are represented by the five sections into which the volume is organized. Parts I through IV—Cognition and Emotion, Unconscious Emotional Processing: Perception of Visual Stimuli, Unconscious Emotional Behavior, and The Experience of Emotion—offer an up-to-date review of research relevant to different conscious and unconscious components of emotion. Part IV, Perspectives on the Conscious–Unconscious Debate, specifically discusses which emotion processes are conscious and unconscious and provides various perspectives on how these processes configure to produce an "emotion episode." To bring further coherence and clarity to the volume, the authors were asked to answer the following three questions either within the text of their chapter or in the boxes within the chapters. The first question addressed the definition of emotion ("What is the scope of your proposed model? When you use the term *emotion*, how do you use it? What do you mean by terms such as *fear, anxiety,* or *happiness*?"). The second question addressed how the concept of consciousness is understood ("Define your terms: *conscious, unconscious, awareness.* Or say why you do not use the terms."). The third question asked authors to consider how conscious and unconscious emotion-related processes are configured in their chapter

("Does your model deal with what is conscious, what is unconscious, or their relationship? If you do not address the issue of consciousness specifically, can you speculate on the relationship between what is conscious and unconscious? Or if you do not like the conscious–unconscious distinction, or if you do not think this is a good question to ask, can you say why?").

The three overarching questions and the major themes of the volume emerged at the end of a 3-day conference held in the Auvergne region of France in September 2003, at which all authors presented the substance of their chapters. The most remarkable aspect of the conference was discovering the similarity in concerns across theorists. Rather than a set of unrelated talks by neuroscientists, social psychologists, animal behaviorists, cognitive psychologists, and philosophers, the talks revealed enormous areas of commonality among the contributors. In fact, the conference confirmed our belief that the field is "ready" for a systematic attempt to integrate the various themes of research on conscious and unconscious processes in emotion. In what follows, we give a short preview of the major themes of the five sections and the sixteen chapters. As we preview the chapters, we hope that the reader will notice the coherence of the message that emerges from the book, despite the diversity of topics and the authors' differing disciplinary orientations.

THE CHAPTERS

Cognition and Emotion

Part I of the volume deals with the interaction between processes that have been conventionally called *emotion* and *cognition*. Together, these three chapters begin to characterize the possible relationships between thinking and feeling and, in so doing, sketch a broad framework for understanding the emergence and interplay of conscious and unconscious processes in emotional responding. Clarifying this relationship sets the stage for chapters that directly address how conscious and unconscious processes might interact to produce an experience that can be reported.

In Chapter 2, Paul N. Niedenthal, Lawrence W. Barsalou, François Ric, and Sylvia Krauth-Gruber introduce an idea that appears in several chapters (e.g., Anthony P. Atkinson & Ralph Adolphs, Chapter 7; Daniel Lundqvist & Arne Öhman, Chapter 5; Beatrice de Gelder, Chapter 6; Lisa Feldman Barrett, Chapter 11; Jesse J. Prinz, Chapter 15)—that (1) perceiving someone else's emotion, (2) having an emotional response or a subjective feeling state, and (3) using emotion knowledge in conceptual tasks, all draw on fundamentally the same process that relies on somatosensory and motor representations (or embodiments). Niedenthal and colleagues review considerable evidence in support of the notion that emotional processing is embodied. First, they review research showing that individuals embody the emotional gestures of other people, including facial expressions, posture, and vocal affect. They then build on these findings to argue that imitative behavior produces a corresponding state in the perceiver, leading to the general suggestion that embodied knowledge produces felt emotional states. They summarize evidence in support of the idea that both facial and postural poses facilitate the experience of emotions. The reverse is also true. Having participants imagine emotionally evocative situations to induce an emotional state produces changes in the body, although those changes are often nonspecifically associated with pleasant and unpleasant affect rather than distinct profiles of discrete emotions of anger, sadness, fear, and so on. Finally, Niedenthal et al. discuss how physical actions (e.g., arm flexion or extension, posing facial muscles) influence how well participants identify positive and negative information, how they evaluate stimuli (whether they like an ideograph or find a cartoon funny), and how well they remember details from an evocative story. Taken together, these behavioral results validate the plausibility of an embodiment view of emotional processing.

In the next section of their chapter, Niedenthal and colleagues explain how embodied representations can constitute the core conceptual content of emotion knowledge. The general point is that the body provides a fundamental way of representing knowledge about emotion. Such a view of emotional processing, they contend, allows theorists to identify more precisely which processes are, or can be, unconscious and which are conscious. In particular, Niedenthal et al. return to William James's notion that parts of embodied emotion are unconscious, or can be so, until attention is directed to them. Subjective feelings of emotion, such as the perception of bodily changes, are always conscious. In this, Niedenthal et al. agree with other contributors (e.g., Barrett, Chapter 11) that individual and cultural differences in emotion can best be conceptualized in terms of the representations that guide the direction and interpretation of the content of conscious perception.

In Chapter 3, Elizabeth A. Phelps begins with the observation that the neural systems believed to underlie "emotional" processes overlap extensively with those that are involved in "cognition," leading to questions of whether or not these are really separate processing domains. Phelps echoes a point advanced several years ago by Lane, Nadel, Allen, and Kaszniak (2000), which is consistent with other contributors to this volume, all of whom suggest that the neural architecture involved with emotional processing overlaps significantly with that which is related to cognitive processing (Atkinson & Adolphs, Chapter 7; Jeremy R. Gray, Alexandre Schaefer, Todd S. Braver, & Steven B. Most, Chapter 4; Phelps, Chapter 3;

Piotr Winkielman, Kent C. Berridge, & Julia L. Wilbarger, Chapter 14). Specifically, Phelps's chapter focuses on the functions of the human amygdala, a small structure in the medial temporal lobe that is the centerpiece of many emotion models and that figures prominently in many of the chapters in this volume. Phelps advances the popular view that the amygdala is a brain region whose primary function is linked to emotion. She discusses how the amygdala is intimately involved in directing behavioral responses to the emotional significance of a stimulus in a way that is unconscious, unintentional, and may be independent from the process that generates conscious experience of emotion. Her review of her recent research on instructed fear (i.e., the valenced consequences of a stimulus are conveyed through language rather than direct experience) indicates that the amygdala also plays a role in the expression of fears that are learned symbolically (via involvement of the hippocampus) and that depend on awareness and interpretation in a way that is reminiscent of the rule-based processing discussed by Eliot R. Smith and Roland Neumann (Chapter 12). Finally, Phelps discusses how the amygdala influences attention and perception (a point underscored in several other chapters as well) and modulates long-term memory by modulating the storage of hippocampal-dependent memories. As a result of these modulatory mechanisms, individuals are more likely to become aware of emotional events as they occur.

In Chapter 3, Gray, Schaefer, Braver, and Most discuss how affect functions to resolve "control dilemmas"—that is, situations in which the organism is prepared to do more than one thing. First, they propose how affect can resolve control dilemmas that may be conscious; for example, approach–avoidance conflicts. Although a person may be strongly motivated to both approach and withdraw from something, presumably because multiple processing systems for positive and negative affect exist within the brain (Cacioppo, Gardner, & Bernston, 1999), it is impossible to do so simultaneously. Gray and colleagues also review recent findings from their laboratory that suggest that approach-related affective states (e.g., amusement) enhance verbal working memory, whereas withdrawal-related states (e.g., anxiety) enhance spatial working memory. These findings are broadly consistent with the idea that threat can enhance visual processing, presumably because it is important to know where a threat is located.

Second, Gray and colleagues discuss how affect can resolve unconscious control dilemmas, such as those that involve selective attention. For example, individuals demonstrate the phenomenon of attentional capture when threatening information preferentially draws their attention. Current affective states, mood, or chronic affective styles might help to resolve such instances, freeing individuals from the constraints of the immediate features of the external environment. The general idea that runs throughout this chapter, then, is that affect impacts thought and behavior by "tuning" the more cognitive parts of the system to prioritize some functions over others, perhaps when other forms of conflict management, such as contention scheduling, fail to work. Gray et al. suggest (as do others in this volume, e.g., Louis C. Charland, Chapter 10; Barrett, Chapter 11) that affect is a type of valuation function that allows the individual to regulate the influence of internal and external constraints (i.e., the demands of the situation as well as the subjective importance of the event).

Unconscious Emotional Processing: Perception of Visual Stimuli

Part II of the volume describes the mechanisms implicated in the act of perceiving an emotional episode in another person. The chapters in this section (Lundqvist & Öhman, Chapter 5; de Gelder, Chapter 6; and Atkinson & Adolphs, Chapter 7) emphasize the early perceptual contributions to emotional responding (in contrast to the relatively later, more conceptual processing that involves knowledge and memory; e.g., Niedenthal et al., Chapter 2) and fill in some of the detail that other chapters draw on when discussing the interplay of the two (e.g., Phelps, Chapter 3; Smith & Neumann, Chapter 12; and Klaus R. Scherer, Chapter 13).

The three chapters included in this section have several points in common. Most importantly, all discuss the time-line for assessing the evaluative significance of a visual stimulus (primarily the processing of static faces, because that is the focus of most research). These chapters address the early processes that allow a person (1) to code the evaluative significance of visual stimuli, or (2) to detect fear, depending on the underlying assumptions. The early or "low" pathway (involving the superior colliculus and pulvinar nucleus of the thalamus) unconsciously conveys low-frequency information to the amygdala for the initial coding of evaluative significance. This mechanism mediates affective reactions to a stimulus even before it is registered in consciousness, and allows people with blindsight to code the affective significance of things they cannot consciously see. De Gelder, in particular, reviews the literature that investigates the existence of such a pathway, and whether there are additional sensory contributions to blindsight, such as subjective feelings. This pathway is activated within the first 100 milliseconds of evaluative processing. By approximately 300 milliseconds, higher-frequency visual information is conveyed via a later or "high" pathway that provides object-identification information to the visual cortex. This information combines with feedback from the amygdala to the visual cortex, which modulates sensory processing by directing attention to those aspects of the environment that are most salient to the organism for dealing with threatening information. It is via these connections that the amygdala evaluates facets of the affective significance of complex objects (such as faces).

De Gelder and Atkinson and Adolphs (Chapters 6 and 7) are similar in other respects as well. Both discuss whether the scientific findings on emotion perception of static faces generalizes to understanding dynamic facial and body movements. In daily life, information from the face is processed in the context of information coming from other modalities, such as body movements, voice, and so on. Although scientific investigations tend to focus on how organisms process information from one sensory system at a time (usually the visual system in humans, the auditory system in rats), information processing in everyday life is typically multimodal. Thus this is an important emerging area of research in understanding emotion perception. Both chapters also discuss how perception might interact with the subjective experience of emotion or feelings. De Gelder suggests that feelings help guide people with blindsight. Atkinson and Adolphs point out overlap in neural areas involved in emotion perception and those correlated with the subjective experience of emotion, suggesting that the two processes may inform one another. This emphasis on embodiment in perception and experience of emotion is a unifying theme in many of the chapters.

Lundqvist and Öhman (Chapter 5) begin their chapter by identifying an assumption that is largely agreed upon by emotion researchers (although there are alternative points of view, e.g., Michael J. Owren, Drew Rendall, and Jo-Anne Backorowski, Chapter 8; Barrett, Chapter 11). These authors argue that humans emit stereotypic behaviors that encode and signal the presence of specific emotions, and that this ability evolved in concert with efficient routines for automatically decoding facial signals. Evolution has equipped humans with an expressive face to send emotional signals, as well as a highly efficient system for decoding these signals and therefore recognizing threatening versus friendly faces. Lundqvist and Öhman review research in which faces depicting emotional configurations, presented under conditions that prevent their representation in conscious awareness, evoke psychophysical and neural responses that reflect nonspecific emotional (some might say *affective*) activation. The emotional expression on a face (threatening or friendly) regulates subsequent visual processing in a preattentive way. As a result, threatening faces (when compared to friendly faces) stand out more from the background and are easier to detect. Moreover, Lundqvist and Öhman outline how specific features of the face preattentively direct subsequent processing. In particular, eyebrows are important for conveying affective importance (followed by mouth and eyes). They go on to provide a model for facial signal decoding that integrates LeDoux's (1996) research on the subcortical route for evaluation of incoming sensory information with Haxby, Hoffman, and Gobbini's (2000) model of face processing. Early sensory processing extracts information about the threat or safety value of facial signal in a preattentive way, and then directs the way that facial information is subsequently processed in the inferior occipital gyrus and superior temporal sulcus.

Unconscious Emotional Behavior

Part III of the volume deals more directly with emotion-related behaviors. Both chapters (Owren, Rendall, & Bachorowski, Chapter 8, and Mark E. Bouton, Chapter 9) discuss emotional behaviors in a way that is consistent with the basic assumption of appraisal theories of emotion: Stimuli do not have intrinsic value; rather, the meaning of a stimulus is determined by a particular organism in a particular context at a particular point in time. Both highlight the importance of context in determining the value of a stimulus, and in doing so, are consistent with other contributions to this volume (e.g., Barrett, Chapter 11). Both chapters have the potential to change how scientists define *meaning*, by suggesting that what a stimulus means depends on the organism's affective response to it. Furthermore, both suggest that affective meaning is, for most part, unconscious (although conscious feelings that derive from the initial assessment of affective meaning can play a role in meaning making, e.g., Gerald L. Clore, Justin Storbeck, Michael D. Robinson, & David B. Centerbar, Chapter 16).

In Chapter 8, Owren, Rendell, and Bachorowski introduce a somewhat different set of assumptions about unconscious emotion processing than those discussed in the chapters on emotion perception. Rather than assuming that a person emits behavior that encodes his or her emotional state, such that his or her emotions can be decoded and recognized by another person, or that threat information can be extracted from behavioral signals, Owren and colleagues suggest that the meaning of any signal (e.g., a sound or visual image) is determined by the affective change it induces in the perceiver. In particular, Owren and colleagues propose that affect induction may play a key role in the communicative value of mammalian vocalizations. Instead of viewing mammalian vocalizations as a sort of symbol-like language (where one call means there is a predator, another call means that there is food, and so on), Owren and colleagues argue that sounds act on the nervous system, either directly because of their intrinsic acoustic properties, or indirectly because people have learned that certain sounds (e.g., the distinctive features of a person's voice) consistently predict threat or reward. Repeated pairings of individually distinctive sounds with positive or negative outcomes give the sounds themselves come to have predictive value for subsequent affective outcomes.

In these ways, mammals can influence the affective states and behaviors of others by the sounds that they make, and they do so in a way that can be disconnected from their own internal state. For example, a parent can speak to a child in a soothing tone (despite his or her own fatigue or frustration) and hug or help the child in repeated occasions, such that the parent's voice comes to have affective meaning for the child. Another example: A presidential candidate can discuss policies that will have negative consequences for you and your family; in a short time, the very sound of his or her voice becomes aversive. As these two examples illustrate, the vocalizer's signals may have affective consequences that are consciously and deliberately chosen, or that can be unintended. Either way, however, the affective consequences of the signal for the listener are often unconscious and automatic in that the listener has no initial control over the effects of the incoming signal. Owren and colleagues build on this argument to suggest that affect induction is one way that affective communication takes place: through a completely implicit mechanism on both sides of the communication.

Although a vocalization need not always reflect the internal state of the sender, at times it certainly can reflect that state, resulting in a completely unconscious form of affective communication. If a sender's affective state leads to a particular kind of expressive behavior (e.g., to yell at a child), this behavior can have a negative affective impact on the receiver (based on the acoustic properties of the sound, or because the receiver has learned that punishment will follow). This transaction, then, constitutes a completely unconscious process in which the affective state of one person is communicated to and impacts the affective state of another. Such a process also suggests a plausible mechanism for understanding how affective states can be shared. In clinical psychology, there is a saying that people often end up making others feel the way they do. Perhaps this is one mechanism (even the main mechanism) by which this contagion takes place.

In Chapter 9, Bouton directly addresses issues of classical conditioning and emotional response. In doing so, he provides an important grounding for other chapters in this volume (such as Owren et al., Chapter 8) that appeal to some form of classical conditioning in explaining how a stimulus comes to evoke a response. Bouton reviews important findings from his research in animal learning and discusses how they may be instructive for emotion theory. He discusses how emotion-related behaviors deal with a given evocative unconditioned stimulus, and reviews literature to demonstrate that the constellation of behavior elicited depends on contextual factors. Context can be defined in several ways: (1) as distance from a motivational object (a predator or food), (2) as the interoceptive state at the time of learning, and (3) in terms of time (e.g., the duration of the conditioned stim-

ulus, or, said another way, the time between the appearance of the conditioned stimulus and the appearance of the unconditioned stimulus, which,
in turn, evokes the emotional response).

Bouton further discusses how specific types of context influence an
emotional response to the conditioned stimulus. First, he presents evidence
that one form of emotional responding—anxiety—results from the direct
association between the context (i.e., conditioned stimuli [CS] of long duration) and the unconditioned stimulus (US). In doing so, he links anxiety to
the phenomenon of reinstatement (in which an extinguished response
returns if the animal is merely reexposed to the US alone) and suggests that
anxiety (i.e., responses to CS of long duration) is mediated by the bed
nucleus of the stria terminalis (BNST, part of the extended amygdala) and
the hippocampus. In fact, reinstatement effects may be a form of background contextual conditioning that is mediated by the hippocampus (Phillips & LeDoux, 1994).

Second, Bouton suggests that another form of emotional responding—
panic—results from an association between the context and retrieval of particular CS–US pairings. Here, context works as cue to retrieve current
meaning of a CS after it has been conditioned in one context and extinguished in another. The context controls whether the organism responds
negatively to the CS (because the CS–US association is retrieved from
memory) or not (because the CS–no US association is retrieved). Said
another way, context can directly determine which meaning of the CS is
retrieved after extinction. In doing so, Bouton links panic to the phenomenon of renewal (in which a change of context after extinction can cause a
robust return of conditioned responding) and suggests that this form of
responding is amygdala mediated, although it is possible that areas of the
medial prefrontal cortex might be involved (Milad & Quirk, 2002; Morgan,
Romanski, & LeDoux, 1993).

The Experience of Emotion

The next two chapters deal with how conscious and unconscious processes
contribute to the experience of emotion. For the average person, emotional
feelings are the most salient and defining feature of "having" an emotion.
Although there is more to emotion than just the subjective component, the
experience of emotion is a psychological phenomenon that is worthy of scientific investigation in its own right.

In Chapter 10, Charland presents readers with a provocative look at
the nature of valenced feelings. He marshals an argument, primarily on
philosophical grounds, that pleasant and unpleasant (hedonic) feelings are

not an intrinsic property or quality of raw (first-order) emotion experience (as claimed by Barrett, Chapter 11; Cacioppo et al., 1999; Russell, 2003), but are rather created by evaluating and interpreting the emotion experience when that experience is represented in second-order awareness. In other words, valence is not a property of feeling but an interpretation of a feeling as good or bad. Charland argues that valence is laden with personal meaning and is inseparably tied to an experience of the personal significance of what emotion experience means for us at a particular point in time. In Charland's view, valence is an appraisal of first-order, raw feelings (which he defines according to Lambie & Marcel, 2002). Valence does not exist prior to reporting on feeling—it is a property of self-report. In this way, valence, as a property of second-order experience, is probably a function of attention. Charland's view provides a counterpoint that should cause emotion researchers to pause before too quickly accepting the now popular view that stimuli are evaluated for their ability to predict threat or safety, thereby inducing an affective response by a preattentive, automatic, or implicit means of processing (Lundqvist & Öhman, Chapter 5; de Gelder, Chapter 6; Atkinson & Adolphs, Chapter 7; Barrett, Chapter 11; Winkielman, Berridge, & Wilbarger, Chapter 14). His view also challenges the idea that the meaning of a stimulus is defined by the affective reaction that it induces (Owren, Rendell, & Bachorowski, Chapter 8). Furthermore, Charland highlights the important observation that raw feelings (whatever their content, be it pleasure–displeasure, arousal–activation, anger, sadness, fear, etc.) can be judged on moral grounds, on how expected or unexpected they were, on how socially appropriate they are, and so on. Therefore, it is important to distinguish the contents of initial raw feelings from subsequent judgments of their desirability (e.g., Barrett, 1996), even if those judgments then go on to influence raw feelings in a recursive way.

In Chapter 11, Barrett begins with a critical examination of a guiding assumption within many scientific models of emotion (and one that appears in several chapters in this volume): People experience emotion because people have "emotions"—internal mechanisms that, once triggered, cause observable changes in behavior and feeling. She questions the view that the experience of emotion issues from separate mechanisms for anger, sadness, fear, and so on, and outlines an alternative hypothesis. Specifically, she suggests that the basic building blocks for emotional life are affective (i.e., involve core positive and negative affect) and conceptual (i.e., involve processes of categorization and interpretation). Barrett builds upon Russell's (2003; Russell & Barrett, 1999) idea of core affect by suggesting that evaluative processing produces an ongoing stream of neurophysiological change (i.e., change in a person's homeostatic state) that can evoke evolutionarily tuned behaviors for dealing with stimuli of significant value. These changes are then available for representation (although not necessarily) in awareness as feelings of pleasure–displeasure and activation–deactivation. She also argues that the experience of emotion is psychologically constructed via the same processes that influence the experience of color and people's experience of each other. Conceptual knowledge about emotion (i.e., emotion categories that are acquired in childhood and vary across cultures) shapes the perception of core affect into an experience of emotion in much the same way that category knowledge about people shapes our perceptions of other people's behavioral actions into meaningful acts. Simply put, then, people experience an emotion when they categorize an instance of affective feeling.

With this framework, Barrett suggests that the content and structure of category knowledge about emotion determine the content of what people feel. She argues that conceptualizing involves sensory–motor representations (drawing on Barsalou's situated conceptualization view, as discussed in Niedenthal et al., Chapter 2), such that conceptual knowledge about emotion can seamlessly shape the perception of core affect into the experience of an emotion. In her view, the experience of emotion is a perceptual act, guided by embodied conceptual knowledge about emotion. The result is a model of emotion experience that has much in common with the social-psychological literature on person perception and with literature on embodied conceptual knowledge as it has recently been applied to social psychology (e.g., Niedenthal et al., Chapter 2). What differentiates her model from these existing models of emotion experience is the emphasis on categorization processes as constituting a core mechanism driving the differentiation of emotion experience. Like other contributors to this volume, Barrett situates her theory in William James's original ideas about the embodiment of experienced emotion.

Perspectives on the Conscious–Unconscious Debate

The final section of this volume is devoted to examining various issues that relate to conscious and unconscious emotion. First, each chapter discusses the ways in which conscious and unconscious processes configure to produce an emotional response (however it is defined). Second, each critically examines the idea that feelings are presumed to have a causal status with regard to emotion, questioning whether feelings really are the main mediators between emotion and behavior. Finally, several of the chapters ask the provocative question about whether it is meaningful to talk about "unconscious" emotion.

Smith and Neumann (Chapter 12) frame many existing models of emotion in a general dual-process framework. First, they discuss an associative system that records information slowly and builds up representations based on a large sample of experiences, and that produces "schematic processing" by filling in information quickly and automatically in a preconscious, pattern-completion sort of way. Associative processing operates automatically and preconsciously to structure people's conscious experience, with little dependence on attention or cognitive resources. Smith and Neumann argue that associative processing also serves an alarm function, and this idea provides a framework for integrating material from other chapters that discusses the role of the amygdala in affect or emotion generation. Second, they discuss a rule-based system that is involved in a kind of emotion generation in which events can be learned quickly, even after a single trial, that requires attention and other cognitive resources for its operation, and that is often associated with a sense of subjective effort.

By discussing emotion in dual-process terms, Smith and Neumann integrate the science of emotion into a larger framework that makes contact with other major theories of the human mind. Importantly, they point out that emotion theorists should resist the tendency to refer to associative processing as emotion elicitation, and to rule-based processing as emotion regulation. In addition to the more automatic forms of emotion generation, it is possible to "think" oneself into an emotion by remembering a past event or by imagining something yet to happen. In fact, remembering prior emotional events and imagining hypothetical events are two of the most popular ways of inducing emotion in the lab. Similarly, there are both rule-based forms of regulation (e.g., such as the reappraisal strategy investigated by Gross (1999, 2002) and Ochsner, Bunge, Gross, and Gabrieli (2002) and associative forms of regulation (as in contextual conditioning and extinction, as discussed by Bouton, Chapter 9).

In Chapter 13, Scherer discusses how unconscious and conscious processes configure to produce an emotional response, and concludes that the majority of emotional work is done by unconscious processes. He suggests that the emotion process for an individual begins with evaluating the significance of a stimulus event. By evaluation, Scherer means something more complex that a simple "good for me/bad for me" judgment. Rather, he suggests that people automatically judge the stimulus event according to a set of appraisal rules or criteria (e.g., novelty, agreeableness, goal conduciveness, and so on). These appraisals of stimulus meaning result in differentiated emotion. In his view, appraisals also cause specific preparatory responses associated with proprioceptive information that, when synchronized with conceptual knowledge about emotion, produces a conscious experience of emotion.

Scherer's model, as a type of appraisal model, is rooted in the view that the meaning of a stimulus for a given person in a given context at a particular point in time elicits an emotional response, such that the character of that response is dictated by the contextual constraints. In principle, Scherer's view admits great flexibility in emotional responding, although he organizes emotional responses into the familiar set of "basic" categories. In this, as in several other points, Scherer's model bears some similarity to those of other theorists in this volume. He argues that emotional responses occur only when a stimulus has significant consequences in relation to a person's needs, goals, or values; in this way emotion may be a sign of a potential control dilemma, as characterized by Gray et al. in Chapter 4. At the heart of Scherer's model are two types of processing mechanisms that determine the emotional value of a stimulus—pattern matching and rule-based inference—and these are emblematic of the dual-process foundation of many emotion models (as discussed by Smith & Neumann, Chapter 12). Finally, Scherer proposes the intriguing idea that an identifiable emotional response results from a sort of perceptual binding that takes place when several types of information are synchronized. In this, he foreshadows the importance of understanding how cross-modal processing proceeds in emotional responding.

In Chapter 14, Winkielman, Berridge, and Wilbarger present the argument that affective states can drive behavior in the absence of conscious feeling. First they discuss evolutionary and functional considerations regarding the independence of mechanisms that control basic affective reactions from those of consciousness. They then present a functional neuroanatomical model of unconscious affect, in which they identify the subcortical areas that are essential for triggering basic affective reactions and the cortical systems that support the conscious experience of affect. They suggest a functional decoupling of affect state and affective feelings based on evidence from neuropsychology, neuroscience, and experimental psychology that is consistent with the elicitation–experience distinction drawn by Prinz in Chapter 15. Their view is largely consistent other contributors who address emotion perception (Lundqvist & Öhman, Chapter 5; de Gelder, Chapter 6; Atkinson & Adolphs, Chapter 7), emotion and awareness (Phelps, Chapter 3), and affective responding (Owren et al., Chapter 8; Barrett, Chapter 11), although they stand in contrast to some of the ideas presented in Charland (Chapter 10). Furthermore, Winkielman et al. argue that these findings support the existence of unconscious emotion as well, with the argument that mechanisms responsible for differentiated emotion responding (e.g., fear, anger, disgust) can function in organisms that differ widely in their capacity for conscious experience and often do not require elaborated cortical processing. This position is in contrast to other that of other contributors (Barrett, Chapter 11; Clore, Storbeck, Robinson, & Centerbar, Chapter 16) who allow for unconscious affect but not unconscious emotion as coordinated packets of distinctive responses. Finally, Winkielman et al. present a functional discussion of when and why an affective state is likely to be represented in awareness (or not). The basic idea is that to be conscious, affect needs to be represented by a hierarchical system of subcortical and cortical networks as well as integrated with higher-order categorical processes.

Prinz, in Chapter 15, also discusses two types of pathways in emotion processing that are similar to, but do not overlap with, the associative and rule-based processes discussed by Smith and Neumann (Chapter 12) and Scherer (Chapter 13). First, Prinz argues that some paths are involved in emotion elicitation of which a person is not aware. Similar to Scherer, Prinz argues that these paths produce a small set of "basic" emotion categories that can be distinguished by their behavioral and autonomic patterns (although there may be some heterogeneity within a category). Yet, no single somatic component corresponds to an emotional state on its own. Rather, Prinz echoes Scherer in suggesting that some sort of integration is necessary. Second, he argues that a separate path is involved in the conscious perception of these embodied states. He draws an analogy between emotion processing and visual processing, where emotion elicitation is more like early visual processing, and the conscious experience of emotion is more like mid-level visual processing in which patterns of responses are perceived. As suggested by other authors contributing to this volume, perception requires attention, although attention need not be effortful or intentional. All told, Prinz outlines a model of emotion that is similar to that of William James and consistent with other views of embodied emotional processing that are discussed in this volume.

In the concluding chapter, Clore, Storbeck, Robinson, and Centerbar call attention to and question seven of the assumptions ("sins") that ground much of the existing research on emotion and that characterize many (although certainly not all) of the perspectives offered in this volume. Each challenge does find common ground, however, with at least one other contribution in this volume. First, Clore et al. question whether emotion can truly be considered implicit or unconscious. They suggest that although most emotional processes are unconscious, there may be no unconscious emotions per se. In this, they agree with Barrett (Chapter 11). Second, Clore et al. question the tendency to treat subcortical processing (i.e., involving the amygdala) in humans as the locus of "real" emotion, with cortical contributions serving only a regulatory function after the fact. In addition, they make the provocative claim that the particular subcortical route discovered by LeDoux, which serves as the centerpiece of emotional processing in many of the chapters in this volume, really has limited influence on emotion-related processing in humans. Third, Clore et al. question the causal status of affective feelings. In their view, an unconscious affective state can have a direct influence on behavior. In this, Clore et al. seem to agree with Barrett (Chapter 11) and Winkielman et al. (Chapter 14). But Clore et al. also allow that unconscious affect can indirectly influence behavior through conscious feeling. In particular, these authors argue that conscious feelings are a potent tool for ensuring that explicit judgments and choices are consistent with the judgments and choices that are derived from unconscious affect. In this sense, feelings can be used to resolve any control dilemmas (Gray et al., Chapter 4) that may be in evidence. Moreover, Clore et al. suggest that feelings of arousal play a role in attention and that unconscious components of arousal play a role in memory. To some extent, this view agrees with points made by Phelps (Chapter 3).

Fourth, Clore et al. argue against the notion that preferences precede inferences, instead arguing that evaluative processing is a special case of semantic processing. Fifth, they argue against the idea that expressive actions (such as arm flexions) have direct, fixed effects on affective state. Instead, they suggest that affect is elicited by a mind in context, and they review data showing how the influence of a physical action on affect depends on the contextual meaning of an action. This view seems entirely consistent with Owren et al. (Chapter 8), and also with contemporary views of embodied conceptual processing, such those advanced by Niedenthal et al. (Chapter 2) and Barrett (Chapter 11) who see embodied processes as largely driven by contextual considerations. Sin #6 addresses the common wisdom that the amygdala is adequate to trigger emotion. Instead, Clore et al. argue that semantic processing appears to be necessary for affective computations involving visual stimuli. They seem to base this argument on the fact that areas of the visual association cortex (linked with stimulus recognition) are important in the amygdala's response to stimuli. Certainly, the amygdala alone is not sufficient for affective computations, but it would certainly seem necessary, and the difference between the position advanced by Clore et al. and that represented in other chapters in this volume is one of emphasis more than kind.

Finally, Clore et al. argue that appraisal theories have been fundamentally misunderstood; the claims made by appraisal theorists have generally not concerned the processes involved in generating emotion, as intimated by Prinz (Chapter 15) and many other critics. Rather, these theories reveal the structure of emotion—the rules about which emotions are felt when. In this sense, appraisals describe the structure of emotion in terms of its cognitive, perceptual, or situational causes, but not in terms of some temporal flow of processes.

COMING TOGETHER

Due to the exquisite balance of similarity and difference—in focus, in level of analysis, and in mechanistic accounts—we believe that the chapters in this volume contain a research agenda and a set of core themes and integrative theories for future work on emotion and consciousness. It has often been said that the literature on emotion is a group of descriptions of very small pieces of the very large "elephant" that is emotion (e.g., Russell & Barrett, 1999). For this very reason, some researchers prefer to avoid theorizing about emotion altogether, even when developing influential theories of memory, attention, or social cognition. Emerging from this volume, we believe, is a semblance of an elephant.

One reason for the elephant's emergence is that broader models can now account for, and integrate findings across, levels of analysis, so that psychological concepts of thinking and feeling, conscious and unconscious can be biologically grounded. One example of a broad model that emerges from several chapters is the "embodiment" perspective, which explains fundamental and sweeping concepts such as empathy, emotion perception, emotion experience, perspective taking, emotional learning, and conflict resolution with an increasingly similar set of assumptions and mechanisms. A core affect perspective (Russell, 2003) also holds some promise for integrating findings across several key literatures involved with understanding emotion-related processing. This perspective is broadly consistent with the data discussed in many chapters of this volume, and in neurobiological models of emotion-related processing (e.g., Rolls, 1999). Of course, there may be other models, as well.

That being said, many features of the elephant need to be empirically established. Although the contributors to the present volume do not always agree in the content of their arguments, we moved toward agreement on what the central arguments are and how to resolve them. This consensus means, we hope, that future debates in the area of emotion can begin to use the same language and take place within compatible scopes of inquiry—rather than on different planets.

REFERENCES

Aristotle. (1941). On the soul. In R. McKeon (Ed.), *The basic works of Aristotle*. New York: Random House.

Barrett, L. F. (1996). Hedonic tone, perceived arousal, and item desirability: Three components of self-reported mood. *Cognition and Emotion, 10,* 47–68.

Cacioppo, J. T., Gardner, W. L., & Bernston, G. G. (1999). The affect system has parallel and integrative processing components: Form follows function. *Journal of Personality and Social Psychology, 76*, 839–855.

Gross, J. J. (1998). Antecedent- and response-focused emotion regulation: Divergent consequences for experience, expression, and physiology. *Journal of Personality and Social Psychology, 74*, 224–237.

Gross, J. J. (2002). Emotion regulation: Affective, cognitive, and social consequences. *Psychophysiology, 39*, 281–291.

Haxby, J. V., Hoffman, E. A., & Gobbini, M. I. (2000). The distributed human neural system for face perception. *Trends in Cognitive Sciences, 4*, 223–233.

Lambie, J. A., & Marcel, A. J. (2002). Consciousness and emotion experience: A theoretical framework. *Psychological Review, 109*, 219–259

Lane, R. D., Nadel, L., Allen, J. J. B., & Kaszniak, A. W. (2000). The study of emotion from the perspective of cognitive neuroscience. In R. D. Lane & L. Nadel (Eds.), *Cognitive neuroscience of emotion* (pp. 3–11). New York: Oxford University Press.

LeDoux, J. E. (1996). *The emotional brain: The mysterious underpinnings of emotional life.* New York: Simon & Schuster.

Milad, M. R. & Quirk, G. J. (2002). Neurons in medial prefrontal cortex signal memory for fear extinction. *Nature, 240*, 70–74.

Morgan, M. A., Romanski, L. M., & LeDoux, J. E. (1993). Extinction of emotional learning: Contribution of medial prefrontal cortex. *Neuroscience Letters, 163*, 109–113.

Ochsner, K. N., Bunge, S. A., Gross, J. J., & Gabrieli, J. D. E. (2002). Rethinking feelings: An fMRI study of the cognitive regulation of emotion. *Journal of Cognitive Neuroscience, 14*(8), 1215–1229.

Phillips, R. G., & LeDoux, J. E. (1994). Lesions of the dorsal hippocampal formation interfere with background but not foreground contextual fear conditioning. *Learning and Memory, 1*, 34–44.

Rolls, E. T. (1999). *The brain and emotion.* New York: Oxford University Press.

Russell, J. A. (2003). Core affect and the psychological construction of emotion. *Psychological Review, 110*, 145–172.

Russell, J. A., & Barrett, L. F. (1999). Core affect, prototypical emotional episodes, & other things called emotion: Dissecting the elephant. *Journal of Personality and Social Psychology, 76*, 805–819.

PART I

Cognition and Emotion

CHAPTER 2

Embodiment in the Acquisition and Use of Emotion Knowledge

PAULA M. NIEDENTHAL
LAWRENCE W. BARSALOU
FRANÇOIS RIC
SILVIA KRAUTH-GRUBER

The past 50 years have seen an exponential increase in the number of journal and book pages devoted to reports and discussions of research on emotion. Despite the growth of interest in the empirical study of emotion, however, the literature remains largely unintegrated. Researchers have independently studied the processes involved in the perception, interpretation, experience, and use of knowledge about emotion, relying on very different theoretical orientations. In addressing such apparently wide-ranging problems, for example, emotion researchers have tested principles of evolutionary theory with the use of facial expression recognition data and with the use of autonomic nervous system data; they have pursued cognitive theories of emotion and measured reaction times to categorizing words or studied judgments of similarity between words denoting emotional states; and they have evaluated social constructivist theories with the use of linguistic analyses and archival data on social customs. In this chapter, we seek to understand the body of knowledge about emotion with a single mechanistic account. Following the pun present in the preceding sentence, in the present chapter, we introduce the notion of *embodiment* and argue

1. *What is the scope of your proposed model? When you use the term* emotion, *how do you use it? What do you mean by terms such as* fear, anxiety, *or* happiness?

The topic of the chapter is the processing of emotional information and emotion concepts. Our point is that processing emotional information involves a simulation of the corresponding emotional state or cue in the perceiver. Consistent with many basic emotion theorists, emotions are defined as short-term, biologically based patterns of perception, subjective experience, physiology, and action (or action tendencies) that constitute responses to specific physical and social problems posed by the environment.

2. *Define your terms:* conscious, unconscious, awareness. *Or say why you do not use these terms.*

By consciousness we mean the object of attention. Once attention has been directed at an embodied emotion, then it can become a subject of advanced representational processes. As noted at the end of the chapter, this will have many consequences for the subjective experience of emotion.

3. *Does your model deal with what is conscious, what is unconscious, or their relationship? If you do not address this area specifically, can you speculate on the relationship between what is conscious and unconscious? Or if you do not like the conscious–unconscious distinction, or if you do not think this is a good question to ask, can you say why?*

We have suggested that although emotions are embodied, this embodiment need not be conscious. It is also possible that some embodied components of emotion, such as the perceptual patterns that define them, can never be conscious. When conscious attention is directed to the cognitively penetrable

that the acquisition of knowledge about emotion—the perception, recognition, and interpretation of an emotion in the self or other—involves the embodiment of emotional states, and the use of emotion knowledge involves the reenactment of these same states. In other words, we think that (1) perceiving emotions involves embodiment, and (2) using emotion knowledge relies on the very same somatosensory and motor states. The implication of this perspective is that perceiving someone else's emotion, having an emotional response or feeling oneself, and using emotion knowledge in conceptual tasks are all fundamentally the same process.

In the sections that follow, we provide evidence for the following four claims: (1) Individuals embody other people's emotional behavior; (2) embodied emotions produce corresponding subjective emotional states in the individual; (3) imagining other people and events also produces embodied emotions and corresponding feelings; and (4) embodied emotions mediate cognitive responses. After reviewing this evidence, we discuss how theories of embodied cognition can account for these types of effects (we focus largely on Barsalou's [1999a] recent theory of embodied cognition). We end by identifying implications of this approach for understanding conscious and unconscious aspects of emotion.

WHAT IS EMBODIMENT?

By *embodiment* we mean the bodily states that arise (e.g., postures, facial expressions, and uses of the voice [i.e., prosody]) during the perception of an emotional stimulus and the later use of emotional information (in the absence of the emotional stimulus). In the area of emotion the concept of embodiment is associated with the theory of William James (1890/1981), who argued that individuals' perceptions of the bodily states that occur in the presence of emotional events constitute their emotions (really, their feelings), in the sense of "feeling" somatosensory and motor changes. In essence, James defined emotions as the conscious perception of bodily states. Although our aims are somewhat different—we are concerned with the theoretical grounding for emotion concepts—we come full circle and return to James in this chapter. We propose that the *bodily states*, or embodiments of emotion, can be, and often are, unconscious, and that the *feeling states* are conscious. If we consider that embodiments can be unconscious until consciously attended to and manifested as feelings, then the general debate about whether emotion is conscious or unconscious becomes, in our mind, more tenable, and the various disagreements on this point (e.g., see Winkielman, Berridge, & Wilbarger, Chapter 14; Clore, Storbeck, Robinson, & Centerbar, Chapter 16) can be reconciled. It is, above all, necessary to decide whether an emotion is a *bodily state*, a *feeling state*, or both.

INDIVIDUALS EMBODY OTHERS' EMOTIONAL GESTURES AND BEHAVIORS

In this first section we review empirical evidence for the claim that people embody the emotional behaviors of others. These behaviors may include, but are not limited to, facial expressions, postures, and vocal parameters that convey emotion. Here we present evidence concerning the ubiquity of imitation; in the next section we discuss the relations between imitation and subjective emotional state. There is evidence suggesting that such imitation is automatic, in that it does not have to be conscious or intentional. However, it is clear that goals, such as the goal to empathize, can enhance or suppress the tendency or the effort put into imitation.

Embodiment of Facial, Postural, and Vocal Expressions of Emotion

Probably the most extensive evidence for the embodiment of others' emotional behavior involves the facial and vocal expressions of emotion. In several frequently cited studies, Dimberg (1982, 1990) showed that 8-second presentations of slides of angry and happy faces elicited facial electromyographic (EMG) responses in perceivers that corresponded to the perceived expressions. For example, zygomatic activity (which occurs when individuals smile) was higher when participants viewed a happy, compared to an angry, face. In addition, corrugator activity (which occurs when individuals frown) was elevated when participants viewed an angry face, and it decreased when participants viewed a happy face. Furthermore, these effects were obtained when the faces were presented subliminally (Dimberg, Thunberg, & Elmehed, 2000).

Vaughan and Lanzetta (1980) used a vicarious conditioning paradigm in which participants viewed the videotaped facial expression of pain displayed by a confederate (unconditioned stimulus) while working on a paired-association learning task. The pain expression that always followed a target word of the same word category (flower or tree names) produced a similar facial response in the observer during the confederate's pain expression, as indicated by EMG activity (for related findings, see Bavelas, Black, Lemery, & Mullett, 1987).

Embodiment of positive facial expressions was demonstrated by Bush, Barr, McHugo, and Lanzetta (1989). In their study participants viewed two comedy routines. In one, smiling faces had been spliced into the film concurrent with sound-track laughter. Half of the participants were instructed to inhibit their facial expressions. The half whose expressions were spontaneous—that is, in whom mimicry was permitted—displayed greater zygomatic and oricularis activity during the spliced segments than during the segments without smiling faces. Research by Leventhal and colleagues (Leventhal & Mace, 1970; Leventhal & Cupchik, 1975; Cupchik & Leventhal, 1974) similarly showed that exposure to the expressive displays of others produces mimetic responses in observers (and see Chartrand & Bargh, 1999).

McHugo and colleagues studied the embodiment of more complex expressive behaviors (including facial expression, gaze direction, and bodily posture) of political leaders on observers' facial reactions as a function of their prior attitudes. In one study (McHugo, Lanzetta, Sullivan, Masters, & Englis, 1985), participants watched televised news conferences of then-President Ronald Reagan. Independent of their prior attitudes, participants showed increased brow activity (contraction of the corrugator supercilii muscle) in response to Reagan's negative expressions and reduced cheek activity (low zygomatic major activity) during Reagan's positive expressions.

Finally, emotional embodiment has been shown for emotional prosody. In a recent study by Neumann and Strack (2000), participants listened to recorded speeches that were read in either a sad or a happy voice. Under the pretext that the experimenters were interested in whether memory for the content of a speech is improved by the simultaneous reproduction of it by the listener, the participants had to repeat the content of the speech aloud as they listened to it. Thus the participants were focused on the content of the speech that they were instructed to repeat, not on the prosody of the speaker. Different participant-judges later rated the emotional prosody of the initial participants as they repeated the speech. Results showed that participants embodied the prosody of the speakers when shadowing their speech, even though prosody was completely irrelevant to task performance, and they were unaware of the influence on their own prosody.

In sum, a large number of studies over the last 30 years has documented the ubiquity of facial, postural, and prosodic embodiment. These studies all show that individuals partly or fully embody the emotional expressions of other people, and some of the results also show that this process is either very subtle, and likely to occur outside of consciousness, or unmoderated by contextual factors, suggesting that such embodiment is highly automatic in nature. Why would the embodiment of others' facial, bodily, and vocal expressions of emotion be so automatic and so ubiquitous? In the present view, imitation is the mechanism by which observers come to comprehend the emotions of others. But, of course, this premise would only make sense if the imitation produced a corresponding state in the observer (for a discussion, see Décety & Chaminade, 2003; Zajonc, Adlemann, Murphy, & Niedenthal, 1987). Indeed, much research has tested this notion, and it is to such work that we turn next.

EMBODIMENT OF OTHERS' EMOTIONS PRODUCES EMOTIONAL STATES

In some of the studies described in the previous sections, researchers measured not only the embodiment of others' emotional gestures, but also the occurrence of corresponding emotional states in the perceiver. For example, in the study by Vaughan and Lanzetta (1980), participants not only imitated the confederate's painful expressions, they also responded to the confederate's pain expression as if they were in pain (as indicated by an increase in autonomic arousal). Furthermore, in a follow-up study, Vaughan and Lanzetta (1981) found that the vicarious emotional responses elicited by observing the confederate's painful expression could be modified by the opportunity for embodiment, in particular, by the instruction to suppress or amplify facial expression during the confederate's shock period. Consistent with an embodiment account, participants in the amplify condition who embodied the expressions of pain showed higher autonomic arousal compared to both no-instruction participants and participants in the inhibition condition who had to suppress their facial expressions.

Feedback effects of mimicked facial expression on participants' emotional experience were also found in a study by Hsee, Hatfield, Carlson, and Chemtob (1990). Participants were secretly filmed while watching a videotaped interview of a fellow student who described either one of the happiest or one of the saddest events in his or her life, and who displayed the corresponding expressive behavior (i.e., happy or sad facial expressions, gestures, posture, tone of voice). Participants not only embodied the emotional expressions of the target person they viewed (evaluated by judges who rated the videotaped facial expressions of the participants), but also their own emotions were affected by the emotional expression they mimicked.

Finally, neuroscientific evidence that imitated emotion gestures produce emotions was found by Hutchison and colleagues, who examined the activation of pain-related neurons in patients (Hutchison, Davis, Lozano, Tasker, & Dostrovsky, 1999). Importantly, they found that not only were such neurons also activated when a painful stimulus was applied to the patient's own hand, but the same neurons were also activated when the patient watched the painful stimulus applied to the experimenter's hand. This finding was interpreted as evidence of an embodied simulation in the perceiver of what was happening to the perceived person (see Gallese, 2003, for summaries of related research).

The studies just reviewed provide correlational evidence that people's embodiments of others' emotional gestures are accompanied by congruent emotional states or responses. However, except for a few demonstrations in which mimicry was experimentally inhibited or facilitated, it cannot be concluded from the studies that embodiment *causes* emotional states. We next review research that suggests that emotion-specific embodied states, such as facial expressions, vocal expressions, and bodily postures, can produce the corresponding emotion or at least modulate the ongoing emotional experience.

Effects of Facial Embodiment:
Tests of the Facial Feedback Hypothesis

Most of the research that demonstrates the influence of embodied emotions on emotional state was conducted with the aim of testing the facial feedback hypothesis, according to which feedback from facial musculature has direct or moderating effects on emotional state (for a review of findings and mechanistic accounts, see Adelmann & Zajonc, 1989; McIntosh, 1996). In canonical facial feedback studies, participants' facial expressions were manipulated by the experimenter's demand to pose (facilitate) or hide (inhibit) their spontaneous emotional expression, by using a muscle-to-muscle instruction that specified the facial muscle to contract, or by nonemotional tasks that allowed the experimenter to guide the production of facial expressions without cueing the emotional meaning of the expression. In many such studies, the opportunity to experience emotion was presented in the form of a variety of emotional stimuli, such as painful electric shocks, pleasant and unpleasant slides and films, odors, or imagery, and the moderation of the emotion by facial expression was assessed. Findings demonstrated that the intensity and quality of the participants' manipulated facial expression affected the intensity of their self-reported emotional feelings as well as their autonomic responses.

For example, in three experiments, Lanzetta, Cartwright-Smith, and Kleck (1976) demonstrated that manipulated facial expression affected the intensity of emotional reactions during the anticipation and reception of electric shocks. In Study 1 participants received an initial set of shocks (baseline sequence) that varied in intensity, and rated the aversiveness of each received shock. Shock intensity was announced by a shock signal slide. For the second set of shocks, participants were instructed to hide their facial display in response to anticipating the shocks announced by the slide. The inhibition instruction caused low- and medium-intensity shocks to be experienced as less painful, but did not decrease the painfulness of high-intensity shocks. In a follow-up study the same basic procedure was used, but this time expression-inhibition as well as expression-exaggeration instructions were given in the manipulation sequence. Participants who were asked to simulate anticipating and receiving no shocks (inhibition instruction) reported experiencing the shocks as less aversive and painful compared to participants who simulated intense shocks (exaggeration instruction). Similar results were found in a study by Kopel and Arkowitz (1974).

Kleck, Vaughan, Cartwright-Smith, Vaughan, Colby, and Lanzetta (1976) manipulated participants' facial expressions by social means. The presence of an observer during the receipt of either no-, low-, or medium-intensity shocks attenuated participants' facial expressivity (natural inhibition) and produced lower self-rated painfulness of shocks compared to the alone condition. Using pleasant and unpleasant slides as emotion-eliciting stimuli, Lanzetta, Biernat, and Kleck (1982) induced contextual inhibition of facial expression by the means of a mirror installed in front of the participants. The mirror had attenuating effects on both participants' expressivity and the self-reported intensity of felt pleasantness–unpleasantness. Similar attenuating as well as facilitating effects of facial expression, manipulated by suppression–exaggeration instructions, were also found with pleasant and unpleasant films (Zuckerman, Klorman, Larrance, & Spiegel, 1981) and odors (Kraut, 1982).

Such modulating effects of facial expressions were also found in studies that used less obvious facial manipulations. In Laird (1974), participants contracted specific facial muscles involved in smile or frown expressions while watching positive and negative slides (Study1) or humorous cartoons (Study 2). "Smiling" participants felt happier while viewing positive slides, whereas "frowning" participants felt angrier while viewing negative slides. Incongruent expressions were shown to attenuate their feelings (see also Rutledge & Hupka, 1985).

Although most of this research demonstrates that facial expressions modulate emotions induced by emotional stimuli, several studies have shown that facial expressions can also initiate corresponding emotional experience in the absence of any emotional stimulus. For instance, using a muscle-to-muscle instruction procedure similar to Laird's (1974), Duclos et al. (1989) instructed participants to adopt facial expressions of fear, anger, disgust, or sadness while listening to neutral tones. Participants then rated their feelings on several emotion scales. Self-reported fear and sadness were highest in the fear and sadness expression trials, respectively, and higher than in the other three expression trials. Equally high anger and disgust ratings were found in the anger and disgust expression trials, which were higher than in the other two expressing trials. Finally, evidence for the emotion-initiating power of facial expressions was found in other studies in which emotion-specific facial expressions, manipulated by muscle-to-muscle instructions, resulted in self-reports of the associated emotion (Duncan & Laird, 1977, 1980), especially for participants whose faces best matched the prototypical emotional expression (Ekman, Levenson, & Friesen, 1983; Levenson, Ekman, & Friesen, 1990), and for participants who were more responsive to their inner bodily cues than to external situational cues (Duclos & Laird, 2001; see also Soussignan, 2002).

Effects of Postural Embodiment

Sir Francis Galton (1884) believed that people's attitudes and feelings are reflected in their bodily postures. In an anecdotal way, he suggested that observing the bodily orientation of people during a party could reveal their attraction or "inclination" to one another. Bull (1951) was one of the first to examine the relation between bodily posture and emotional experience. In one study she induced the emotions of disgust, fear, anger, depression, and joy through hypnosis and found that participants automatically adopted the corresponding bodily postures. Furthermore, when asked to adopt emotion-specific postures, participants reported experiencing the associated emotions.

Since the work of Bull, several experimental studies have directly explored the impact of bodily posture on emotional experience. For example, Duclos et al. (1989) studied the impact of emotion-specific bodily postures on participants' feelings. All participants had to listen to the same series of neutral tones, which were not intended to induce specific emotions but were presented as part of a multiple-tasks procedure. In an unobtrusive way, they were also asked to adopt bodily postures associated with anger, fear, or sadness. As expected, posture facilitated the emotional experience of the corresponding emotion. Participants reported feeling sadder in the sad posture, more fearful in the fear posture, and angrier in the angry posture.

In Stepper and Strack (1993) participants' bodily posture was manipulated in an unobtrusive way by either having them adopt a conventional working position or one of two ergonomic positions (upright or slumped posture) when receiving success feedback concerning their performance on an achievement task. Participants who received success feedback in the slumped posture felt less proud and reported being in a worse mood than participants in the upright position and participants in a nonmanipulated control group, who did not differ from one another (see also Riskind & Gotay, 1982).

Flack, Laird, and Cavallaro (1999) examined both separate and combined effects of facial expression and bodily posture related to anger, sadness, fear, and happiness on corresponding emotional experience. Replicating the results of Duclos et al. (1989), they found specific effects of expressive behavior on participants' self-reported emotional feelings. Participants always felt the specific emotion they were enacting either with their face or with their body posture. Furthermore, they found that combined effects of matching facial and bodily expressions produced stronger corresponding feelings.

Effects of Vocal Embodiment

In a series of experiments Hatfield, Hsee, Costello, Weisman, and Denney (1995) instructed participants to listen to tapes with sound patterns that they then had to reproduce into a telephone. The sounds were designed to convey the characteristics associated with specific emotions (joy, love, fear, sadness, anger, neutral). Participants' self-reported emotions were affected by the specific sounds they produced. This result demonstrated that emotion-specific tone of voice amplifies the corresponding emotional feeling. Siegman, Anderson, and Berger (1990), in turn, showed that vocal expression can be used, like facial or postural expression, to regulate or control one's emotion. Participants who were instructed to discuss an anger-provoking topic in a slow and soft voice felt less angry and their heart rate slowed. Those who had to speak loudly and rapidly felt angrier and became more physiologically aroused.

Summary

Taken together, the studies reviewed in this section demonstrate that people's expressive behavior not only facilitates but can also produce the corresponding emotional experience. Facial expressions, bodily posture, and vocal expressions have emotion-specific, facilitative effects on self-reported emotional feelings, as well as effects on other measures of emotional experience. Facial, postural, and vocal embodiments not only modulate ongoing emotional experience but also facilitate the generation of the corresponding emotions. These findings strongly suggest that the embodiment or simulation of others' emotions provides the meaning of the perceived event. Perhaps, then, this is a general rule. Perhaps emotional meaning is the partial or full embodied simulation of an emotion. If this were the case, then simulation in the absence of a triggering affective perception or stimulus would involve embodied responses. Furthermore, simulating a particular emotion would affect the ease of processing the symbols associated with affective meanings. It is to the evidence for these two proposals that we turn next.

AFFECTIVE IMAGERY IS ACCOMPANIED BY EMOTION PROCESSES

Numerous studies have used imagery related to simulations of past experiences to manipulate emotional states in the laboratory (e.g., Bodenhausen, Kramer, & Süsser, 1994; Schwarz & Clore, 1983; Strack, Schwarz, & Gschneidinger, 1985; Wegener, Petty, & Smith, 1995). However, in these studies, it is not clear whether the required imagery activated emotion processes or only primed information merely associated with specific emotion words, which then guided subsequent judgments that constituted a dependent variable of interest (Innes-Ker & Niedenthal, 2002; Niedenthal, Rohmann, & Dalle, 2003).

Research designed to test just this question has indeed found that physiological changes resulting from imagery parallel those obtained in the presence of the stimuli eliciting the same emotion. For instance, Grossberg and Wilson (1968) asked participants to imagine themselves in various situations. One half of the situations had been evaluated by each participant as fearful, and the other half were rated as neutral. Results indicated that significant changes in heart rate and skin conductance between baseline (as measured for each individual at the beginning of the experimental session) and presentation of the situation (read by an experimenter) were similar for neutral and fearful situations. However, the increase in physiological responses between presentation and simulation were more marked for fearful situations than for neutral (see also Lang, Kozak, Miller, Levin, & McLean, 1980; Vrana, Cuthbert, & Lang, 1989).

In a related experiment, Gollnisch and Averill (1993) extended these results to other emotions. They asked participants to imagine situations that involve fear, sadness, anger, or joy. Measures included heart rate, electrodermal activity, and respiration. Mean levels of heart rate were significantly higher during imagery than baseline but did not differ as a function of emotion. Mean respiratory rates increased significantly during imagery in comparison with baseline (as measured in 2-minute pretrial rest period), but only for fear, anger, and joy; sadness produced a decrease in respiratory rates. Skin conductance was unresponsive to the manipulation (Gehricke & Fridlund, 2002; Gehricke & Shapiro, 2000).

Vrana and Rollock (2002; see also Vrana, 1993, 1995) presented participants with emotional imagery scenarios related to joy, anger, fear, or neutral. Participants were asked to imagine they were actually in the scene, participating actively in it. As expected, facial expression (as measured by EMG activity at zygomatic and corrugator facial muscles) differed as a function of emotional tonality of the scenario (see also Dimberg, 1990). Corrugator activity was greater during fear and anger simulation than during neutral and joy scenarios. In contrast, zygomatic activity was greater during joy than during any other scenario.

Differences between imagery of sadness versus joy situations were also found. For instance, Gehricke and Fridlund (2002) found that the simulation of joy situations led to greater EMG activity in the cheek region than simulations of sad situations, whereas the reverse was true for EMG activity in the brow region.

Finally, similar results were found when participants were asked to imagine fictitious persons (Vanman, Paul, Ito, & Miller, 1997) or to think about persons whose descriptions were designed to covertly resemble those of significant others participants liked or disliked (Andersen, Reznik, & Manzella, 1996).

In sum, a sizable literature now demonstrates that when emotional events are simulated using imagery, and in the absence of the initial stimulus, individuals reenact or relive the emotions, or partial feelings of emotion, as indicated by a number of different measures of emotion. If it is the case that the mental processing of past experience can produce embodied emotion, then we can ask whether the process of embodying emotions interacts with the processing of emotional meaning per se. In the next section we show that this is indeed the case.

EMBODIED EMOTIONS MEDIATE COGNITIVE RESPONSES

A growing body of research has demonstrated that embodied emotions influence cognitive responses to emotional information. In the following section, we present evidence of such an impact on stimulus identification, stimulus evaluation, and recall.

Stimulus identification

Neumann and Strack (2000, Experiment 1) instructed participants to indicate as quickly as possible whether adjectives presented on a computer screen were positive or negative. While performing the task, participants either pressed the palm of their nondominant hand on the top of the table (extension condition) or used their palm to pull up on the underside of the table (flexion condition). These motor movements were manipulated because they are associated with positive affect and approach (arm flexion) and with negative affect and avoidance (arm extension; e.g., Cacioppo, Priester, & Berntson, 1993). Arm flexion facilitated the identification of positive information, whereas arm extension facilitated the identification of negative information. These results suggest that affective movement facilitates the encoding of affective information of the same valence.

This kind of effect could be the basis of facial expression recognition (Zajonc & Markus, 1984; Zajonc, Pietromonaco, & Bargh, 1982). Indeed, Wallbott (1991) proposed that imitation of facial expression facilitates its recognition. He instructed participants to identify the emotion expressed in a series of face pictures. While performing the task, participants' faces were covertly videotaped. Two weeks later, each participant was asked to watch the videotape of him- or herself while he or she performed the identification task, and to guess the identification of the facial expression being judged (which was, of course, not visible). The participants identified the emotion expressed in the pictures above chance level by seeing only their own facial expression while performing the task. These results are compatible with the idea that participants had partially simulated others' facial expression while performing the identification task and that this simulation provided emotional cues for identifying the emotion presented in the picture (see also Niedenthal, Brauer, Halberstadt, & Innes-Ker, 2001; Adolphs, Damasio, & Tranel, 2002; Atkinson & Adophs, Chapter 7, for convergent neuropsychological evidence).

Evaluation

Evaluation responses also seem to be mediated by embodied emotions (but for an alternative view, see Clore et al., Chapter 16). Cacioppo and colleagues (1993), for example, exposed participants to neutral Chinese ideographs, and participants rated each one on a liking scale. Participants performed the task while pressing their palm on the top (arm extension) or pulling it up from the underside (arm flexion) of the table. The ideographs were judged as more pleasant during arm flexion than during arm extension. Subsequent studies demonstrated that participants associated arm flexion with an approach motivational orientation, but only when they performed the musculature contraction, not when they merely watched someone else performing it.

Using a different type of embodiment manipulation, Strack, Martin, and Stepper (1988) found that participants instructed to hold a pencil between their front teeth, thus unobtrusively expressing a smile, evaluated cartoons as funnier, compared with participants asked to hold a pencil between their lips, without touching the pencil with their teeth (which produced a frown expression), or participants instructed to hold the pencil in their nondominant hand (a control condition).

Ohira and Kurono (1993) asked participants to exaggerate their (negative) facial expressions while reading a text presenting a target person as somewhat hostile, under the cover story of transmitting nonverbal information to a person who was supposedly on the other side of a one-way mirror. These participants later judged the target more negatively than participants who had been asked to conceal their facial expressions or who were not given instructions concerning their facial expressions.

Memory

Laird, Wagener, Halal, and Szegda (1982) asked participants to read passages related either to anger or happiness. After an interpolated task, participants were instructed to recall as much information as possible about the presented stories while contracting specific facial muscles so that they expressed either a happy or an angry face (importantly, the instructions did not refer to happiness or anger). Participants expressing an angry face recalled more of the angry passages than participants expressing a happy face, whereas the reverse was true for happy passages. A second experiment generalized these findings to fear, anger, and sadness, thus ruling out the possibility that frowning leads to better recall of any negative information.

Moreover, by controlling facial expressions at encoding, Laird et al. were able to rule out another interpretation in terms of state-dependent retrieval. That is, a possible account of the Experiment 1 findings is that participants reading, for instance, angry passages had felt anger, and that the manipulation of a facial expression of anger produced the same state, which then served as a retrieval cue (i.e., an example of state-dependent retrieval). In Experiment 2, they found that the facial expression at recall still affected memory performance in an emotion-congruent manner when controlling for the facial expression at encoding; that is, participants maintained the same emotion expression throughout the experiment.

Schnall and Laird (2003) also demonstrated that such effects could be obtained even when (1) the facial expression is not maintained at time of recall, and (2) when recall implied an autobiographical event that required long-term memory. Consistent with these findings, Riskind (1983) found that participants who expressed smiles were faster at recalling pleasant autobiographical memories and took longer to recall unpleasant memories than participants who expressed a sad face.

Similar results were found when emotional gestures other than facial expressions were manipulated. Förster and Strack (1996) instructed participants to listen to positive and negative adjectives while performing either horizontal head movements (shaking, associated with negative attitude), vertical movements (nodding, associated with agreement), or circular movements (control condition), following a procedure designed by Wells and Petty (1980). They found that recognition of positive words was better when the presentation of these words was associated with vertical movements (nodding), whereas recognition of negative words was better when presentation of these words was associated with horizontal movements (head shaking; see Förster & Strack, 1997, 1998, for replications).

We have reviewed existing findings that suggest that individuals embody others' emotions, that such embodiment causes corresponding emotions in the perceiver, and that embodiment seems to be involved in facilitating and inhibiting the cognitive processing of emotional information more generally. In the next section we describe a recent theory of conceptual processing that can, we think, account for the ensemble of findings and the way we have linked and interpreted them to this point.

THEORETICAL ACCOUNTS
OF EMBODIED EMOTION EFFECTS

How do we explain the roles of embodiment in emotional phenomena? What implications do these phenomena have for the emotion concepts that people use to interpret emotional experience? The standard answer to such questions is that amodal knowledge structures represent emotion concepts, and embodied states are peripheral appendages that either trigger or indicate the activation of the amodal structures. An alternative account is that embodiments constitute the core conceptual content of emotion concepts. That is, rather than serving as peripheral appendages to emotion concepts, embodiments constitute their core meanings. We address each of these two approaches in turn.

Amodal Accounts of Embodied Emotion Effects

The Transduction Principle

The amodal view of emotion concepts dominates the cognitive sciences and reflects a much wider view of knowledge. The key assumption underlying this view is the transduction principle, namely, the idea that knowledge results from transducing modality-specific states in perception, action, and introspection into amodal data structures that represent knowledge (Barsalou, 1999). To understand how the transduction principle works, first consider the modality-specific states that initiate the transduction process. Such states arise in sensory systems (e.g., vision, audition, taste, smell, touch), the motor system (e.g., action, proprioception), and introspection (i.e., mental states such as emotions, affects, evaluations, motivations, cognitive operations, memories).

The representation of these states can be thought of in two ways. First, these states can be viewed as patterns of neural activation in the respective brain systems. Consider the perception of a rose, which might produce patterns of neural activation in the visual, olfactory, and somatosensory systems. Reaching to touch the rose might produce neural activation in motor and spatial systems. Introspectively, the rose might produce neural activation in the amygdala. Together, these neural states constitute the brain's immediate response to the rose. At a second level of representation, some of this neural activation may produce conscious states. Certainly, though, much of the underlying neural processing remains unconscious. For example, people may be unaware of the low-level processing in vision that extracts shape information, or the low-level processing in action that generates an arm movement. Nevertheless, some aspects of these neural states become realized as conscious images in experience. Two points to be noted, then, are (1) that the modality-specific states activated during a specific experience occur at both neural and experiential levels, and (2) the mapping between them is not one to one.

According to the transduction principle, knowledge about the world, the body, and the mind result from redescribing the types of modality-specific states, illustrated by the example of the rose, with amodal knowledge structures. Thus, in such accounts, modality-specific states themselves do not represent knowledge, but the amodal data structures transduced from them do. Knowledge about roses does not consist of the modality-specific states that they produce in perception, action, and introspection. Instead, knowledge about roses resides in amodal knowledge structures that describe these states.

Examples of Amodal Representations

Most of the dominant theories in cognitive science represent knowledge in this manner. For example, a list representing features of a rose might look like:

Rose
petals
pollen
thorns
fragrance

Although words represent features in the theoretical notation, a key assumption is that amodal symbols actually represent each word in human memory, where there is a close correspondence between words and their amodal counterparts. For lack of a better notation, theorists generally use words to represent the content of amodal representations. Importantly, however, amodal symbols are assumed to constitute the underlying conceptual content in memory. During the processing of category members, these symbols are transduced from modality-specific states to represent their features. Later, when people need to communicate something about the category, they access the words associated with the symbols to do so.

A second important class of amodal theories integrates various types of conceptual relations with features to produce more complex representations (Barsalou & Hale, 1993). Theories in this category include semantic memory models, predicate-calculus representations of knowledge, frames, and production systems. Not only do such theories represent elemental features of categories, they also represent a variety of important relations between them. Rather than representing _pollen_ and _fragrance_ as independent features of roses, these theories might add the following relation between them:

Cause (pollen, fragrance)

Analogous to features, the relations between features are represented amodally. Specifically, as the relations arise in modality-specific states, amodal symbols for them are transduced, which then become bound to amodal symbols for the features that they integrate.

Finally, some (but certainly not all) connectionist theories implement the transduction principle. Feed-forward network theories offer one example. In feed-forward networks, a first layer of input units performs perceptual processing, extracting and representing features on a modality. The feature representations are then transduced into a second representation in the network's hidden units, which is typically interpreted as a conceptual representation. Conceptual representations are amodal for two reasons. First, random weights are set initially on the connections linking the input and hidden units; this step is necessary for implementing learning. The consequence, though, is a significant degree of arbitrariness between input- and hidden-level representations. Second, the activation patterns on the hidden units redescribe the input patterns, such that the hidden unit patterns have a linear relationship to the output units (in contrast, the input patterns have a nonlinear relationship). For these reasons, the hidden units that represent conceptual knowledge are transductions of perceptual states, much like the transductions that underlie more traditional knowledge structures. However, connectionist architectures that use a common set of units to represent perceptual and conceptual states do not exhibit transduction.

Representing Emotion Concepts Amodally

The dominant approach to representing emotion knowledge similarly rests on the transduction principle (Bower, 1981; Johnson-Laird & Oatley, 1989; Ortony, Clore, & Foss, 1987). According to these theories, various types of amodal knowledge structures are transduced from emotional experience to represent emotion concepts. Furthermore, representing knowledge of an emotion in the absence of experiencing it involves activating the appropriate amodal representation. Once this representation is active, it describes various domains of information relevant to the emotion, thereby producing inferences about it.

In general, knowledge about emotion falls into three general domains. First, people have knowledge about the situations that elicit emotions. Thus, seeing a smiling baby produces positive affect, whereas seeing a vomiting baby produces negative affect. Second, people have knowledge about the actions that are relevant when particular emotions are experienced. Thus, a smiling baby elicits approach responses, whereas a vomiting baby produces avoidance, at least initially. Third, people have knowledge about the introspective states associated with the "hot" component of emotions, including both valence and arousal information (e.g., Barrett, Chapter 11; Feldman, 1995). Thus, smiling babies produce warm, mildly aroused feelings, whereas vomiting babies produce negative, highly aroused feelings. Most importantly, amodal theories of emotion assume that amodal knowledge structures represent all three aspects of emotional experience. When people need to consult their knowledge of emotion, they activate and process such structures.

Embodiment in Amodal Theories

According to amodal theories, embodied states are peripheral appendages linked to amodal knowledge structures. Thus a positive emotion, such as happiness, might be linked with embodied states for producing the relevant facial expressions, postures, arm movements, vocal expressions, and so forth. Importantly, however, these embodied states do not constitute core emotion knowledge. Instead, each embodied state is linked to an amodal symbol that represents it. The embodied state of smiling, for example, is linked to an amodal symbol for smiling in the concept of happiness. When knowledge about happiness is processed, the amodal symbol for smiling becomes active, thereby carrying the inference that happiness includes smiling. Notably, however, embodied smiling is not necessary to represent the conceptual relation between smiling and happiness. Instead, actual smiling is only a peripheral state that can either trigger the concept for happiness or can result from its activation, mediated by the amodal symbol for smiling.

Amodal theories similarly peripheralize all other content in emotion concepts. The perception of another person smiling is represented by the same amodal symbol that represents the action of smiling, not by neural states in the visual system as it perceives smiling—which differ from neural states in the motor system that execute smiling. Similarly, the value and arousal of introspective emotional states are represented by amodal symbols, not by the neural states that underlie the modality-specific states. Thus, the modality-specific states that occur in emotion during action, perception, and introspection are peripheral appendages linked to core amodal symbols that stand for them. When these appendages are experienced, they can ultimately trigger an emotion concept via the intervening amodal symbols. When emotion concepts become active, they can ultimately trigger these appendages, again via the amodal symbols that intervene.

Modal Accounts of Embodied Emotion Effects

The Reenactment Principle

Whereas the transduction principle underlies amodal theories of knowledge, the reenactment principle underlies modal theories. According to the reenactment principle, the modality-specific states that arise during per-

ception, action, and introspection are partially captured by the brain's association areas (Damasio, 1989). Again consider the neural activation that
arises in the brain's visual, motor, olfactory, and affective systems when
interacting with a rose. While these states are active, association areas partially capture them, storing them away for future use. Conjunctive neurons
in association areas intercorrelate the active neurons both within and
between modalities, such that a partial record of the brain's processing state
becomes established as a memory. Later, when information about the rose
is needed, these conjunctive neurons attempt to reactivate the pattern of
neural states across the relevant modalities. As a result, the neural state of
processing is reenacted to represent the modality-specific states that the
brain was in while processing the rose. By no means is the reenactment
complete or fully accurate. Indeed, partial reenactment is almost certainly
the norm, along with various types of distortion that could reflect base
rates, background theories, etc. In this view, no amodal symbols are transduced to represent experiences of the world, body, and mind. Instead,
reenactments of original processing states perform this representational
work. For more detailed accounts of this theory, see Barsalou (1999, 2003a,
2003b, in press), and Simmons and Barsalou (2003).

Representing Emotion Concepts Modally

According to this view, modality-specific states represent the content of
concepts, including those for emotion. Consider the three domains of emotion knowledge mentioned earlier: triggering situations, resultant actions,
and introspective states. Reenactments of modality-specific states represent the conceptual content in these domains, not amodal symbols. Thus
reenactments of perceiving smiles visually on other people's faces belong to
the situational knowledge that triggers *happiness*, as do the motor and
somatosensory experiences of smiling oneself. Similarly, reenactments of
valence and arousal states represent these introspective aspects of emotion
concepts, not amodal symbols representing them (for a similar view, see
Barrett, Chapter 11).

In this view, knowledge of the emotion is delivered via actual emotional states, some being conscious and some unconscious; knowledge of an
emotion concept is not seen as a detached description of the respective
emotion. Although these states may not constitute full-blown emotions,
they may typically contain enough information about the original states to
function as representations of them conceptually. Moreover, these partial reenactments constitute the core knowledge of emotional concepts.
Embodied states are not merely peripheral events that trigger emotion
concepts or that result from the activation of emotion concepts. Instead,
embodied states represent the core conceptual content of an emotion.

Explaining Embodiment Effects in Emotion Research

As we saw earlier, embodiment enters ubiquitously into the processing of emotion. Viewing embodied states as the core elements of emotion concepts provides a natural account of these findings. When an embodied emotional response results from perceiving a social stimulus, this embodiment plays a central role in representing the emotional concept that becomes active to interpret the stimulus. For example, when the perception of a smiling baby activates embodied responses for smiling, approach, and positive valence in the self, these embodied states represent the emotional and affective concepts that become active, such as happiness and liking. Embodied states represent these concepts directly, rather than triggering amodal symbols that stand in for them. A similar account explains the embodiment effects reviewed earlier for visual imagery. As a person is imagining a social stimulus, the emotional categories used to interpret it are represented by the embodied states that become active.

A similar account explains the roles of embodiment in triggering emotion concepts and in their subsequent effects on cognitive processing. When a person's body enters into a particular state, this constitutes a retrieval cue of conceptual knowledge. Because modality-specific states represent knowledge, an active modality-specific state in the body or mind triggers concepts that contain the state as elements of their representation, via the encoding specificity principle (e.g., Tulving & Thomson, 1973). As matches occur, the emotion concept that best fits all current retrieval and contextual cues becomes active and dominates the retrieval competition. Furthermore, once an emotion concept dominates, it reenacts other modality-specific aspects of its content on other relevant modalities, thereby producing at least a partial semblance of the emotion. In turn, other cognitive processes, such as categorization, evaluation, and memory, are affected. As an embodied state triggers an emotion concept, and as the emotion becomes active, it biases other cognitive operations toward states consistent with the emotion.

As this brief description illustrates, the embodied approach to emotion offers a plausible and intuitive account of embodiment effects. It is also a productive approach that makes specific predictions, several of which we outline here.

Deep versus Shallow Tasks

The modal account described here predicts that bodily aspects of emotion concepts are simulated only when necessary; that is, in deep, but not in shallow, conceptual tasks. A deep task requires recourse to meaning, whereas a shallow task can be accomplished by simple associative means. According to a strict reading of the amodal models (e.g., Bower, 1981), there should be no simulation—that is, physiological manifestation of the emotion—in shallow or deep conceptual tasks because individuals can simply "read off" amodal feature lists for both tasks. A generous interpretation of an amodal model might yield the prediction that physiological manifestations will occur in both deep- and shallow-feature generation tasks because thinking about the emotion concept automatically activates the highly associated nodes that represent the physiological aspects of the emotion. However, a selective prediction that physiological manifestations of emotion are evoked *only* in deep, but not in shallow, tasks cannot easily be derived from an amodal model. This is because, if anything, physiological nodes are most directly and closely associated with emotion and should be the first to be activated during the use of the emotion concept in a deep or shallow way.

Partial Embodiment

The simulation account predicts that only the needed parts of the bodily representation are simulated (i.e., simulations occur only in the modality required to perform the task). The notion of partial simulation is illustrated by results of recent functional magnetic resonance imaging (fMRI) studies that found a selective activation of relevant parts of the sensory cortex when property verification tasks were performed in different modalities (Kan, Barsalou, Solomon, Minor, & Thompson-Schill, 2003; Kellenbach, Brett, & Patterson, 2001). Again, a strict reading of amodal models does not generate any embodiment predictions, because individuals can simply read off abstract features of emotion concepts. A more generous reading of amodal models would yield the prediction that the processing of emotion concepts should nonspecifically activate the associated sensory basis via top-down links.

Impairment/Facilitation of Sensory–Motor Processing

Finally, the simulation account predicts that manipulations of sensory–motor processing have conceptual consequences. This prediction is supported by studies showing that categorization impairments can result from damage to neural systems representing sensory characteristics of the category (Farah, 1994; Simmons & Barsalou, 2003). Further, several studies show that recognition and categorization of emotion can be impaired by damage to, or blocking of the mechanisms of, somatosensory feedback. Associative models predict no effects (or, at most, nonspecific effects) of such bottom-up manipulations. In short, amodal accounts see embodiment as irrelevant for conceptual processing. At best, they see it as a by-product of associations, not as a *constitutive element of conceptual processing.*

In sum, if these predictions were tested and evidence found in favor of modal models, this evidence would tell us much about the experience and reexperience of emotional states: how individuals ground emotion concepts, how emotion processes can be manipulated in the laboratory (or not), and how emotions and feelings can and cannot be regulated by the individual.

CONSCIOUS AND UNCONSCIOUS STATES OF EMOTION

The perspective presented here has a number of implications for conceptualizing emotion in general and defining its conscious and unconscious processes. First, consistent with William James, we have proposed that embodied states constitute the fundamental way of representing emotional information. For example, when we see a smiling face, we smile, and this response allows us to know the stimulus (see also Atkinson & Adolphs, Chapter 7; de Gelder, Chapter 6). Although James was criticized for not being able to specify why or when the perception of a given event or object would instigate the bodily state of an emotion in the first place, this is a less worrisome criticism now because good support for the notion of inherent affective "programs" (Tomkins, 1962), or bodily responding to signal stimuli, has been reported (e.g., Dimberg, 1986, 1990; Dimberg, Hansson, & Thunberg, 1989); although for a critical view, see Barrett, Chapter 11). Thus, as we have shown in our present review of the relevant research, the perception of certain stimuli, including—and perhaps especially— emotional expressions of other people, automatically produces specific bodily states in the perceiver. It is not necessary for such embodied states of emotion to be conscious, as in imitation for example, or even be available to consciousness. The states may be too subtle to gain consciousness, even if attention is directed to them. And potentially conscious embodiments may not become conscious because competing attentional demands simply win out (e.g., Neumann & Strack, 2000). One interesting implication of the notion of unconscious embodiment as stimulus encoding is that individual variability should be relatively low, within obvious morphological constraints.

When conscious attention is directed to the bodily state, and the bodily state is intense enough be consciously detected, we would suggest, consistent with James, that the individual experiences a *feeling state*. In the attention to, and interpretation of, a feeling state (e.g., in the service of self-report), variability and individual differences, including cultural rules of interpretation, can intervene. In an example of such variability, Laird and his colleagues (e.g., Laird & Crosby, 1974) documented stable individual differences in the extent to which expressive behavior influences feeling states per se (e.g., Laird & Bresler, 1992). Laird notes:

> The differences in impact of behavior seem to reflect the type of cues on which individuals base their emotional experience. People who attend to their own bodily cues, their appearance, and their instrumental actions are more responsive to so-called "personal" or "self-produced" cues. In contrast, individuals who primarily focus on interpretations of the situation and infer responses from what is appropriate in their situation, are responsive to "situational" cues. (Schnall & Laird, 2003, p. 789; see also Feldman, 1995; Barrett, Chapter 11, for further examples and discussion)

Thus, although unconscious embodiments of incoming stimuli may be quite stable and even universal, as noted, subsequent conscious simulations should be quite variable in content because they rely on the represented feeling states; that is, conscious simulations reenact the biases introduced by directing attention to the bodily state and representing it in consciousness as a feeling state. The content of concepts of anger, joy, fear, and so forth, will vary across individuals and situations to the extent that the situation determines selective attention to parts of a represented feeling state or experience and thus helps choose the simulation to be performed.

Distinguishing the bodily state of emotion and the feeling state of emotion is useful in the interpretation of a number of findings that would appear to be inconsistent with the embodiment approach. For example, if biases and individual differences intervene in defining the conscious feeling state, and if the bodily states can occur outside of consciousness, then there is no reason why self-report of feeling states should be highly correlated with bodily states; and, indeed, they are often not correlated (see Barrett, Chapter 11).

Relatedly, in a series of studies, Rimé, Phillipot, and their colleagues examined people's knowledge about the bodily states associated with different emotions, which they call schemata of peripheral changes in emotion (e.g., Rimé, Philippot, & Cisamolo, 1990). Results showed that such schemata, or sets of beliefs, were highly consensual and highly accessible. That is, individuals were in high agreement about the peripheral changes that occur during different emotions. Several studies were then conducted to evaluate the relation between these schemata and actual peripheral changes during an emotional state produced by watching emotionally evocative films. Some experimental participants reported their feelings and peripheral changes during the emotional films, and another set of participants described the contents of their schemata of peripheral changes for the emotions that were said to be evoked by the film (Phillipot, 1997). These two sets of reports were highly correlated, such that reported peripheral changes by one set of individuals were the same as those believed to be produced in the emotional states of interest by another set of individuals. However, further work showed that the reports of peripheral changes by participants who watched the films were less highly correlated with actual peripheral changes. Thus the authors concluded that people tend to report their beliefs about embodied states of emotion rather than an accurate readout of those states. If we separate the notion of bodily states of emotions (as sometimes unconscious) and feeling states (as always the result of conscious attention to the bodily states), we can see that such biases are the norm. The fact that embodied states constitute emotional information processing does not mean that simulations are invariant reproductions of those states.

CONCLUSION

We have reviewed a number of studies that suggest that emotion knowledge is grounded in the somatosensory and motor states to which emotions give rise. We have suggested that the implication of this work is that perceiving someone else's emotion, having an emotional response or feeling a state oneself, and using emotion knowledge in conceptual tasks all rely on the same fundamental processes. As we then demonstrated, recent theories of embodied cognition, which rely on the notions of modal representation of knowledge and the principle of reenactment, account for this accumulated knowledge quite well. Further, such models suggest much about what happens when people process emotional information, and can help generate testable hypotheses about conscious and unconscious states of emotion.

REFERENCES

Adelmann, P., & Zajonc, R. (1989). Facial efference and the experience of emotion. *Annual Review of Psychology, 40,* 249–280.

Adolphs, R., Damasio, H., & Tranel, D. (2002). Neural systems for recognition of emotional prosody: A 3-D lesion study. *Emotion, 2,* 23–51.

Andersen, S. M., Reznik, I., & Manzella, L. M. (1996). Eliciting facial affect, motivation and expectancies in transference: Significant-other representations in social relations. *Journal of Personality and Social Psychology, 71,* 1108–1129.

Barsalou, L. W. (1999). Perceptual symbol systems. *Behavioral and Brain Sciences*, 22, 577–609.

Barsalou, L. W. (2003a). Abstraction in perceptual symbol systems. *Philosophical Transactions of the Royal Society of London: Biological Sciences*, 358, 1177–1187.

Barsalou, L. W. (2003b). Situated simulation in the human conceptual system. *Language and Cognitive Processes*, 18, 513–562.

Barsalou, L. W. (in press). Abstraction as dynamic interpretation in perceptual symbol systems. Invited chapter under review for L. Gershkoff-Stowe & D. Rakison (Eds.), *Building object categories*. Carnegie Symposium Series. Mahwah, NJ: Erlbaum.

Barsalou, L. W., & Hale, C. R. (1993). Components of conceptual representation: From feature lists to recursive frames. In I. Van Mechelen, J. Hampton, R. Michalski, & P. Theuns (Eds.), *Categories and concepts: Theoretical views and inductive data analysis* (pp. 97–144). San Diego, CA: Academic Press.

Bavelas, J., Black, A., Lemery, C., & Mullett, J. (1987). Motor mimicry as primitive empathy. In N. Eisenberg & J. Strayer (Eds.), *Empathy and its development* (pp. 317–338). New York: Cambridge University Press.

Bodenhausen, G. V., Kramer, G. P., & Süsser, K. (1994). Happiness and stereotypic thinking in social judgment. *Journal of Personality and Social Psychology*, 66, 621–632.

Bower, G. H. (1981). Mood and memory. *American Psychologist*, 36, 129–148.

Bull, N. (1951). *The attitude theory of emotion* (Nervous and Mental Disease Monographs, No. 81). New York: Coolidge Foundation.

Bush, L., Barr, C., McHugo, G., & Lanzetta, J. (1989). The effects of facial control and facial mimicry on subjective reactions to comedy routines. *Motivation and Emotion*, 13, 31–52.

Cacioppo, J. T., Priester, J. R., & Berntson, G. G. (1993). Rudimentary determinants of attitudes: II. Arm flexion and extension have differential effects on attitudes. *Journal of Personality and Social Psychology*, 65, 5–17.

Chartrand, T. L., & Bargh, J. A. (1999). The chameleon effect: The perception–behavior link and social interaction. *Journal of Personality and Social Psychology*, 76, 893–910.

Cupchik, G., & Leventhal, H. (1974). Consistency between expressive behavior and the evaluation of humorous stimuli: The role of sex and self-observation. *Journal of Personality and Social Psychology*, 30, 429–442.

Damasio, A. R. (1989). Time-locked multiregional retroactivation: A systems-level proposal for the neural substrates of recall and recognition. *Cognition*, 33, 25–62.

Décety, J., & Chaminade, T. (2003). Neural correlates of feeling sympathy. *Neuropsychologia* (Special issue on social cognition), 41, 127–138.

Dimberg, U. (1982). Facial reactions to facial expressions. *Psychophysiology*, 19, 643–647.

Dimberg, U. (1986). Facial reactions to fear-relevant and fear-irrelevant stimuli. *Biological Psychology*, 23, 153–161.

Dimberg, U. (1990). Facial electromyography and emotional reactions. *Psychophysiology, 27,* 481–494.

Dimberg, U., Hansson, G., & Thunberg, M. (1989). Fear of snakes and facial reactions: A case of rapid emotional responding. *Scandinavian Journal of Psychology, 39,* 75–80.

Dimberg, U., Thunberg, M., & Elmehed, K. (2000). Unconscious facial reactions to emotional facial expressions. *Psychological Science, 11,* 86–89.

Duclos, S., & Laird, J. (2001). The deliberate control of emotional experience through control of expressions. *Cognition and Emotion, 15,* 27–56.

Duclos, S. E., Laird, J. D., Schneider, E., Sexter, M., Stern, L., & Van Lighten, O. (1989). Emotion-specific effects of facial expressions and postures on emotional experience. *Journal of Personality and Social Psychology, 57,* 100–108.

Duncan, I. W., & Laird, J. D. (1977). Cross-modality consistencies in individual differences in self-attribution. *Journal of Personality, 45,* 191–206.

Duncan, I. W., & Laird, J. D. (1980). Positive and reverse placebo effects as a function of differences in cues used in self-perception. *Journal of Personality and Psychology, 39,* 1024–1036.

Ekman, P., Levenson, R., & Friesen, W. (1983). Autonomous nervous system activity distinguishes among emotions. *Science, 221,* 1208–1210.

Farah, M. (1994). Neuropsychological inference with an interactive brain: A critique of the locality assumption. *Behavioral and Brain Sciences, 17,* 43–61.

Feldman, L. A. (1995). Variations in the circumplex structure of mood. *Personality and Social Psychology Bulletin, 21,* 806–817.

Flack, W., Laird, J., & Cavallaro, L. (1999). Separate and combined effects of facial expressions and bodily postures on emotional feelings. *European Journal of Social Psychology, 29,* 203–217.

Förster, J., & Strack, F. (1996). Influence of overt head movements on memory for valenced words: A case of conceptual–motor compatibility. *Journal of Personality and Social Psychology, 71,* 421–430.

Förster, J., & Strack, F. (1997). Motor actions in retrieval of valenced information: I. A motor congruence effect. *Perceptual and Motor Skills, 85,* 1419–1427.

Förster, J., & Strack, F. (1998). Motor actions in retrieval of valenced information: II. Boundary conditions for motor congruence effects. *Perceptual and Motor Skills, 86,* 1423–1426.

Gallese, V. (2003). The roots of empathy: The shared manifold hypothesis and the neural basis of intersubjectivity. *Psychopathology, 36,* 171–180.

Galton, F. (1884). Measurement of character. *Fortnightly Review, 42,*179–185.

Gehricke, J. G., & Fridlund, A. J. (2002). Smiling, frowning, and autonomic activity in mildly depressed and nondepressed men in response to emotional imagery of social context. *Perceptual and Motor Skills, 94,* 141–151.

Gehricke, J. G., & Shapiro, D. (2000). Reduced facial expression and social context in major depression: Discrepancies between facial muscle activity and self-reported emotion. *Psychiatry Research, 95,* 157–167.

Gollnisch, G., & Averill, J. R. (1993). Emotional imagery: Strategies and correlates. *Cognition and Emotion, 7,* 407–429.

Grossberg, J. M., & Wilson, H. K. (1968). Physiological changes accompanying the visualization of fearful and neutral situations. *Journal of Personality and Social Psychology, 10*, 124–133.

Hatfield, E., Hsee, C. K., Costello, J., Weisman, M. S., & Denney, C. (1995). The impact of vocal feedback on emotional experience and expression. *Journal of Social Behavior and Personality, 10*, 293–312.

Hsee, C. K., Hatfield, E., Carlson, J. G., & Chemtob, C. (1990). The effect of power on susceptibility to emotional contagion. *Cognition and Emotion, 4*, 327–340.

Hutchison, W. D., Davis, K. D., Lozano, A. M., Tasker, R. K., & Dostrovsky, J. O. (1999). Pain-related neurons in the human cingulate cortex. *Nature–Neuroscience, 2*, 403–405.

James, W. (1981). *The principles of psychology.* Cambridge, MA: Harvard University Press. (Original work published 1890)

Innes-Ker, Å., & Niedenthal, P. M. (2002). Emotion concepts and emotional states in social judgment and categorization. *Journal of Personality and Social Psychology, 83*, 804–816.

Johnson-Laird, P. N., & Oatley, K. (1989). The language of emotions: An analysis of a semantic field. *Cognition and Emotion, 3*, 81–123.

Kan, I. P., Barsalou, L. W., Solomon, K. O., Minor, J. K., & Thompson-Schill, S. L. (2003). Role of mental imagery in a property verification task: fMRI evidence to perceptual representation of conceptual knowledge. *Cognitive Neuropsychology, 20*, 525–540.

Kellenbach, M. L., Brett, M., & Patterson, K. (2001). Large, colorful, or noisy? Attribute- and modality-specific activations during retrieval of perceptual attribute knowledge. *Cognitive, Affective, and Behavioral Neuroscience, 1*, 207–221.

Kleck, R. E., Vaughan, R. C., Cartwright-Smith, J., Vaughan, K. B., Colby, C. Z., & Lanzetta, J. T. (1976). Effects of being observed on expressive, subjective, and physiological responses to painful stimuli. *Journal of Personality and Social Psychology, 34*, 1211–1218.

Kopel, S., & Arkowitz, H. (1974). Role playing as a source of self-observation and behavior change. *Journal of Personality and Social Psychology, 29*, 677–686.

Kraut, R. E. (1982). Social presence, facial feedback, and emotion. *Journal of Personality and Social Psychology, 42*, 853–863.

Laird, J. D. (1974). Self-attribution of emotion: The effects of expressive behavior on the quality of emotional experience. *Journal of Personality and Social Psychology, 29*, 475–486.

Laird, J. D., & Bresler, C. (1992). The processing of emotional experience: A self-perception theory. In M. S. Clark (Ed.), *Review of personality and social psychology: Vol. 13. Emotion* (pp. 213–234). Newbury Park, CA: Sage.

Laird, J. D., & Crosby, M. (1974). Individual differences in the self-attribution of emotion. In H. London & R. Nisbett (Eds.), *Thinking and feeling: The cognitive alteration of feeling states* (pp. 44–59). Chicago: Aldine.

Laird, J. D., Wagener, J., Halal, M., & Szegda, M. (1982). Remembering what you feel: Effects of emotion on memory. *Journal of Personality and Social Psychology, 42*, 646–657.

Lang, P. J., Kozak, M. J., Miller, G. A., Levin, D. N., & McLean, A. (1980). Emotional imagery: Conceptual structure and pattern of somatovisceral response. *Psychophysiology, 17,* 179–192.

Lanzetta, J., Biernat, J., & Kleck, R. (1982). Self-focused attention, facial behavior, autonomic arousal and the experience of emotion. *Motivation and Emotion, 6,* 49–63.

Lanzetta, J., Cartwright-Smith, J., & Kleck, R. (1976). Effects of nonverbal dissimulation on emotional experience and autonomic arousal. *Journal of Personality and Social Psychology, 33,* 354–370.

Levenson, R., Ekman, P., & Friesen,W. V. (1990). Voluntary facial action generates emotion specific autonomic nervous system activity. *Psychophysiology, 27,* 363–384.

Leventhal, H., & Cupchik, G. C. (1975). The informational and facilitative effects of an audience upon expression and the evaluation of humorous stimuli. *Journal of Experimental Social Psychology, 11,* 363–380.

Leventhal, H., & Mace, W. (1970). The effect of laughter on evaluation of a slapstick movie. *Journal of Personality, 38,* 16–30.

McHugo, G., Lanzetta, J., Sullivan, D., Masters, R., & Englis, B. (1985). Emotional reactions to a political leader's expressive display. *Journal of Personality and Social Psychology, 49,* 1513–1529.

McIntosh, D. (1996). Facial feedback hypotheses: Evidence, implications, and directions. *Motivation and Emotion, 20,* 121–147.

Neumann, R., & Strack, F. (2000). Approach and avoidance: The influence of proprioceptive and exteroceptive cues on encoding of affective information. *Journal of Personality and Social Psychology, 79,* 39–48.

Niedenthal, P. M., Brauer, M., Halberstadt, J. B., & Innes-Ker, Å. (2001). When did her smile drop?: Facial mimicry and the influences of emotional state on the detection of change in emotional expression. *Cognition and Emotion, 15,* 853–864.

Niedenthal, P. M., Rohmann, A., & Dalle, N. (2003). What is primed by emotion concepts and emotion words? In J. Musch & K. C. Klauer (Eds.), *The psychology of evaluation: Affective processes in cognition and emotion* (pp. 307–333). Mahwah, NJ: Erlbaum.

Ohira, H., & Kurono, K. (1993). Facial feedback effects on impression formation. *Perceptual and Motor Skills, 77,* 1251–1258.

Ortony, A., Clore, G. L., & Foss, M. A. (1987). The referential structure of the affective lexicon. *Cognitive Science, 11,* 341–364.

Philippot, P. (1997). Prototypes d'émotion. In J.-P. Leyens & J.-L. Beauvois (Eds.), *L'ère de la cognition.* Grenoble, France: Presses Universitaires de Grenoble.

Rimé, B., Philippot, P., & Cisamolo, D. (1990). Social schemata of peripheral changes in emotion. *Journal of Personality and Social Psychology, 59,* 38–49.

Riskind, J. H. (1983). Nonverbal expressions and the accessibility of life experience memories: A congruency hypothesis. *Social Cognition, 2,* 62–86.

Riskind, J. H., & Gotay, C. C. (1982). Physical posture: Could it have regulatory or feedback effects on motivation and emotion? *Motivation and Emotion, 6,* 273–298.

Rutledge, L., & Hupka, R. (1985). The facial feedback hypothesis: Methodological concerns and new supporting evidence. *Motivation and Emotion, 9,* 219–240.

Schnall, S., & Laird, J. D. (2003). Keep smiling: Enduring effects of facial expressions and postures on emotional experience and memory. *Cognition and Emotion, 17,* 787–797.

Schwarz, N., & Clore, G. L. (1983). Mood, misattribution, and judgments of well-being: Informative and directive functions of affective states. *Journal of Personality and Social Psychology, 45,* 513–523.

Siegman, A., Anderson, R., & Berger, T. (1990). The angry voice: Its effects on the experience of anger and cardiovascular reactivity. *Psychosomatic Medicine, 52,* 631–643.

Simmons, K., & Barsalou, L. W. (2003). The similarity-in-topography principle: Reconciling theories of conceptual deficits. *Cognitive Neuropsychology, 20,* 451–486. [Reprinted in A. Martin & A. Caramazza (Eds.), *The organisation of conceptual knowledge in the brain: Neuropsychological and neuroimaging perspectives* (pp. 451–486). East Sussex, UK: Psychology Press.]

Soussignan, R. (2002). Duchenne Smile, emotional experience and autonomic reactivity: A test of the facial feedback hypothesis. *Emotion, 2,* 52–74.

Stepper, S., & Strack, F. (1993). Proprioceptive determinants of emotional and nonemotional feelings. *Journal of Personality and Social Psychology, 64,* 211–220.

Strack, F., Martin, L. L., & Stepper, S. (1988). Inhibiting and facilitating conditions of the human smile: A nonobtrusive test of the facial feedback hypothesis. *Journal of Personality and Social Psychology, 54,* 768–777.

Strack, F., Schwarz, N., & Gschneidinger, E. (1985). Happiness and reminiscing: The role of time perspective, mood, and mode of thinking. *Journal of Personality and Social Psychology, 49,* 1460–1469.

Tomkins, S. S. (1962). *Affect, imagery, and consciousness: The positive affects.* New York: Springer.

Tulving, E., & Thomson, D. M. (1973). Encoding specificity and retrieval processes in episodic memory. *Psychological Review, 80,* 352–373.

Vanman, E. J., Paul, B. Y., Ito, T. A., & Miller, N. (1997). The modern face of prejudice and structural features that moderate the effect of cooperation on affect. *Journal of Personality and Social Psychology, 73,* 941–959.

Vaughan, K., & Lanzetta, J. (1980). Vicarious instigation and conditioning of facial expressive and autonomic responses to a model's expressive display of pain. *Journal of Personality and Social Psychology, 38,* 909–923.

Vaughan, K., & Lanzetta, J. (1981). The effect of modification of expressive display on vicarious emotional arousal. *Journal of Experimental Social Psychology, 17,* 16–30.

Vrana, S. R. (1993). The psychophysiology of disgust: Differentiating negative emotional contexts with facial EMG. *Psychophysiology, 30,* 279–286.

Vrana, S. R. (1995). Emotional modulation of skin conductance and eyeblink responses to a startle probe. *Psychophysiology, 32,* 351–357.

Vrana, S. R., Cuthbert, B. N., & Lang, P. J. (1989). Processing fearful and neutral sentences: Memory and heart rate change. *Cognition and Emotion, 3,* 179–195.

Vrana, S. R., & Rollock, D. (2002). The role of ethnicity, gender, emotional content, and contextual differences in physiological, expressive, and self-reported emotional responses to imagery. *Cognition and Emotion, 16*, 165–192.

Wallbott, H. G. (1991). Recognition of emotion from facial expression via imitation? Some indirect evidence for an old theory. *British Journal of Social Psychology, 30*, 207–219.

Wegener, D. T., Petty, R. E., & Smith, S. M. (1995). Positive mood can increase or decrease message scrutiny: The hedonic contingency view of mood and message processing. *Journal of Personality and Social Psychology, 69*, 5–15.

Wells, G. L., & Petty, R. E. (1980). The effects of overt head movements on persuasion: Compatibility and incompatibility of responses. *Basic and Applied Social Psychology, 1*, 219–230.

Zajonc, R. B., Adelmann, P. K., Murphy, S. T., & Niedenthal, P. M. (1987). Convergence in the physical appearance of spouses. *Motivation and Emotion, 11*, 335–346.

Zajonc, R. B., & Markus, H. (1984). Affect and cognition: The hard interface. In C. E. Izard, J. Kagan, & R. B. Zajonc (Eds.), *Emotions, cognition, and behavior* (pp. 73–102). Cambridge, UK: Cambridge University Press.

Zajonc, R. B., Pietromonaco, P., & Bargh, J. (1982). Independence and interaction of affect and cognition. In M. S. Clark & S. T. Fiske (Eds.), *Affect and cognition* (pp. 211–227). Hillsdale, NJ: Erlbaum.

Zuckerman, M., Klorman, R., Larrance, D., & Spiegel, N. (1981). Facial, autonomic, and subjective components of emotion: The facial feedback hypothesis versus the externalizer–internalizer distinction. *Journal of Personality and Social Psychology, 41*, 929–944.

CHAPTER 3

The Interaction of Emotion and Cognition

Insights from Studies of the Human Amygdala

Elizabeth A. Phelps

Initial investigations of human affective neuroscience emphasized the identification of neural structures that seem to be specialized for emotion processing (Damasio, 1994; LeDoux, 1996). At the same time, research in cognitive neuroscience explored other brain systems identified as primarily important for cognitive functions (Gazzaniga, Ivry, & Mangun, 1998). These initial efforts paralleled the traditional division between psychological study of emotion and cognition. The cognitive revolution and the development of a subdiscipline of psychology focused on understanding cognition relegated the study of emotion to other domains (Anderson, 1999; Neisser, 1976), particularly social and clinical psychology. Although there have been debates over the years as to the appropriate role of emotion in the study of cognition (Lazarus, 1981; Zajonc, 1980), until recently both psychological and neuroscience research on cognitive function usually failed to consider a role for emotion.

As neuroscience research in human affective processes progresses, however, it has become increasingly apparent that the neural systems of emotion interact extensively with those underlying cognitive processes (see

1. *What is the scope of your proposed model? When you use the term* emotion, *how do you use it? What do you mean by terms such as* fear, anxiety, *or* happiness?

In this chapter, I use the term *emotion* (in most cases) when referring to the reaction to stimuli that elicit a physiological arousal response, usually due to their aversive nature. The amygdala has primarily been shown to play a role in processing stimuli that are arousing; this role has been shown to extend to arousal in response to positive stimuli (e.g., Anderson, Christoff, Panitz, DeRosa, & Gabrieli, 2002), although most studies use negative stimuli. In addition, the amygdala has been shown to process stimuli that convey fear or threat-related signals (e.g., pictures of fear faces), even if these stimuli do not elicit a detectable physiological response. Although the amygdala is often broadly thought of as a critical structure in emotion processing, there is no clear evidence that it plays an important role in other key components of emotion, such as the subjective experience of emotional states (Anderson & Phelps, 2002).

2. *Define your terms:* conscious, unconscious, awarness. *Or say why you do not use these terms.*

I use the term *awareness* throughout my chapter. The primary means used to assess awareness in the studies I report is verbal report; that is, do subjects indicate awareness of an event.

3. *Does your model deal with what is conscious, what is unconscious, or their relationship? If you do not address this area specifically, can you speculate on the relationship between what is conscious and unconscious? Or if you do not like the conscious–unconscious distinction, or if you do not think this is a good question to ask, can you say why?*

I address the conscious–unconcious distinction primarily by referring to indirect (or implicit) and direct (or explicit) means of expression. I address the interaction of the two by providing examples of how an acquired conscious awareness and explicit strategies can influence the indirect expression of emotion (primarily through physiological measures of arousal). I also indicate how the emotional qualities of a event can influence the likelihood that the subject will be aware of that event, either during initial stimulus processing or later, during recollection.

also Gray, Schaefer, Braver, & Most, Chapter 4). These interactions have prompted a reconsideration of the appropriate role of emotion in efforts to understand cognition (Gazzaniga, Ivry, & Mangun, 2002). In this chapter, I review recent insights from affective neuroscience into the interaction of emotion and cognition. I focus on the role of the human amygdala, a small structure in the medial temporal lobe thought to be specialized for emotion, and its interaction with processes of cognition and awareness.

INDEPENDENT SYSTEMS FOR EMOTION
AND COGNITION

The amygdala is an almond-shaped structure in the medial temporal lobe, located just anterior to the hippocampal complex. It was first identified as a brain structure potentially important for emotion when Klüver and Bucy (1939) observed the behavior of monkeys after medial temporal lobe lesions, which included the amygdala, hippocampus, and surrounding cortices. These monkeys displayed a pattern of behavior, called "psychic blindness," marked by odd emotional responses, such as approaching objects that would normally elicit a fear response (e.g., snakes). Approximately 20 years later, Weiskrantz (1956) identified the amygdala as the medial temporal lobe structure whose damage is directly responsible for psychic blindness. Since that time, it has been widely acknowledged that the amygdala is a brain region whose primary function is linked to emotion.

More recent investigations in nonhuman animals have explored the precise role of the amygdala in emotion processing. These studies have mostly investigated the role of the amygdala in emotional learning, using fear conditioning methods, as a model paradigm. In fear conditioning method, a neutral stimulus (e.g., a tone), the conditioned stimulus (CS) acquires emotional properties by being paired with an aversive event (e.g., a foot shock), the unconditioned stimulus (US). After a few pairings, the animal displays a range of fear responses, such as changes in heart rate, blood pressure, startle reflexes, and freezing, to the previously neutral CS. These learned fear responses are conditioned responses (CRs). Using fear conditioning as a model paradigm, researchers have mapped the pathways of fear learning from stimulus input to response output (e.g., Davis, 2000; Kapp, Whalen, Supple, & Pascoe, 1992; LeDoux, 1996). These elegant animal models have identified the amygdala as a critical structure in the acquisition, storage, and expression of fear learning (see LeDoux, 2002, for a review).

Some of the initial efforts to explore the neural systems of emotion processing in the human brain were inspired by these animal models. Findings from studies of fear conditioning in humans are largely consistent with results from other species. In a typical paradigm in humans, a neutral stimulus such as a blue square (the CS) is paired with a mild shock to the wrist (the US). After a few pairings the blue square itself elicits physiological indications of fear (the CR), such as an increased skin conductance response (SCR; a measure of mild sweating that occurs with autonomic nervous system arousal). Using functional magnetic resonance imaging (fMRI), activation of the amygdala has been observed during fear conditioning (LaBar, Gatenby, Gore, Le Doux, & Phelps, 1998; Buchel, Moris,

Dolan, & Friston, 1998). The strength of this activation was correlated with the strength of the CR, as assessed by the SCR (LaBar et al., 1998). In addition, patients with amygdala damage fail to show any evidence of a CR, even though they show a normal response to the US, indicating that the amygdala is critical for the expression of *learned* fear responses, not the physiological expression of fear itself (Bechara et al., 1995: LaBar, Le Doux, Spencer, & Phelps, 1995).

Although the findings from fear conditioning in humans are consistent with animal models that identify the amygdala as a critical structure in the acquisition and expression of fear learning, there are some differences between humans and nonhumans with amygdala damage. Even though the human amygdala is critical for the expression of the CR, patients with amygdala damage do not display odd emotional responses similar to those observed by Klüver and Bucy (1939) in monkeys (Anderson & Phelps, 2002). In fact, the famous amnesic patient H.M. had a lesion similar to that of the Klüver–Bucy monkeys; however, the effect he experienced was described as primarily a long-term memory deficit with relatively normal social and emotional responses (Milner, Corkin, & Teuber, 1968). A hint of a possible reason for this difference in emotional behavior between humans and nonhumans with amygdala damage came from the initial studies on fear conditioning in humans. These patients with amygdala lesions, who failed to demonstrate any evidence of a CR, as assessed with physiological measures, showed an intact awareness and understanding of the events of fear conditioning (LaBar et al., 1995; Bechara et al., 1995).

For example, patient S.P., who suffers from bilateral damage to the amygdala, was given a fear conditioning paradigm in which a blue square was paired with a mild shock to the wrist. Unlike normal control subjects, she failed to demonstrate a CR to the blue square, as assessed with SCR. She was shown the data indicating a deficit in the normal expression of a CR and asked to comment on what she believed was the significance of these results.

> "I knew that there was an anticipation that the blue square, at some particular point in time, would bring on one of the volt shocks. But even though I knew that, and I knew that from the very beginning, except for the very first one where I was surprised. That was my response—I knew it was going to happen. I expected that it was going to happen. So I learned from the very beginning that it was going to happen: blue and shock. And it happened. I turned out to be right, it happened!" (in Phelps, 2002, p. 559)

As S.P. indicates in her description of fear conditioning, even though she failed to demonstrate a CR, she had a very good awareness and understanding of the emotional significance of the CS (i.e., the blue square). This awareness most likely would have been sufficient to guide her actions had she been given the option of avoiding the blue square. Studies in patients with hippocampal damage, whose amygdala is intact, show the opposite pattern. That is, they are unable to explicitly report the events of fear conditioning, but they show a normal CR, as assessed physiologically with SCR (Bechara et al., 1995). This double dissociation demonstrates the influence of multiple memory systems—an episodic or declarative memory system, dependent on the hippocampal complex, that underlies an awareness and understanding of learned events, and an emotional learning system, dependent on the amygdala, that is necessary for learned implicit, physiological expressions of emotional experience. It is possible that patients with amygdala damage display relatively normal emotional responses by relying on episodic representations that result in a cognitive awareness and understanding of the emotional significance of events.

These initial studies of fear conditioning following amygdala damage in humans suggest that emotional and cognitive learning systems are represented independently in the human brain. The findings appear to support the tradition of investigating cognitive processes independent of emotion's influence. However, even though this initial research on the human amygdala indicates an independence of emotion and cognition, more recent findings highlight the complex interactions between the neural systems of emotion and those of cognition (see also Gray et al., Chapter 4). In the remainder of this chapter, I review recent research suggesting that even though an amygdala/emotion system can operate independently of cognition and awareness, there are also extensive interactions. Cognitive awareness can influence amygdala function and emotional expression. At the same time, emotion and amygdala processing can influence awareness and a range of cognitive functions. These interactions are bidirectional and suggest a complex relationship between emotion and cognition.

THE INFLUENCE OF COGNITION ON EMOTION

The performance of patients with amygdala damage during fear conditioning shows that the amygdala is not necessary for an awareness and understanding of the emotional significance of a CS (LaBar et al., 1995; Bechara, et al., 1995; Phelps, 2002). These patients, who have an intact hippocampus, are able to remember and explicitly report that the CS predicts the aversive shock. Fear conditioning in which a neutral CS is paired with an aversive US, resulting in an aversive experience (i.e., pain or discomfort), is only one of the means that can be used to learn about the emotional significance of a stimulus. The emotional properties of a stimulus can also be conveyed through verbal instruction without any direct aversive consequence. This type of symbolic communication is typical in everyday human experience (e.g., see Smith & Neumann, Chapter 12). For example, many common fears, such as a fear of flying, are not usually the result of direct experience but rather are acquired through hearing about potential negative consequences of flying.

Given that patients with amygdala damage are able to remember and verbally report the events of fear conditioning, it is unlikely the amygdala is necessary to acquire an episodic representation and awareness of the emotional properties of a stimulus that are conveyed through language. It is unclear if this type of symbolic communication of emotion requires the amygdala at all. This question was addressed using a paradigm of "instructed fear." As in the fear conditioning paradigm described earlier, a blue square is paired with the possibility of a mild shock to the wrist. However, with instructed fear, subjects are simply told a blue square (the threat stimulus) is potentially linked to a shock. Subjects never actually receive a shock.

Previous studies have shown that instructed fear results in a similar physiological expression of fear (i.e., SCR) as fear conditioning (Hugdahl & Öhman, 1977). Simply being told a stimulus predicts a mild shock is enough to elicit a fear response to that stimulus. fMRI was used to determine if this cognitive, episodic representation of the aversive properties of a stimulus could influence the amygdala. Significant activation of the left amygdala was observed in response to presentation of a blue square verbally linked to the possibility of a mild shock (i.e., the threat stimulus) compared to a yellow square that was not linked to threat (i.e., the safe stimulus). The strength of the amygdala response to the threat stimulus predicted the magnitude of the physiological expression of fear, as assessed with SCR (Phelps et al., 2001). These results are similar to those observed with fear conditioning in which amygdala activation to a CS predicted the strength of the CR (LaBar et al., 1998).

The finding that instructed fear leads to amygdala activation suggests that an episodic representation and awareness of the emotional significance of the threat stimulus can influence the amygdala. However, these brain-imaging results do not indicate if the amygdala plays any critical role in the expression of instructed fear. To explore the precise role of the amygdala, patients suffering from unilateral (right and left) and bilateral amygdala damage participated in the instructed fear paradigm. Although all the subjects remembered and verbally reported that the blue square predicted the possibility of shock, patients with left and bilateral amygdala damage failed to show any physiological expression of fear to the threat stimulus. Patients with right amygdala damage and normal controls demonstrated physiological responses consistent with fear to the blue square (Funayama, Grillon, Davis, & Phelps, 2001). These results indicate that awareness of the aversive properties of a stimulus, acquired symbolically without direct aversive experience, can influence the amygdala (primarily, the left amygdala), which in turn mediates the physiological expression of fear.

The instructed fear studies demonstrate one method by which cognition and awareness can influence amygdala function. In everyday human life, many of our fears are the result of our interpretation of the significance of events. Whether a specific threat is real and imminent or unrealistic and unlikely, humans can use imagination and interpretation to induce a fear response. The instructed fear studies indicate that symbolically represented fears that are imagined and anticipated, but never experienced, rely on similar neural mechanisms for expression as fears acquired through direct aversive experience.

With instructed fear, cognitive interpretation and imagination result in a fear response. It is also possible to use cognitive control and interpretation to diminish a fear response. This is one of the principles guiding cognitive therapies for psychological disorders. For instance, in anxiety disorders a fear response, which may be appropriate in some situations, is expressed in inappropriate or maladaptive circumstances. Cognitive therapy focuses on changing the thought patterns related to the generation of a maladaptive anxiety response in an effort to change this behavior. This type of emotion regulation is important not only in controlling unwanted fear responses but also normal social interaction and emotional function. If the amygdala plays a role in the expression of fears that are learned symbolically and depend on awareness and interpretation for expression, then it is possible the amygdala response is also altered by cognitive strategies that diminish a fear response.

In an effort to examine the effect of emotion regulation strategies on the amygdala, fMRI was used during a study of reappraisal, an emotion regulation technique in which the significance of a potentially ambiguous event is interpreted, or reappraised, to alter its emotional connotation. For instance, if subjects were shown a picture of women crying outside of a church, a possible interpretation would be that the women are at a funeral for a loved one. However, if subjects were instructed to reappraise the scene so that the emotional reaction is less negative, they might imagine instead that the women are at a wedding and their tears are joyful. Previous research has shown that this type of reappraisal instruction can significantly alter the emotional state of the subjects (Gross, 2002). A study by Ochsner, Bunge, Gross, and Gabrielli (2002) asked subjects to reappraise the emotional significance of negative scenes during fMRI. Reappraisal not only significantly diminished the rating of negative affect for the scenes but also reduced the amygdala response, relative to scenes they were instructed to attend to without reappraising them (see also Schaffer, Jackson, Davidson, Kimbers, & Thompson-Schill, 2002). In addition to the amygdala, a region of the left dorsolateral prefrontal cortex (DLPFC) showed greater activation on reappraise versus attend trials. This DLPFC region is similar to that observed during executive control tasks in working memory (Smith & Jonides, 1999), consistent with the notion that reappraisal engages cognitive control mechanisms. The amygdala and DLPFC were inversely correlated across subjects. That is, those subjects who showed greater DLPFC engagement during reappraisal also showed a greater reduction in amygdala activation to the negative scenes.

More recently, a study by Delgado and colleagues (2004) instructed subjects to use an active emotion regulation strategy to diminish conditioned fear responses. The emotion regulation strategy diminished the physiological expression of the CR as well as amygdala activation to the CS. Consistent with Ochsner et al. (2002), a similar pattern of activation was observed in the DLPFC (i.e., greater activation to reappraise vs. attend). These results demonstrate that explicit cognitive strategies and control mechanisms can alter the amygdala response during tasks that range from viewing negative scenes to fear conditioning.

The studies of instructed fear and emotion regulation indicate that even if cognitive awareness and understanding of the emotional properties of a CS are not necessary for conditioned fear, there are a number of ways that cognition and awareness can influence the amygdala and emotional responses. Symbolic communication and awareness of the potentially aversive properties of an event can result in the expression of an emotional response that is dependent on the amygdala. In addition, cognitive control mechanisms can be used to help execute emotion regulation strategies, which can diminish an amygdala response to an emotional scene or a CS. These findings suggest that the independence of the amygdala function and cognitive awareness observed in fear conditioning may not reflect the importance of cognitive mechanisms of emotional learning or the complexity of emotional expressions that are typical in everyday human experience.

THE INFLUENCE OF EMOTION ON COGNITION

The influence of cognitive mechanisms on amygdala function indicates that this subcortical structure can be influenced by symbolic representations, cognitive control, and conscious interpretation. However, the relation between the amygdala and cognitive awareness also goes the other way.

Emotion, through the amygdala, can influence cognitive mechanisms and conscious awareness of events and stimuli. Two primary means have been identified by which the amygdala alters cognitive awareness: (1) The amygdala modulates long-term retention of memory, so that over time we are more likely to be aware of emotional events; and (2) the amygdala influences attention and perception (Lundqvist & Öhman, Chapter 5; de Gelder, Chapter 6; Atkinson & Adolphs, Chapter 7) so that emotional events are more likely to reach awareness.

Memories for emotional events seem to have a vividness and persistence that other memories lack. It has been suggested that one adaptive function of emotion is to enhance the storage of episodic memories so that events that are linked to an emotional response, and are potentially more important for survival, are not forgotten (McGaugh, 2000). It is widely acknowledged that emotion enhances episodic memory for events (Christianson, 1992). The result is that over time, we are more likely to remember and be aware of emotional events than neutral events. This modulation of long-term memory and awareness for emotional events is, in part, due to the amygdala's modulation of the storage of hippocampal-dependent memories.

The hippocampal complex is necessary for initial encoding of episodic or declarative memory. After encoding, there is a period of time during which the disruption of the hippocampus impairs memory retention, suggesting that the hippocampal complex is also critical for the long-term storage, or *consolidation*, of memories. Eventually, however, episodic memories can be retrieved independent of the hippocampal function, at which point they are thought to be consolidated (see Squire, Clark, & Bayley, 2004, for a review). In an elegant series of studies in rats, McGaugh and colleagues demonstrated that the release of stress hormones with arousal engages a mechanism by which the amygdala modulates the consolidation, or storage, of hippocampal-dependent memories (see McGaugh, 2000, for a review). The amygdala is not necessary for the normal formation or storage of episodic memories; it simply influences how well these memories are stored when there is an emotional arousal reaction to the event.

A series of lesion, phamacological, and brain-imaging studies in humans supports these animal models, suggesting that the amygdala plays a role in the enhanced retention of hippocampal-dependent episodic memory for emotional events. For example, it has been demonstrated that patients with amygdala damage, in contrast to normal controls, fail to show enhanced memory for arousing events (Cahill, Babinsky, Markowitsch, & McGaugh, 1995). In normal control subjects, the memory advantage for emotional events is more pronounced over time, indicating that emotional events are not forgotten at the same rate as neutral events (Kleinsmith & Kaplan,

1963), consistent with enhanced consolidation or storage of memories with arousal. Patients with amygdala damage, unlike normal controls, show similar forgetting curves for arousing and neutral stimuli (LaBar & Phelps, 1998). When normal control subjects are given beta-blockers, which block the action of stress hormones on the amygdala, these subjects perform similarly to patients with amygdala lesions in that they no longer demonstrate a memory advantage for arousing stimuli after a delay (Cahill, Prins, Weber, & McGaugh, 1994). Finally, a number of brain-imaging studies have shown that amygdala activation during the encoding of emotionally arousing events is predictive of the ability to retrieve these events at a later time (Cahill et al., 1996; Canli, Zhao, Brewer, Gabrielli, & Cahill, 2000; Hamann, Ely, Grafton, & Kilts, 1999). These findings, using a range of techniques in humans, support animal models that outline a mechanism by which the amygdala enhances the storage or retention of emotional events with arousal.

By modulating the storage or retention of events with emotion, the amygdala alters the stimuli that are available to awareness over time. Most events encountered in our daily lives are forgotten. For instance, it would be difficult for most people to accurately recollect what they had for dinner a week ago, unless this dinner was significant for some reason. Emotion helps ensure that events are not forgotten. Although there may be other means by which emotion enhances episodic memory that are not amygdala dependent (see Phelps et al., 1998), a wide range of research suggests that the human amygdala is at least partially responsible for the enhanced long-term retention and awareness of events that elicit an arousal response.

In addition to modulating the long-term retention and storage of emotional events, the amygdala can also affect memory by altering the initial stage of memory processing—encoding. Findings from a number of studies suggest that emotion can change the processing of stimuli when they are first encountered by influencing attention. Emotion has been shown to both capture and facilitate attention. Attention paradigms that require the processing of nonemotional aspects of a stimulus, such as the emotional version of the Stroop task in which subjects report the color of an emotional word (Pratto & John, 1991), often report that emotion impairs performance by making it difficult to disengage from the emotional stimulus (Fox, Russo, Bowles, & Dutton, 2001). However, other studies have shown that in situations with limited attentional resources, emotional stimuli are more likely to reach awareness, suggesting that emotion can also facilitate attention. A classic example of the facilitation of attention with emotion is the cocktail party effect. It is possible to selectively inhibit the processing of irrelevant stimuli (e.g., conversations among others at a cocktail party) unless an emotionally relevant stimulus (e.g., your name) is presented. In this case, the attentional bottleneck is selec-

tively reduced to allow processing and awareness of an emotionally significant event (see Lachman, Rachman, & Butterfield, 1979, for a review). It has
been suggested that this facilitation of attention with emotion may be dependent on the amygdala (Whalen, 1998).

To assess if the human amygdala plays a role in the enhanced awareness of emotional events in situations with limited attentional resources,
the performance of patients with amygdala damage was examined using the
attentional blink paradigm (Anderson & Phelps, 2001). This is a rapid serial
visual presentation (RSVP) paradigm in which a series of words is presented rapidly. On each trial, 15 words are presented at a rate of approximately 100 milliseconds per word. At this rate, it is very difficult for subjects to report the words because they go by so quickly. However, if
subjects are instructed to ignore most of the words and focus only on two of
the 15 words that are presented in a different-colored ink (i.e., green vs.
black ink), they are often able to selectively attend to these words and
report them at the end of each trial—although the ability to report the second word (Target 2) presented in green ink is somewhat dependent on the
location of this word in the list. When Target 2 is presented several words
after the first target word (Target 1), subjects were usually able to report it.
However, if Target 2 is presented only two or three words after Target 1
(called the early lag period), the ability to identify and report Target 2 is
diminished. This is the classic attentional blink effect (Chun & Potter,
1995). Noticing and encoding Target 1 creates a temporary refractory
period during which it is difficult to notice and encode Target 2. In other
words, it is as if attention "blinked."

Using this attentional blink paradigm, Anderson and Phelps (2001)
showed that emotion enhanced the likelihood that Target 2 would be
detected in the early lag period. When Target 2 was an emotionally arousing word, normal subjects were much less likely to miss it when it was presented in the early lag period. In other words, emotion attenuated the
attentional blink effect, indicating a facilitation of attention with emotion.
Patients with amygdala damage, however, failed to show the normal attenu-
ation of the attentional blink with emotion. Unlike normal controls, these
patients were equally likely to miss Target 2 presented in the early lag
period when it was emotion or neutral. These results demonstrate that the
amygdala plays a critical role in the facilitation of attention with emotion.

The mechanism by which the amygdala might facilitate attention and
awareness for emotional events has been suggested by brain-imaging studies in humans and anatomical studies in nonhuman primates. A number of
brain-imaging studies have demonstrated enhanced activation of visual
processing regions in response to emotional stimuli (Anderson et al., 2003;
Kosslyn et al., 1996; Morris, Buchel, & Dolan, 2001; Vuilleumier, Armony,

Driver, & Dolan, 2001). Some of these studies have reported that this modulation of activation in visual regions with emotion is correlated with the amygdala response (Morris et al., 2001) or linked to amygdala function (Vuilleumier et al., 2004). These findings support proposed models that suggest that the amygdala modulates the sensitivity of perceptual processing with emotion (Kapp, Supple, & Whalen, 1994; Weinberger, 1995; Whalen, 1998).

Anatomical studies in primates have shown that the amygdala has reciprocal connections with cortical visual areas (Amaral, Behniea, & Kelly, 2003). The amygdala has been shown to respond to the emotional significance of an event quickly and prior to awareness (LeDoux, 1996; Whalen et al., 1998). It is hypothesized that this early amygdala response may result in feedback to visual-processing regions, which in turn enhances further perceptual processing. A number of cortical visual-processing regions has been shown to be enhanced with emotion and modulated by amygdala function, including early visual regions such as the extrastriate cortex (Morris et al., 2001, Vuilleumier et al., 2004). Consistent with the hypothesis that emotion influences even the earliest stages of perception, a recent study found that emotion enhances contrast sensitivity (Ling, Phelps, Holmes, & Carrasco, 2004), a primary visual function known to be coded in the early visual cortex. Although there is no direct evidence that the human amygdala alters a specific perceptual process, the findings from a range of imaging, anatomical, and behavioral studies are consistent with the hypothesis that the facilitation of attention with emotion may be the result of the amygdala's modulation of perception.

The amygdala's influence on attention and perception suggests that the initial processing of emotional stimuli is enhanced relative to neutral stimuli. This enhanced awareness for emotional stimuli with limited attentional resources may also lead to greater memory encoding, resulting in both greater immediate and later awareness with emotion. By altering memory storage, attention, and perception with emotion, the amygdala helps to ensure that emotionally significant events receive priority in cognitive processing and awareness.

CONCLUSION

In this chapter I have outlined how some of the neural mechanisms of emotion and cognition, which can operate independently, also have complex interactions. A cognitive awareness of the emotional significance of events and conscious application of emotion regulation strategies can influence amygdala function and emotional expression, suggesting two means by which cognition alters emotion. In addition, the emotion, via the amygdala, influences cognition by mediating the long-term retention and awareness of emotional events, as well as immediate stimulus processing, by modulating attention and perception. Although it is possible to study the behavioral and neural mechanisms of emotion and cognition independently, this research suggests that independent investigations of emotion and cognition may result in an incomplete and inaccurate view of normal emotion and cognitive processes. The neural systems of emotion and cognition are both independent and interdependent. A comprehensive understanding of either emotion or cognition requires a consideration of the complex interactions between the two.

REFERENCES

Amaral, D. G., Behniea, H., & Kelly, J. L. (2003). Topographic organization of projections from the amygdala to the visual cortex in the macaque monkey. *Neuroscience, 118*(4), 1099–120.

Anderson, A. K., Christoff, K., Panitz, D., DeRosa, E., & Gabrieli, J. D. (2003). Neural correlates of the automatic processing of threat facial signals. *Journal of Neuroscience, 23*(13), 5627–5633.

Anderson, A. K., & Phelps, E. A. (2001). The human amygdala supports affective modulatory influences on visual awareness. *Nature, 411,* 305–309.

Anderson, A. K., & Phelps, E. A. (2002). Is the human amygdala critical for the subjective experience of emotion? Evidence of intact dispositional affect in patients with amygdala lesions. *Journal of Cognitive Neuroscience, 14,* 709–720.

Anderson, J. K. (1999). *Cognitive psychology and its implications* (5th ed.). San Francisco: Freeman.

Bechara, A., Tranel, D., Damasio, H., Adolphs, R., Rockland, C., & Damasio, A. R. (1995). Double dissociation of conditioning and declarative knowledge relative to the amygdala and hippocampus in human. *Science, 269,* 1115–1118.

Buchel, C., Moris, J., Dolan, R. J., & Friston, K. J. (1998). Brain systems mediating aversive conditioning: An event-related fMRI study. *Neuron, 20,* 947–957.

Cahill, L., Babinsky, R., Markowitsch, H. J., & McGaugh, J. L. (1995). The amygdala and emotional memory. *Science, 377,* 295–296.

Cahill, L., Haier, R. J., Fallon, J., Alkire, M. T., Tang, C., Keator, D., Wu, J., & McGaugh, J. L. (1996). Amygdala activity at encoding correlated with long-term, free recall of emotional information. *Proceedings of the National Academy of Sciences, 93,* 8016–8021.

Cahill, L., Prins, B., Weber, M., & McGaugh, J. L. (1994). β-adrenergic activation and memory for emotional events. *Nature, 371,* 702–704.

Canli, T., Zhao, Z., Brewer, J., Gabrielli, J. D. E., & Cahill, L. (2000). Event-related activation in the human amygdala associates with later memory for individual emotional experience. *Journal of Neuroscience, 20,* 1–5.

Christianson, S. A. (1992). *The handbook of emotion and memory: research and theory*. Mahwah, NJ: Erlbaum.

Chun, M. M., & Potter, M. C. (1995). A two-stage model for multiple target detection in rapid serial visual presentation. *Journal of Experimental Psychology: Human Perception and Performance, 21*, 109–127.

Damasio, A. R. (1994). *Descarte's error*. New York: Putnam.

Davis, M. (2000). The role of the amygdala in conditioned fear and anxiety. In J. P. Aggleton (Ed.), *The amygdala: A functional analysis* (2nd ed., pp. 213–287). New York: Oxford University Press.

Delgado, M. R., Trujillo, J. L., Holmes, B., Nearing, K. L., LeDoux, J. E. & Phelps, E. A. (2004, April). *Emotion regulation of conditioned fear: The contributions of reappraisal*. Eleventh annual meeting of the Cognitive Neuroscience Society, San Francisco.

Fox, E., Russo, R., Bowles, R., & Dutton, K. (2001). Do threatening stimuli draw or hold attention in visual attention in subclinical anxiety? *Journal of Experimental Psychology: General, 130*, 681–700.

Funayama, E. S., Grillon, C. G., Davis, M., & Phelps, E. A. (2001). A double dissociation in the affective modulation of startle in humans: Effects of unilateral temporal lobectomy. *Journal of Cognitive Neuroscience, 13*, 721–729.

Gazzaniga, M. S., Ivry, R. B., & Mangun, G. R. (1998). *Cognitive neuroscience: The biology of the mind*. New York: Norton.

Gazzaniga, M. S., Ivry, R. B., & Mangun, G. R. (2002). *Cognitive neuroscience: The biology of the mind* (2nd ed.). New York: Norton.

Gross, J. J. (2002). Emotion regulation: Affective, cognitive, and social consequences. *Psychophysiology, 39*, 281–291.

Hamann, S. B., Ely, T. D., Grafton, S. T., & Kilts, C. D. (1999). Amygdala activity related to enhanced memory for pleasant and aversive stimuli. *Nature Neuroscience, 2*(3), 289–293.

Hugdahl, K., & Öhman, A. (1977). Effects of instruction on acquisition and extinction of electrodermal responses to fear-relevant stimuli. *Journal of Experimental Psychology: Human Learning and Memory, 3*(5), 608–618.

Kapp, B. S., Supple, W. F., & Whalen, P. J. (1994). Stimulation of the amygdaloid central nucleus produces EEG arousal. *Behavioral Neuroscience, 108*, 81–93.

Kapp, B. S., Whalen, P. J., Supple, W. F., & Pascoe, J. P. (1992). Amygdaloid contributions to conditioned arousal and sensory information processing. In J. P. Aggleton (Ed.), *The amygdala: Neurobiological aspects of emotion, memory and mental dysfunction* (pp. 229–254). New York: Oxford University Press.

Kleinsmith, L. J., & Kaplan, S. (1963). Paired-associate learning as a function of arousal and interpolated interval. *Journal of Experimental Psychology, 65*(2), 190–193.

Klüver, H., & Bucy, P. C. (1939). Preliminary analysis of functions of the temporal lobes in monkeys. *Archives of Neurology and Psychiatry Chicago, 42*, 979–1000.

Kosslyn, S. M., Shin, L. M., Thompson, W. L., McNally, P. J., Rauch, S. L., Pitman, R. K., & Alpert, N. M. (1996). Neural effects of visualizing and perceiving aversive stimuli: A PET investigation. *Neuroreport, 7*, 1569–1576.

LaBar, K. S., Gatenby, C., Gore, J. C., LeDoux, J. E., & Phelps, E. A. (1998). Human amygdala activation during conditioned fear acquisition and extinction: A mixed trial fMRI study. *Neuron, 20,* 937–945.

LaBar, K. S., LeDoux, J. E., Spencer, D. D., & Phelps, E. A. (1995). Impaired fear conditioning following unilateral temporal lobectomy in humans. *Journal of Neuroscience, 15,* 6846–6855.

LaBar, K. S., & Phelps, E. A. (1998). Role of the human amygdala in arousal mediated memory consolidation. *Psychological Science, 9,* 490–493.

Lachman, R., Lachman, E., & Butterfield, E. C. (1979). *Cognitive psychology and information processing.* Hillsdale, NJ: Erlbaum.

Lazarus, R. S. (1981). A cognitivist's reply to Zajonc on emotion and cognition. *American Psychologist, 36*(2), 222–223.

LeDoux, J. E. (1996). *The emotional brain: The mysterious underpinnings of emotional life.* New York: Simon & Schuster.

LeDoux, J. E. (2002). *The synaptic self: How our brain became who we are.* New York: Viking-Penguin.

Ling, S., Phelps, E., Holmes, B., & Carrasco, M. (2004, May). *Emotion potentiates attentional effects in early vision.* Abstract presented at the Vision Sciences Society, annual meeting, Sarasota, FL.

McGaugh, J. L. (2000). Memory—a century of consolidation. *Science, 287,* 248–251.

Milner, B., Corkin, S., & Teuber, H. L. (1968). Further analysis of the hippocampal amnesic syndrome: 14-year follow-up study of H. M. *Neuropsychologia, 6,* 216–234.

Morris, J. S., Buchel, C., & Dolan, R. J. (2001). Parallel neural responses in amygdala subregions and sensory cortex during implicit fear conditioning. *Neuroimage, 13,* 1044–1052.

Neisser, U. (1976). *Cognition and reality: Principles and implications of cognitive psychology.* San Francisco: Freeman.

Ochsner, K. N., Bunge, S. A., Gross, J. J., & Gabrielli, J. D. E. (2002). Rethinking feelings: An fMRI study of the cognitive regulation of emotion. *Journal of Cognitive Neuroscience, 14,* 1215–1229.

Phelps, E. A. (2002). Emotions. In M. S. Gazzaniga, R. B. Ivry, & G. R. Mangun (Eds.), *Cognitive neuroscience: The biology of mind* (2nd ed., pp. 537–576). New York: Norton.

Phelps, E. A., LaBar, D. S., Anderson, A. K., O'Conner, K. J., Fulbright, R. K., & Spencer, D. S. (1998). Specifying the contributions of the human amygdala to emotional memory: A case study. *Neurocase, 4,* 527–540.

Phelps, E. A., O'Connor, K. J., Gatenby, J. C., Grillon, C., Gore, J. C., & Davis, M. (2001). Activation of the left amygdala to a cognitive representation of fear. *Nature Neuroscience, 4,* 437–441.

Pratto, F. & John, O. P. (1991). Automatic vigilance: The attention grabbing power of negative social information. *Journal of Personality and Social Psychology, 61,* 380–391.

Schaefer, S. M., Jackson, D. C., Davidson, R. J., Kimberg, D. Y., & Thompson-Schill, S. L. (2002). Modulation of amygdalar activity by the conscious regulation of negative emotion. *Journal of Cognitive Neuroscience, 14,* 913–921.

Smith, E. E., & Jonides, J. (1999). Storage and executive processes in the frontal lobes. *Science, 283,* 1657–1661.

Squire, L. R., Clark, R. E., & Bayley, P. J. (2004). Medial temporal lobe function and memory. In M. S. Gazzaniga (Ed.), *The cognitive neurosciences III* (pp. 691–708). Canbridge, MA: MIT Press.

Vuilleumier, P., Armony, J. L., Driver, J., & Dolan, R. J. (2001). Effects of attention and emotion on face processing in the human brain: An event-related fMRI study. *Neuron, 30,* 829–841.

Vuilleumier, P., Richardson, M., Armony, J., Driver, J., & Dolan, R. (2004). Distant influences of amygdala lesion on visual cortical activation during emotional face processing. *Nature Neuroscience, 7,* 1271–1278.

Weinberger, D. R. (1995). Retuning the brain by fear conditioning. In M. S. Gazzaniga (Ed.), *The cognitive neurosciences* (pp. 1071–1090). Cambridge, MA: MIT Press.

Weiskrantz, L. (1956). Behavioral changes associated with ablation of the amygdaloid complex in monkeys. *Journal of Comparative Physiological Psychology, 49,* 381–391.

Whalen, P. J. (1998). Fear, vigilance, and ambiguity: Initial neuroimaging studies of the human amygdala. *Current Directions in Psychological Science, 7*(6), 177–188.

Whalen, P. J., Rauch, S. L., Etcoff, N. L., McInerney, S. C., Lee, M. B., & Jenike, M. A. (1998). Masked presentations of emotional facial expressions modulate amygdala activity without explicit knowledge. *Journal of Neuroscience, 18*(1), 411–418.

Zajonc, R. B. (1980). Feeling and thinking: Preferences need no inferences. *American Psychologist, 35*(2), 151–175.

CHAPTER 4

Affect and the Resolution of Cognitive Control Dilemmas

JEREMY R. GRAY
ALEXANDRE SCHAEFER
TODD S. BRAVER
STEVEN B. MOST

Many people find the topic of emotion–cognition interactions to be intriguing, as if personally relevant and familiar, yet mysterious nonetheless. In some ways this mirrors that of scientific knowledge. The effects of emotion on cognition are clearly important but are not fully understood, despite clear evidence for a number of important phenomena, including effects on memory, attention, and decision making (Ashby, Isen, & Turken, 1999; Christianson, 1992; Dalgleish & Power, 1999; Dolan, 2002; Eich, Kihlstrom, Bower, Forgas, & Niedenthal, 2000; Forgas, 2001; Isen, 1993; Lane & Nadel, 2000; Lerner, Small, & Loewenstein, 2004; Oatley & Johnson-Laird, 1987; Phelps, Chapter 3; Power & Dalgleish, 1997; Salovey, Mayer, & Caruso, 2002). The aim of this chapter is to articulate an empirically grounded framework for understanding emotion–cognition interactions in mechanistic terms, organized around the concept of *control dilemmas.*

We focus on affective influences on the exertion of cognitive control and on the direction of selective attention, both of which can be understood in terms of control dilemmas. We do not aim to provide a falsifiable theory so much as a meta-theory: a unified conceptual framework within which to better compare and contrast—and hence potentially understand—re-

1. *What is the scope of your proposed model? When you use the term* emotion, *how do you use it? What do you mean by terms such as* fear, anxiety, *or* happiness?

As used in this chapter the term *emotion* refers to prototypical emotional episodes (Russell & Barrett, 1999): emotion in the heat of the moment, a "complex set of interrelated subevents concerned with a specific object" (Russell & Barrett, 1999, p. 806), accompanied by a subjective feeling (or core affect, Russell & Barrett, 1999) that is at least accessible to awareness, even if not always at the forefront of one's consciousness. Not everything affective qualifies as emotion, such as preferences and motivationally significant stimuli that need not be subjectively experienced, as well as stimuli that have the potential to evoke emotion (e.g., a photograph of a loved one). Although emotion is often accompanied by facial and other expressions, these are not considered here.

2. *Define your terms:* conscious, unconscious, awareness. *Or say why you do not use these terms.*

3. *Does your model deal with what is conscious, what is unconscious, or their relationship? If you do not address this area specifically, can you speculate on the relationship between what is conscious and unconscious? Or if you do not like the conscious–unconscious distinction, or if you do not think this is a good question to ask, can you say why?*

Our meta-theory does not deal explicitly with consciousness, so we do not attempt to define it. In part, we argue that emotional states (which tend to be conscious or accessible to consciousness, but need not be; see Winkielman, Berridge, & Wilbarger, Chapter 14) should interact with high-level executive processes (which also tend to be conscious, but also need not be). We also argue that affect can interact with components of selective attention, both endogenous (controlled) and exogenous (automatic). To the extent that consciousness is functional, in the sense of having causal consequences, an intriguing candidate for the function of consciousness is to give one part of the system access to global control of the whole system. Each part of the system typically has only limited control of a local subsystem and can provide only a weak bias on the whole system. Informational discrepancies or violations of expectation may be critical as triggering or gating events and, as such, are important for understanding the contents of consciousness (although in themselves, say little about the nature of consciousness; Gray, 1995).

markably varied phenomena. We seek empirical and theoretical constraints on theory building. The meta-theory does not depend on a theory or definition of consciousness.

In diverse subdisciplines of psychology, and increasingly in neuroscience and behavioral economics, considerable research has investigated the influences of emotion and related phenomena—both conscious and unconscious—on cognition. Is there a way to refer to and potentially systematize such diverse effects and influences? A promising possibility is to consider people as complex systems, in particular, as complex control systems whose overall function is self-regulation (Carver & Scheier, 1990; Tomarken & Keener, 1998).

A self-regulating system that is complex enough or flexible enough to do more than one thing needs some way of settling on (or otherwise "deciding") what is the best thing to do. Flexibility is useful, but it is a double-edged sword: Being able to do more than one thing opens the door to having more than a single viable option—and hence to being conflicted about which option is best. Thermostats are paradigmatic control systems that are too simple be conflicted. People can be conceptualized as control systems that, in comparison to a thermostat, are vastly more complex and conflicted (Carver & Scheier, 1990; Dollard & Miller, 1950; Miller, 1944). By a conflict or control dilemma we mean a situation involving inherent tradeoffs in the control of behavior, situations that at the extreme feel subjectively like "damned if you do, damned if you don't." By *inherent* we mean logically or structurally inescapable, such as the speed versus the accuracy of a response, taken in the sense of Marr's (1982) computational level of analysis. That is, conflict is a necessary consequence of optimizing competing goals or constraints. (In the intended sense, conflict is also pervasive in economic analyses of human behavior; for example, conflict between market equity and market efficiency.) Conflict can occur at many mechanistic levels within a control system. Although many control dilemmas can be largely or completely unconscious, they can also be conscious. States of conflict can be subjectively experienced as very unpleasant and even debilitating. Although the affective consequences of conflict are important clinically and theoretically (Carver & Scheier, 1990), they are not central to our interest in the relation between emotion and control dilemmas. Rather, we focus on the role of emotion and affect external to the dilemma as playing a role that can help resolve the dilemma.

In this chapter *cognitive control* refers to the regulation of thought, feeling, and behavior by actively maintained, internal representations of context information, such as a goal or other information that, when held actively in mind, changes the way in which other information is processed (Braver, Cohen, & Barch, 2002). Active goals can bias processing, leading to changes in thoughts, feeling, and behavior. Cognitive control (also referred to as executive processes or executive attention) is typically deliberate and effortful (Norman & Shallice, 1986; Posner & DiGirolamo, 1998; Posner & Snyder, 1975; Shiffrin & Schneider, 1977; Smith & Jonides, 1999). For example, trying to remember a new phone number just long enough to dial it is effortful and requires cognitive control. In contrast, automatic control is often seemingly effortless or automatic (Bargh, 1994; Shiffrin & Schneider, 1977); for example, doing something that is highly practiced, such as dialing a phone number one dials every day. Behavior is still controlled by associative links between pressing one digit and the next in the series; it is just not controlled at each step by an actively maintained representation. In short, the process is more ballistic. That is, the cognitive control of thought, feeling, and behavior differs from stimulus-based control of thought, feeling, and behavior because it involves actively maintained internal representations. There is no requirement that a goal be conscious, or even accessible to awareness, just that it be actively maintained.

In this chapter we elaborate the idea that a general function of affect is to help resolve control dilemmas. Some control dilemmas involve cognitive control, whereas other do not. Dilemmas can exist between one form of controlled processing and another, between one form of automatic processing and another, and between controlled versus automatic processing. Various theorists have suggested that emotion and affect help assign value or prioritize processing (Dolan, 2002; Oatley & Johnson-Laird, 1987; Simon, 1967; Tomarken & Keener, 1998; Tucker & Williamson, 1984). In behavioral economics risk is increasingly viewed as affective, rather than purely cognitive, in nature (Loewenstein & Prelec, 1993; Rottenstreich & Hsee, 2001). Emotion can serve as an interrupt signal that preempts ongoing processing and redirects behavior to more urgent demands (Oatley & Johnson-Laird, 1987; Simon, 1967). And emotion can serve as a signal that one's progress toward a goal is better than expected (leading to positive affect) or worse than expected (leading to negative affect; Carver & Scheier, 1990). Conscious emotion, in the form of emotional states, may be a way to convert diverse, fairly abstract contextual cues into an overall assessment of the situation and into an embodied, coordinated response, with the overall control system more optimally tuned to respond as effectively as possible. One function of emotional states may be to modulate cognitive processing in a situation-specific way, setting priorities among conflicting alternatives or tradeoffs. In some sense, emotion serves as a valuation function, regulating the overall mental economy in a way that takes into account both situational (external environment) factors as well as internal constraints on value or subjective importance. A control system dynamically adjusts the behavior of its constituent parts to maintain the integrity, homeostasis, or stability of the whole system, in accord with the internal and external "market forces." Emotion and cognition are two parts of the overall system. Emotion may influence thought and behavior, in part, by influencing how cognitive parts of the system control thought and behavior. In an integrated system, at some point the distinction between control-by-emotion and control-by-cognition breaks down, and there is just control (Gray, Braver, & Raichle, 2002). Both affective and cognitive forces are at work, exerting control over behavior, yet it is impossible to draw a hard and fast line demarcating where one stops and the other begins. They conjointly control behavior. A subthesis of this chapter is that such integration is especially important during control dilemmas.

Consider an example. There is often a tension between the short-term and the long-term effects of a given choice or action: "Damned *now* if you do, damned *later* if you don't" (or vice-versa). Such temporal dilemmas are inherent in many real-world situations, such as buying on credit, and in various self-control tasks, including delay of gratification (Mischel, Shoda, & Rodriguez, 1989), distributed choice (Herrnstein, Loewenstein, Prelec, & Vaughan, 1993; Herrnstein, Prelec, & Vaughan, 1986), and other equally fiendish scenarios (e.g., Heatherton, Herman, & Polivy, 1991; Leith & Baumeister, 1996). Emotion might help to resolve the control dilemma in favor of one outcome or another, by helping to tip the balance. When people are genuinely threatened, they may *need* to choose what is better in the short term, even if it means incurring a larger long-term cost (Gray, 1999). An emotional state may help people act in what would ordinarily be an impulsive way. Consistent with this logic, threat-related emotional states can bias people to prioritize immediate gains, even at an overall cost, such that they repeatedly chose a smaller–sooner reward over a larger–later one (Gray, 1999). In children, stress tends to impair ability to delay gratification (see Metcalfe & Mischel, 1999), whereas induced positive mood appears to enhance delay of gratification (Fry, 1977). This example is meant to illustrate a control dilemma (short-term vs. long-term conflict) in which emotion provides a way to tip the balance (acting impulsively, delaying gratification) in ways that could be adaptive. Beyond short-term versus long-term conflicts, there are myriad ways in which people feel conflicted. Emotion might help to resolve some of these dilemmas.

POTENTIALLY CONSCIOUS CONTROL DILEMMAS: EMOTION AND COGNITIVE CONTROL

In this section we first consider a control dilemma that has been extensively considered and investigated, namely, approach–withdrawal conflict, and then turn to other forms of conflict. We do not claim that such conflict is always conscious, but we do consider it likely that such conflict is potentially conscious or accessible to awareness.

Approach–Withdrawal Conflict

It is impossible to simultaneously approach and withdraw from something, and yet it is possible to be strongly motivated to do both—creating a state of profound conflict. In this section we consider approach–withdrawal conflict, viewing it as a fundamental way for people to be conflicted. Approach–withdrawal emotions are those such as enthusiasm or desire (approach motivated) and fear and anxiety (withdrawal related; Davidson, 1995; Sutton & Davidson, 1997). Many theorists consider approach and withdrawal motivation to be basic or fundamental dimensions, with other aspects of motivation being elaborations of, or otherwise built upon, these two (Carver, Sutton, & Scheier, 2000; Frijda, 1999; Gray, 2002; Lang, Bradley, & Cuthbert, 1990; Miller, 1944).

Approach- and withdrawal-motivated emotions are action oriented or goal directed (Carver et al., 2000; Davidson, 1998). These emotions are subjectively experienced as urgent. Because they are goal directed, these emotions might be expected to influence the cognitive and neural mechanisms that support action control and goal-directed behavior, including cognitive control and the lateral prefrontal cortex (Gray, 2001; Gray et al., 2002; Heller, 1990; Tomarken & Keener, 1998). A key idea of the control dilemma perspective is that emotional states can prioritize some (cognitive) functions over others. That is, when there is a conflict over which of two mutually exclusive options to exercise in a given situation (e.g., which of two strategies), only one of which can be implemented at a time, we argue that a given emotion may be able to enhance one of them; enhancing both does not resolve the dilemma. The idea we explore is that emotion helps commit the overall system to a particular, coherent mode of operation (Oatley & Johnson-Laird, 1987). One important source of evidence for this perspective is demonstrations of emotion's selective effects on cognition, including working memory and cognitive control tasks (Gray, 2001; Gray et al., 2002), frontal lobe tasks (Bartolic, Basso, Schefft, Glauser, & Titanic-Schefft, 1999), and reasoning tasks (Markham & Darke, 1992; Palfai & Salovey, 1993). Selectivity demonstrates that the underlying cognitive and neural architecture is suitable for the overall perspective we propose. Identifying selective effects of emotion does not show that the effects are adaptive—which would require further evidence.

To provide methodologically rigorous evidence for selectivity, we asked participants to watch short videos (to induce an emotional state) and then perform a computerized "three-back" working memory task (to tax cognitive control; Gray, 2001). The three-back task is like a challenging (but not terribly exciting) video game, in which participants need to keep a list of three items in mind. Every few seconds participants have to update their mental list, adding a new item and dropping the oldest, and pressing a button to indicate if the old one matched the new one. Most people find the task very demanding. Working memory, or the active maintenance and manipulation of information in mind, can greatly tax cognitive control, especially when both maintenance and manipulation are required. For methodological reasons, we used both verbal and nonverbal versions of the working memory task. The key prediction was that a given emotional state would influence some tasks but not others, and that the profile of how tasks were influenced would depend on the emotional state. The specific direction of the effect was predicted on the basis of prefrontal hemispheric asymmetries for both approach–withdrawal emotion (e.g., Davidson, 1995; Harmon-Jones & Allen, 1997; Harmon-Jones & Sigelman, 2001; Sutton & Davidson, 1997) and for verbal–nonverbal cognition (e.g., Hellige, 1993; Kelley et al., 1998). The two asymmetries are typically investigated separately, but two untested theoretical positions suggested that emotional asymmetries and cognitive asymmetries could interact (Heller, 1990; Tomarken & Keener, 1998). Specifically, approach-related states should activate the left prefrontal cortex (PFC) and enhance processing that depends on that region (e.g., verbal), whereas withdrawal-related states should activate the right PFC and enhance processing that depends on that region (e.g., nonverbal).

We tested this hypothesis in behavioral studies (Gray, 2001) and a functional magnetic resonance imaging (fMRI) study (Gray et al., 2002). The key behavioral effect we found is that an approach-related state (amusement, from 10-minute comedy videos) enhanced verbal working memory performance but impaired spatial working memory performance. In contrast, a withdrawal-related state (anxiety, from 10-minute horror videos) had exactly the opposite effect. That mild anxiety actually enhanced performance on the spatial task is a counterintuitive finding. Moreover, task-related brain activity was modulated by induced emotions in a manner that was not only consistent with these effects; in addition, the magnitude of the effect of emotion on brain activity predicted the magnitude of the effect on behavior. First, we discuss the behavioral data and then the fMRI data.

A planned analysis of individual differences suggested that the behavioral effect was due to induced approach- and withdrawal-related emotional states specifically. The more emotionally engaged with the film clips a person became (as indicated by self-reported ratings afterward), the stronger the experienced emotional state and the stronger the effect on performance. Critically, individual differences in self-reported personality, and specifically approach and withdrawal disposition as assessed using Behavioral Inhibition and Activation scales (BIS–BAS; Carver & White, 1994), predicted which people would experience which effects more strongly. The key result was that individual differences in approach–withdrawal emotional reactivity (BIS–BAS) predicted how strongly the emotion induction would influence task performance. That is, the strength of the behavioral effect covaried with individual differences in approach and withdrawal motivation, and this relation was not explained by performance in a neutral condition. The behavioral effect and the validation using BIS–BAS measures provided a methodologically rigorous test of the idea that induced emotional states have selective effects on cognitive control or executive function, broadly construed.

A further question concerns the specific direction of the observed effect: That is, why should mild anxiety enhance spatial working memory, but mild amusement enhance verbal working memory? The data reveal a selective effect but, of themselves, do not indicate why the effect should be in the direction observed. There are several possible reasons why this particular direction might be adaptive, not simply accidental. We have previously discussed this effect in terms of weak biases on computational efficiency, acting in a hemisphere-specific manner (Gray & Braver, 2002b). Several weak biases acting in concert could give rise to an overall, and perhaps even substantial, computational advantage to having different cognitive functions lateralized, with emotional enhancement of some, but not other, functions achieved in a hemisphere-specific manner. We briefly discuss two potential types of lateralized cognitive biases that could account for the behavioral data: sustained attention and fine motor control.

Sustained attention and orienting might be more critical in withdrawal-related than approach-related states to facilitate vigilance for a potential threat and rapid orienting to the occurrence of an actual threat. Because nearly all creatures face the threat of predation, there is strong selection pressure to evolve strategies to reduce the danger (Lima & Dill, 1990). Although these forms of attention would be useful in approach-related states, they seem unlikely to be as critical as they are in withdrawal states. Consistent with a hemisphere-based account, neural networks for sustained attention and attentional orienting are relatively right lateralized (Cabeza & Nyberg, 2000; Pardo, Fox, & Raichle, 1991). Fine versus gross movement control could be more important in approach versus withdrawal states, respectively. Fine motor control is left lateralized (e.g., left hemisphere control of the right hand; Hellige, 1993) and could be more important in approach-related behaviors (e.g., precise grasping). Coordination of large muscles groups would be more critical for withdrawal (e.g., escaping by running). Several weak biases acting collectively could produce an overall computational advantage for colateralization of cognitive control functions to enable selective regulation by approach–withdrawal states. This account is speculative yet consistent with computational principles and neurobiological evidence about hemispheric specialization, and it makes testable predictions.

Another possible interpretation that we have begun to explore depends on the idea that there are two modes of cognitive control: proactive and reactive (Braver, Gray, & Burgess, in press). A proactive mode is what we have described above simply as cognitive control: the active maintenance of context information to bias subsequent information processing. In addition, we hypothesize that the cognitive system can exert control through the use of a reactive, rather than a proactive, control strategy. We posit that reactive control occurs following (rather than prior to) the occurrence of some imperative event. Prior to this event, the system remains relatively unbiased and thus relatively free to be driven by bottom-up inputs. Reactive control mechanisms are engaged only as needed, rather than consistently, and on a "just-in-time" basis, rather than in advance of their required usage. Finally, when control depends upon the use of context information, the activation of such information by reactive mechanisms occurs transiently rather than in a sustained fashion, and thus decays quickly. As a consequence, in situations when the same context must be accessed repeatedly, full reactivation of the information must occur each time it is needed.

It may be the case that the proactive and reactive systems are fully independent and thus may both be engaged simultaneously. Nevertheless, there is likely to be a bias favoring one type of control strategy over the other. Such a bias could result from stable individual differences, task demands, or—most relevant for this chapter—induced emotion. Specifically, when participants engage in a verbal working memory task, they may spontaneously adopt a proactive mode, given the relative ease of actively maintaining just a few words. Conversely, when they engage in a nonverbal working memory task, participants may adopt a reactive mode, given the relative difficulty of actively maintaining large amounts of visuospatial information. Approach-related emotional states may bias the system toward a proactive control mode, in part, to sustain a representation of a potential reward actively in mind and guide behavior toward obtaining that reward. Threat-related emotional states may bias the system toward a reactive mode; threats are typically encountered suddenly rather than slowly, with long anticipation. It seems likely that there is no perfect mapping of the emotional state onto the control mode (e.g., one can envision rumination producing a proactive, sustained anticipatory anxiety). The point for present purposes is that the effect of induced emotion on verbal and nonverbal working memory performance (Gray, 2001; Gray et al., 2002) may, we speculate, be explainable in terms of effects on proactive and reactive control, rather than on verbal and nonverbal processing specifically. Even if this account should eventually fall short, we suggest that it is worth trying to understand emotion–cognition interactions in terms of effects on underlying computational processes, and not particular tasks.

In an fMRI study using the same behavioral paradigm, we provided what is, to our knowledge, the first evidence for selectivity of emotional influences on cognitive control using functional brain imaging (Gray et al., 2002). Although there has been a great deal of work on emotion–cognition interaction (see Phelps, Chapter 3), little or none of it has examined whether emotion can have selective effects on cognitive brain activity. To our knowledge, there are no imaging studies that can be reinterpreted as evidence for such integration, because the minimum experimental design requirements have not been met. Single-task studies (e.g., of emotion and verbal fluency; Baker, Frith, & Dolan, 1997) cannot show selectivity, because showing selectivity requires having at least two tasks, one of which is influenced by emotion and the other is not.

Using the same methods as the behavioral studies, we found that induced emotion modulated task-related neural activity within the lateral prefrontal cortex, a region of the brain that is critical for cognitive control (Braver et al., 2002; Miller & Cohen, 2001). The most salient finding was that some brain areas showed a selective effect, with the influence of a particular emotion (amusement, anxiety) depending on the type of cognitive control task (verbal, nonverbal), thereby meeting formal criteria for integration. Moreover, how strongly the emotion induction modulated brain activity was correlated with how strongly the emotion modulated task performance—a finding that is consistent with a causal role of this brain area in influencing behavior. The mere existence of a region with this highly specific profile of activity suggests that emotional states and higher cognition are truly integrated. At some point of processing, functional specialization is lost and emotion and cognition conjointly and equally contribute to the control of thought and behavior. The fMRI data make this point compellingly: Integration occurs not merely somewhere in the brain, but does so specifically in areas that are known from much other work to be critical for cognitive control.

Emotion and Inhibitory Control

When considering how emotion interacts with cognitive control, inhibitory control seems to warrant close attention; yet, to our knowledge, it has been the subject of limited investigation. Because inhibitory control is necessary in situations of conflict between an intended thought, feeling, or behavior and a prepotent or dominant one, effects of emotion on inhibitory control might be particularly relevant to a control dilemma perspective. We note that such high-conflict situations might also involve consciousness, although we are agnostic about a necessary role for consciousness. Inhibition may also be a consequence of emotional response—for example, freezing behavior or other behaviors that suppress active motor responses.

Inhibitory control is the cognitive capability responsible for deliberately suppressing dominant, automatic thoughts or motor responses in order to replace them with responses more adapted to the individual's current goals. For clarity, inhibitory control should be distinguished from behavioral inhibition, as used by Gray (1982) to indicate a system characterized by a sensitivity to signals of punishment, nonreward, and novelty aimed at avoiding aversive outcomes. Inhibitory control should also be distinguished from Kagan's (e.g., Kagan, Reznick, & Snidman, 1988) use of the term *inhibition* to describe socially inhibited (shy) children. This section focuses solely on inhibitory control in the first sense.

A classic example of inhibitory control is instantiated in the Stroop task, in which participants are instructed to name the ink color of color words (MacLeod, 1991; Stroop, 1935). There are typically three conditions in a Stroop task: an incongruent condition in which the subject has to name ink colors that are different from the color word (e.g., the word RED in green ink), a congruent condition (RED in red ink), and a control condition in which the words are not color names or are replaced by non-word symbols. The classic result is slower reaction times in the incongruent condition. The interpretation of this effect is that reading a word is an automatic skill (i.e., highly overlearned). When subjects try to name the color of a word, it is practically impossible for them to avoid reading the word, despite the fact that reading the word interferes with the main task. To respond as instructed, participants have to inhibit the automatic word reading in order to successfully accomplish the task (Hughdahl & Stormark, 2002; MacLeod, 1991). Thus there is a control dilemma: a direct conflict between automatic processing (reading the word) and controlled processing (naming the color). The effect is so strong that the unintended slowing can be readily perceived by the participant.

Inhibition appears to be a basic, core aspect of executive control that is involved in most executive tasks (Miyake et al., 2000; Zacks & Hasher, 1994) and is an important function of the prefrontal cortex (Diamond & Goldman-Rakic, 1989; Fuster, 1997). Top-down inhibitory control of dominant responses is an omnipresent process during the self-regulation of emotion, when involuntary emotional responses have to be suppressed and overridden by controlled responses more adapted to the individual's goals (Ochsner, Bunge, Gross, & Gabrieli, 2002; Schaefer et al., 2003).

Most everyday life situations in which inhibitory control is required involve emotions, to a certain extent. Indeed, inhibitory control is enacted in situations in which a choice has to be made between at least two conflicting responses. Inhibitory control processes suppress the response that is incongruent with the individual's current goals and prioritize the congruent response. This implies that the utilization of inhibitory control is a necessary consequence of the appraisal of the goal—(in)congruency of a given situation. Goal incongruency is a strong potential cause of emotional activation (Carver & Scheier, 1990; Frijda, 1986; Higgins, 1987; Johnson & Multhaup, 1992; Lazarus, 1991; Power & Dalgleish, 1997; Scherer, 2001). (Note that goal incongruency or expectation mismatch may trigger more elaborate processing and conscious awareness (Gray, 1995). Therefore, inhibitory processes are likely to be activated conjointly with an emotional activation in natural situations, thereby increasing the need to understand their potential interactions.

There are at least three main sources of empirical contributions to the understanding of the interactions between emotion and inhibitory control. First, several studies have tried to assess the inhibition of emotional contents, mostly using the emotional Stroop task. Second, several studies assessed the performance of emotionally disordered patients in inhibitory control tasks. Third, at least two studies have investigated how affective manipulations influence performance on cognitive control tasks that require inhibition.

In the emotional Stroop paradigm, participants are asked to name the ink color of emotional words compared to neutral words (for an excellent review, see Williams, Mathews, & MacLeod, 1996). The prototypical result is that the time needed to name negative or positive words is increased in comparison to neutral words, though the effect is more reliable if the words used refer to a personal concern of the subjects (Hughdahl & Stormark, 2002). However—and importantly—it is not clear that inhibitory control processes are the critical factor in the emotional Stroop effects. Indeed, there are no clear incongruent or congruent conditions in this paradigm, because the words are not color words. Hence it can be argued that there is no conflict between two competing responses of the same category. The emotional Stroop results might be best understood as the results of an attentional bias toward emotional information (Hughdahl & Stormark, 2002).

Another method of investigating the interaction between emotion and inhibitory control is to assess the impact of long-term emotional states and dispositions on inhibitory performance. Disposition can be investigated by examining performance of either normal participants or emotionally disordered patients on inhibitory tasks. Several studies tried to assess the performance of patients with emotional disorders on inhibition tasks. A reliable finding seems to be the impairment of inhibitory control in depressed patients. For instance, Lemelin and colleagues (Lemelin, Baruch, Vincent, Everett, & Vincent, 1997; Lemelin et al., 1996) found that depressed patients were impaired in the standard Stroop task and in a visuospatial interference test, suggesting that these patients had impaired inhibitory control. Similar results have been reported for bipolar depressed patients in their depressive phase (Ali et al., 2000; Jones, Duncan, Mirsky, Post, & Theodore, 1994). Further, Murphy and colleagues (1999) found that the reaction times of depressed patients were slower when attempting to inhibit a response in a go/no-go task, which requires withholding a response.

An impairment of inhibitory control also seems to be a consistent finding in patients with obsessive–compulsive disorder (OCD), a debilitating anxiety disorder. For instance, Hartston and Swertlow (1999) found that patients with OCD were impaired in their performance on the Stroop task. Bannon, Gonsalvez, Croft, and Boyce (2002) found the same result using a Stroop task and a go/no-go task; Rosenberg, Dick, O'Hearn, and Sweeney (1997) found an impairment of response inhibition in patients with OCD, using an antisaccade task. Interestingly, the impairment of response inhibition in patients with OCD remained significant even after controlling for schizotypal and depressive symptoms (Aycicegi, Dinn, Harris, & Erkmen, 2003).

Other emotional disorders also seem to be associated with a dysfunction of inhibitory control. For instance, Wood, Mathews, and Dalgleish (2001) found that high-trait-anxious individuals were impaired in their ability to inhibit the inappropriate meaning of a homograph. Further, Stein, Kennedy, and Twamley (2002) found that women suffering from posttraumatic stress disorder (PTSD) were impaired in their performance on the Stroop Color–Word Test and in a set-shifting task. Moreover, Murphy and colleagues (1999) found that manic patients committed more errors than depressed and controls in a go/no-go task.

Overall, the data seem to indicate that emotional disorders are associated with impairments of inhibitory control. However, it is not yet clear which processes are responsible for this pattern of results. Indeed, at least two main alternative explanations can account for the association between emotional disorders and inhibitory impairment. The first account emphasizes an impairment of inhibition as causing the emotional disorders by impairing capacities that regulate emotion. The second account emphasizes that depressed or anxious moods are associated with more rumination (negative repetitive thoughts) that creates a working memory load and depletes attentional resources (Watkins & Brown, 2002).

A direct test of the interaction between affect and inhibitory control would consist of assessing the performance of normal subjects in an inhibition test just after the induction of an emotional state. To our knowledge, only two studies have explicitly adopted this procedure, and they obtained contradictory results. First, Kuhl and Kazen (1999) assessed standard Stroop color naming after a brief exposure to affectively valenced words. They found that the color–word interference disappeared after exposure to positive words, compared to neutral and negative words, with no differences between neutral and negative words. This is a remarkable result, although it is not clear whether the effect is caused by an actual emotional state or the priming of emotional semantic categories that have been activated by the emotional words. Even still, exposure to positive affective stimuli enhanced performance. Second, Phillips, Bull, Adams, and Fraser (2002) assessed Stroop performance after a mood induction procedure by recollection of positive versus neutral memories. They found that the recollection of positive memories impaired Stroop performance in a standard version of the task (naming the ink color of incongruent color words), and that this impairment was more pronounced when the subjects had to alternate between word and color naming. Hence this study's results argue for a deleterious effect of positive emotion on inhibitory control. One of the main differences between these two studies is the mood induction procedure (MIP) used. Although memory recollection might have been more effective than using affectively valenced words to elicit an actual emotional state, the task of recollecting an emotional autobiographical memory may have increased the occurrence of thoughts related to the remembered event or mood-related thoughts, thereby depleting the working memory resources necessary to successfully achieve the Stroop task.

More generally, to understand emotional modulation of inhibitory control, several conceptual and methodological issues need to be better understood. For instance, direct tests of the emotional modulation of inhibitory control should take into account the different processing characteristics of MIP and their possible effects on the inhibition task. In addition, it would be worthwhile to explore the effects of other emotional properties than valence (e.g., emotional arousal, specific emotional appraisals) on inhibitory control. Future studies should also consider the possibility that cognitive control encompasses several dissociable processing components that play different roles in inhibitory control processes, and that may be differentially affected by emotion. Indeed, some distinctions have been proposed in the literature between conflict detection and maintenance processes (Botvinick, Braver, Barch, Carter, & Cohen, 2001; Braver & Cohen, 2000; Kerns et al., 2004), and between reactive and proactive control (see previous section; Braver et al., in press).

POTENTIALLY UNCONSCIOUS CONTROL DILEMMAS: AFFECTIVE INFLUENCES ON SELECTIVE ATTENTION

In this section we shift from considering emotion as a quasi-executive form of control that shapes cognition, to considering affective influences on selective attention. We do not claim that such influences are always unconscious, but we do consider it likely that they are often unconscious or not accessible to awareness. Selective attention has multiple components, including some that are controlled and some that are automatic, and for this reason is potentially a very interesting paradigm in which to examine relations among emotion, control, and consciousness.

Although the word *control* implies the operation of explicit, goal-driven mechanisms, control dilemmas themselves can occur whenever the cognitive system must "choose" between two or more comparable options. In such cases, selective attention can shift the weight allotted to certain signals, biasing the paths taken in the course of cognitive processing (Desimone & Duncan, 1995). Notably, selective attention is not always under deliberate or effortful control; just as people can often direct attention voluntarily, attention can also be captured without a person's volition (Yantis & Jonides, 1984). The former type of attentional allocation is often referred to as *endogenous, voluntary,* or *top-down*; the latter is often referred to as *exogenous, automatic,* or *bottom-up*. Evidence from a number of studies suggests that differences in manner of allocation reflect the operation of separable components of attention. For example, relatively automatic attentional shifts tend to be linked with a transient time-course, in which maximum facilitation of processing at the attended location is reached within about 150 milliseconds, but declines soon thereafter. In contrast, voluntary shifts can be sustained: Maximum facilitation is reached after about 300 milliseconds and can be maintained for extended periods of time (Müller & Rabbitt, 1989; Nakayama & Mackeben, 1989). In addition, different neural networks are implicated in the different types of attention shifts, with automatic shifts associated with heightened right-lateralized activity in the temporoparietal and inferior frontal cortices, and voluntary shifts associated more with activity in the intraparietal and superior frontal cortices (Corbetta & Shulman, 2002). Finally, it has been suggested that exogenously and endogenously allocated attention might have different consequences for the binding of visual features (Briand & Klein, 1987) as well as for conscious awareness of a stimulus (Most, Scholl, Clifford, & Simons, 2005).

Regardless of distinctions between different components, attention by its very nature involves the resolution of competing demands. The distinction between relatively automatic and voluntary attentional shifting, plus a growing literature on individual differences and attentional biases to emotional information, make an examination of selective attention potentially fruitful for exploring control dilemmas at multiple levels of cognitive processing.

Evolutionary arguments have highlighted the adaptive nature of biases to attend to emotional information (e.g., Lundqvist & Öhman, Chapter 5;

Öhman & Mineka, 2001). When unexpected sources of danger or self-relevance appear, it is almost always in one's best interest to attend to them right away (cf. Simon, 1967). Consistent with this hypothesis, several studies have demonstrated that potentially threatening stimuli capture attention more readily than nonthreatening stimuli. For example, it is easier to detect a discrepant angry face among happy faces than vice versa (Öhman, Lundqvist, & Esteves, 2001; Lundqvist & Öhman, Chapter 5). Furthermore, such effects can be very specific; stimuli that are evocative to one person can seem bland to another—and attentional biases often reflect such idiosyncrasies. In one study, patients with specific phobias were asked to engage in a visual search for pictures of snakes, spiders, or flowers and mushrooms in a computer display (Öhman, Flykt, & Esteves, 2001). In this paradigm, the time it takes to locate a target typically varies as a function of the number of distracters in the display: The greater the number of distracters, the longer the search time. Attentional biases to a stimulus are inferred when people consistently direct attention to that stimulus first, in which case search time is generally unaffected by the number of distracters present (Treisman & Gelade, 1980). When participants searched for spider or snake targets among flower and mushroom distractors, not only were they faster to find the target than when searching for flowers or mushrooms among snakes and spiders, but this was especially true when the target was specific to the participant's phobia (i.e., a snake for people with snake phobia or a spider for those with spider phobia). Importantly, the speed of finding the fear-relevant targets (but not the fear-irrelevant targets) was relatively unaffected by the number of distractors in the display—a pattern that suggests strong attentional biases for fear-relevant stimuli (Öhman, Flykt, et al., 2001).

Given that people appear predisposed to attend to emotional stimuli, emotional or mood states and chronic affective styles might help to mediate such attentional biases. Some of the strongest evidence in support of this possibility comes from research on emotional disorders (McNally, 1996). For example, in a dot-probe task, clinically anxious individuals were faster than both healthy controls and clinically depressed individuals to respond to probes, when the probes appeared at locations previously occupied by threat cues rather than locations previously occupied by neutral cues (MacLeod, Mathews, & Tata, 1986). Similarly, people with PTSD, as well as particular phobias and anxieties, have difficulty ignoring information relevant to their disorders, as demonstrated by interference in the emotional Stroop paradigm. In this task, people were slower to name the colors of words when the words themselves were emotional rather than neutral. Again, these effects can be quite specific. Thus war veterans with PTSD were especially slow in response to words such as *body-bags* (McNally,

Kaspi, Riemann, & Zeitlin, 1990), whereas socially anxious individuals were selectively slower in response to socially relevant words such as *party* (Hope, Rapee, Heimberg, & Dombeck, 1990; McNally et al., 1990).

Notably, in both the emotional Stroop and dot-probe paradigms, the emotional nature of the stimuli is irrelevant to the assigned task. This stands in contrast with the search paradigm (e.g., Lundqvist & Öhman, Chapter 5; Öhman, Flykt, et al., 2001), in which subjects actively search for a target that differs from the surrounding stimuli along an emotion-relevant dimension. By emphasizing distinctions between paradigms in which people actively search for an emotional stimulus and those in which subjects must suppress emotional information, researchers might begin to delineate levels of attentional control that are most affected by emotion-related states or traits. Potentially, these levels could map onto distinctions between relatively automatic and voluntary components of attention—and, if only loosely, onto unconscious and conscious processes (cf. Bishop, Duncan, Brett, & Lawrence, 2004).

As insights from the clinical and psychophysical literatures continue to converge, our understanding of how affect influences attentional control is likely to grow more precise. For example, although the emotional Stroop and dot-probe paradigms initially revealed attentional biases broadly defined, more recent experiments have sought to pinpoint the mechanisms underlying these biases. Indeed, the simple act of orienting attention can be broken down into at least three components: disengaging from one stimulus, shifting attention, and engaging with a new stimulus (Posner & Petersen, 1990). Recent studies have suggested that the biases revealed via the dot-probe (and perhaps the emotional Stroop) might reflect difficulty in disengaging from emotional information rather than biases to shift attention to such information in the first place (Fox, Russo, Bowles, & Dutton, 2001). In these experiments, threatening and nonthreatening faces or words were used as cues indicating the likely location of a target. All cues appeared before the target in one of two potential target locations. *Valid* cues correctly indicated the target location; *invalid* cues incorrectly indicated the target location. High-anxious subjects were slower to respond to the target if the cue was invalid but threatening. However, the emotionality of the cues did not seem to affect response time when the cues were valid. This pattern of results suggests that the differences in response times reflected difficulty disengaging from the threatening cues rather than faster allocation of attention to them. Interestingly, these effects were seen only in high-anxious, not low-anxious, subjects (Fox et al., 2001). Such findings contribute to our understanding of which particular components of attention are likely to be especially influenced by emotion. Further understanding of the rich interactions between attention and emotion can give us not only insight into the organizational structure of emotion-based attentional biases but also serve as a model for understanding how emotional systems can help organize the functioning of other cognitive domains as well.

LOOKING TO THE FUTURE (WITH ANTICIPATION!)

By elaborating several examples, our aim has been to articulate more broadly a meta-theoretical perspective on the function of emotion and affect. We propose that a very general function of affect is to help resolve control dilemmas inherent in being an autonomous (yet highly social), self-regulating control system—er, that is, a human being. We are cautiously optimistic that a control dilemma perspective might be useful beyond the examples given here, by providing coherence to a field poised to make major advances. There are many other ways in which people—and self-regulating systems, more generally—can be conflicted. Some types of mental conflict may be severe enough that the conflict becomes conscious or otherwise initiates processing that strongly influences the contents of consciousness. Yet other conflicts may be resolved without so much as raising a metaphorical ripple on the surface of the mind, and these may be more the norm than the exception, given that a large proportion of the control of human behavior operates expertly without consciousness.

To hint at the broader relevance of a control dilemma perspective, beyond the examples considered above, we note several tradeoffs that have been suggested to be influenced by emotion and affect. First, a substantial literature converges on the idea that negative moods promote more systematic processing and positive moods promote heuristic processing (e.g., Bless & Schwarz, 1999; Bolte, Goschke, & Kuhl, 2003; Palfai & Salovey, 1993). The conflict appears to be between whether to engage cognitive control mechanisms (analytic processing) or not (heuristic processing). Heuristic and analytic processing may often preclude each other, leading to control conflict, although it has been suggested that they need not always conflict (Isen, 1993).

Second, a related distinction and possible control dilemma is between global and local attentional focus. One can typically attend either to the "forest" or the "trees" in a given situation—so how does one's inner homunculus decide to which to attend? An early theoretical account suggested that emotion narrows the range or scope of attention (Easterbrook, 1959). Recent work on strategic memory encoding in OCD has suggested a bias toward seeing the details ("trees") rather than the gestalt ("forest"; Savage et al., 1999; Savage et al., 2000). Conversely, positive affect appears to result in a bias toward a global attentional focus (Gasper & Clore, 2002).

Third, a computational tradeoff between distractibility and perseveration (Braver & Cohen, 2000) has been suggested to be influenced by affect (Dreisbach & Goschke, 2004). Specifically, a brief presentation of positive images during a task-switching paradigm led to increased switch costs (perseveration) compared to when the images were affectively neutral, and to decreased switch-costs (distractibility) when the images were affectively positive.

Fourth, anxiety can influence speed versus accuracy (Leon & Revelle, 1985). Specifically, high-trait-anxious participants performing a difficult geometric analogies task under time-stress did not simply perform worse on the task than low-trait-anxious control participants. Instead, a detailed analysis revealed that the trait-anxious participants performed faster, but less accurately, than the controls.

Fifth, effects of emotion on risk taking have been explored (e.g., Isen, Nygren, & Ashby, 1988; Johnson & Tversky, 1983), and these effects are likely amenable to a conflict analysis in terms of risk–reward tradeoffs.

And sixth, consistent with the idea that emotions are not merely personal phenomena but are also strongly social in nature (e.g., Frijda, 1999), a major function of emotion might be to help reduce social conflicts, for example, self-interest versus group (prosocial or collective) interest (Isen, 1970; Isen & Levin, 1972). In the prisoner's dilemma task, an experimental situation that explicitly presents participants with a conflict between personal and group interest, aspects of emotion and mood could help sustain a bias toward cooperation (Gray & Braver, 2002a; Rilling et al., 2002).

Finally, although we are advocating a general perspective, we emphasize (strongly!) that it is important to make distinctions among affective phenomena. One cannot safely assume that effects of emotion proper on cognition are the same as effects of mood, stress, pain, and various emotional psychopathologies. Risk, motivation, reward, and punishment are also categorically different constructs and cannot safely be lumped together or with emotional states in an "emotion-related" conceptual bin. In addition, as many theorists and investigators have emphasized, emotional and mood states are likely to depend in important ways on individual differences, including variation within a normal range and to extremes that are pathological (e.g., Barrett, Chapter 11; Costa & McCrae, 1980; Davidson, 1998; Larsen & Ketelaar, 1991). The states may differ not simply in intensity (e.g., depressed mood vs. sadness) but possibly in qualitatively and mechanistically different ways.

In sum, many effects of emotion on various tradeoffs have been explored and documented. The larger computational perspective—of emotion as helping to resolve control dilemmas—is more general and, to our knowledge, has not been explored previously as a unifying framework. We are cautiously optimistic that a control dilemma perspective can help us better understand effects of emotion, mood, and affective stimuli on cognition. It will be particularly exciting to further investigate such a perspective in relation to conscious and unconscious processes. Consciousness is intriguing but does not lend itself readily to empirical investigation. Potential relationships among consciousness, emotion, and cognitive control are anything but simple. And yet these relationships are profoundly relevant to human nature and human experience. Consciousness, emotion, and cognitive control may covary to a significant extent. Moreover, they may covary for functionally adaptive reasons related to enhancing global control and, if the present argument is on the right track, to the resolution of control dilemmas.

ACKNOWLEDGMENTS

Some of the research described in this chapter was supported by a grant from the National Science Foundation, and preparation of the chapter was supported by a grant from the National Institute of Mental Health.

REFERENCES

Ali, S. O., Denicoff, K. D., Altshuler, L. L., Hauser, P., Li, X. M., Conrad, A. J., et al. (2000). A preliminary study of the relation of neuropsychological performance in neuroanatomic structures in bipolar disorder. *Neuropsychiatry, Neuropsychology and Behavioral Neurology, 13,* 20–28.

Ashby, F. G., Isen, A. M., & Turken, A. U. (1999). A neuropsychological theory of positive affect and its influence on cognition. *Psychological Review, 106,* 529–550.

Aycicegi, A., Dinn, W. M., Harris, C. L., & Erkmen, H. (2003). Neuropsychological function in obsessive–compulsive disorder: Effects of comorbid conditions on task performance. *European Psychiatry, 18,* 241–248.

Baker, S. C., Frith, C. D., & Dolan, R. J. (1997). The interaction between mood and cognitive function studied with PET. *Psychological Medicine, 27,* 565–578.

Bannon, S., Gonsalvez, C. J., Croft, R. J., & Boyce, P. M. (2002). Response inhibition deficits in obsessive–compulsive disorder. *Psychiatry Research, 110,* 165–174.

Bargh, J. A. (1994). The Four Horsemen of automaticity: Awareness, efficiency, intention, and control in social cognition. In R. S. Wyer, Jr., & T. K. Srull (Eds.), *Handbook of social cognition* (2nd ed., pp. 1–40). Hillsdale, NJ: Erlbaum.

Bartolic, E. I., Basso, M. R., Schefft, B. K., Glauser, T., & Titanic-Schefft, M. (1999). Effects of experimentally-induced emotional states on frontal lobe cognitive task performance. *Neuropsychologia, 37,* 677–683.

Bishop, S., Duncan, J., Brett, M., & Lawrence, A. D. (2004). Prefrontal cortical function and anxiety: Controlling attention to threat-related stimuli. *Nature Neuroscience, 7*, 184–188.

Bless, H., & Schwarz, N. (1999). Sufficient and necessary conditions in dual-process models: The case of mood and information processing. In S. Chaiken & Y. Trope (Eds.), *Dual-process theories in social psychology* (pp. 423–440). New York: Guilford Press.

Bolte, A., Goschke, T., & Kuhl, J. (2003). Emotion and intuition. *Psychological Science, 14*, 416–421.

Botvinick, M. M., Braver, T. S., Barch, D. M., Carter, C. S., & Cohen, J. C. (2001). Conflict monitoring and cognitive control. *Psychological Review, 108*, 624–652.

Braver, T. S., & Cohen, J. D. (2000). On the control of control: The role of dopamine in regulating prefrontal function and working memory. In S. Monsell & J. Driver (Eds.), *Attention and performance XVIII* (pp. 713–738). Cambridge, MA: MIT Press.

Braver, T. S., Cohen, J. D., & Barch, D. M. (2002). The role of the prefrontal cortex in normal and disordered cognitive control: A cognitive neuroscience perspective. In D. T. Stuss & R. T. Knight (Eds.), *Principles of frontal lobe function* (pp. 428–448). Oxford, UK: Oxford University Press.

Braver, T. S., Gray, J. R., & Burgess, G. C. (in press). Explaining the many varieties of working memory variation: Dual mechanisms of cognitive control. In A. R. A. Conway, C. Jarrold, M. J. Kane, A. Miyake, & J. N. Towse (Eds.), *Variation in working memory*. New York: Oxford University Press.

Briand, K. A., & Klein, R. M. (1987). Is Posner's "beam" the same as Treisman's "glue"? On the relation between visual orienting and feature integration theory. *Journal of Experimental Psychology, 13*(2), 228–241.

Cabeza, R., & Nyberg, L. (2000). Imaging cognition II: An empirical review of 275 PET and fMRI studies. *Journal of Cognitive Neuroscience, 12*, 1–47.

Carver, C. S., & Scheier, M. F. (1990). Origins and functions of positive and negative affect: A control-process view. *Psychological Review, 97*, 19–35.

Carver, C. S., Sutton, S. K., & Scheier, M. F. (2000). Action, emotion, and personality: Emerging conceptual integration. *Personality and Social Psychology Bulletin, 26*, 741–751.

Carver, C. S., & White, T. (1994). Behavioral inhibition, behavioral activation, and affective responses to impending reward and punishment: The BIS/BAS scales. *Journal of Personality and Social Psychology, 67*, 319–333.

Christianson, S. A. (Ed.). (1992). *Handbook of emotion and memory*. Hillsdale, NJ: Erlbaum.

Corbetta, M., & Shulman, G. L. (2002). Control of goal-directed and stimulus-driven attention in the brain. *Nature Reviews Neuroscience, 3*, 201–215.

Costa, P. T., & McCrae, R. R. (1980). Influence of extraversion and neuroticism on subjective well-being: Happy and unhappy people. *Journal of Personality and Social Psychology, 38*, 668–678.

Dalgleish, T., & Power, M. J. (Eds.). (1999). *Handbook of cognition and emotion*. New York: Wiley.

Davidson, R. J. (1995). Cerebral asymmetry, emotion, and affective style. In R. J.

Davidson & K. Hugdahl (Eds.), *Brain asymmetry* (pp. 361–387). Cambridge, MA: MIT Press.

Davidson, R. J. (1998). Affective style and affective disorders: Perspectives from affective neuroscience. *Cognition and Emotion, 12,* 307–330.

Desimone, R., & Duncan, J. (1995). Neural mechanisms of selective visual attention. *Annual Review of Neuroscience, 18,* 193–222.

Diamond, A., & Goldman-Rakic, P. S. (1989). Comparison of human infants and rhesus monkeys on Piaget's A-not-B task: Evidence for dependence on dorsolateral prefrontal cortex. *Experimental Brain Research, 74,* 24–40.

Dolan, R. J. (2002). Emotion, cognition, and behavior. *Science, 298,* 1191–1194.

Dollard, J., & Miller, N. E. (1950). The dynamics of conflict: Their implications for therapy. In J. Dollard & N. E. Miller (Eds.), *Personality and psychotherapy* (pp. 352–368). New York: McGraw-Hill.

Dreisbach, G., & Goschke, T. (2004). How positive affect modulates cognitive control: Reduced perseveration at the cost of increased distractibility. *Journal of Experimental Psychology: Learning Memory and Cognition, 30,* 343–353.

Easterbrook, J. A. (1959). The effect of emotion on cue utilization and the organization of behavior. *Psychological Review, 66,* 183–201.

Eich, E., Kihlstrom, J. F., Bower, G. H., Forgas, J. P., & Niedenthal, P. M. (2000). *Cognition and emotion.* New York: Oxford University Press.

Forgas, J. P. (Ed.). (2001). *Handbook of affect and social cognition.* Mahwah, NJ: Erlbaum.

Fox, E., Russo, R., Bowles, R., & Dutton, K. (2001). Do threatening stimuli draw or hold visual attention in subclinical anxiety? *Journal of Experimental Psychology: General, 130,* 681–700.

Frijda, N. H. (1986). *The emotions.* London: Cambridge University Press.

Frijda, N. H. (1999). Emotions and hedonic experience. In D. Kahneman, E. Diener, & N. Schwarz (Eds.), *Well-being: The foundations of hedonic psychology* (pp. 190–210). New York: Russell Sage Foundation.

Fry, P. S. (1977). Success, failure, and resistance to temptation. *Developmental Psychology, 13,* 519–520.

Fuster, J. (1997). *The prefrontal cortex* (3rd ed.). New York: Lippincott-Raven.

Gasper, K., & Clore, G. L. (2002). Attending to the big picture: Mood and global versus local processing of visual information. *Psychological Science, 13,* 34–40.

Gray, J. A. (1982). *The neuropsychology of anxiety: An inquiry into the functions of the septo-hippocampal systems.* Oxford, UK: Oxford University Press.

Gray, J. A. (1995). The contents of consciousness: A neuropsychological conjecture. *Behavioral and Brain Sciences, 18*(4), 659–722.

Gray, J. R. (1999). A bias toward short-term thinking in threat-related negative emotional states. *Personality and Social Psychology Bulletin, 25,* 65–75.

Gray, J. R. (2001). Emotional modulation of cognitive control: Approach–withdrawal states double-dissociate spatial from verbal two-back task performance. *Journal of Experimental Psychology: General, 130,* 436–452.

Gray, J. R. (2002). Does a prosocial–selfish distinction help explain the biological affects? Comment on Buck (1999). *Psychological Review, 109,* 729–738.

Gray, J. R., & Braver, T. S. (2002a). Cognitive control in altruism and self-control: A social cognitive neuroscience perspective. *Behavioral and Brain Sciences, 25,* 260.

Gray, J. R., & Braver, T. S. (2002b). Integration of emotion and cognitive control: A neurocomputational hypothesis of dynamic goal regulation. In S. C. Moore & M. R. Oaksford (Eds.), *Emotional cognition* (pp. 289–316). Amsterdam: Benjamins.

Gray, J. R., Braver, T. S., & Raichle, M. E. (2002). Integration of emotion and cognition in the lateral prefrontal cortex. *Proceedings of the National Academy of Sciences USA, 99,* 4115–4120.

Gross, J. J. (2002). Emotion regulation: Affective, cognitive, and social consequences. *Psychophysiology, 39,* 281–291.

Harmon-Jones, E., & Allen, J. J. (1997). Behavioral activation sensitivity and resting frontal EEG asymmetry: Covariation of putative indicators related to risk for mood disorders. *Journal of Abnormal Psychology, 106*(1), 159–163.

Harmon-Jones, E., & Sigelman, J. (2001). State anger and prefrontal brain activity: Evidence that insult-related relative left-prefrontal activation is associated with experienced anger and aggression. *Journal of Personality and Social Psychology, 80,* 797–803.

Hartston, H. J., & Swerdlow, N. R. (1999). Visuospatial priming and Stroop performance in patients with obsessive compulsive disorder. *Neuropsychology, 13,* 447–457.

Heatherton, T. F., Herman, C. P., & Polivy, J. (1991). Effects of physical threat and ego threat on eating behavior. *Journal of Personality and Social Psychology, 60*(1), 138–143.

Heller, W. (1990). The neuropsychology of emotion: Developmental patterns and implications for psychopathology. In N. Stein, B. L. Leventhal, & T. Trabasso (Eds.), *Psychological and biological approaches to emotion* (pp. 167–211). Hillsdale, NJ: Erlbaum.

Hellige, J. B. (1993). *Hemispheric asymmetry.* Cambridge, MA: Harvard University Press.

Herrnstein, R. J., Loewenstein, G. F., Prelec, D., & Vaughan, W., Jr. (1993). Utility maximization and melioration: Internalities in individual choice. *Journal of Behavioral Decision Making, 6,* 149–185.

Herrnstein, R. J., Prelec, D., & Vaughan, W., Jr. (1986). *An intrapersonal prisoner's dilemma.* Paper presented at the 19th Symposium on the Quantitative Analysis of Behavior, Harvard University, Boston.

Higgins, E. T. (1987). Self-discrepancy: A theory relating self and affect. *Psychological Review, 94,* 319–340.

Hope, D. A., Rapee, R. M., Heimberg, R. G., & Dombeck, M. J. (1990). Representations of the self in social phobia: Vulnerability to social threat. *Cognitive Therapy and Research, 17,* 177–189.

Hughdahl, K., & Stormark, K. M. (2002). Emotional modulation of selective attention: Behavioral and psychophysiological measures. In R. J. Davidson, K. R. Scherer & H. H. Goldsmith (Eds.), *Handbook of affective sciences* (pp. 276–291). New York: Oxford University Press.

Isen, A. M. (1970). Success, failure, attention, and reaction to others: The warm glow of success. *Journal of Personality and Social Psychology, 15,* 294–301.

Isen, A. M. (1993). Positive affect and decision making. In M. Lewis & J. Haviland (Eds.), *Handbook of emotions* (pp. 261–277). New York: Guilford Press.

Isen, A. M., & Levin, P. F. (1972). Effects of feeling good on helping: Cookies and kindness. *Journal of Personality and Social Psychology, 21,* 382–388.

Isen, A. M., Nygren, T. E., & Ashby, F. G. (1988). Influence of positive affect on the subjective utility of gains and losses: It is just not worth the risk. *Journal of Personality and Social Psychology, 55,* 710–717.

Johnson, E., & Tversky, A. (1983). Affect, generalization, and the perception of risk. *Journal of Personality and Social Psychology, 45,* 20–31.

Johnson, M. K., & Multhaup, K. S. (1992). Emotion and MEM. In S. A. Christianson (Ed.), *The handbook of emotion and memory* (pp. 33–66). Hillsdale, NJ: Erlbaum.

Jones, B. P., Duncan, C. C., Mirsky, A. F., Post, R. M., & Theodore, W. H. (1994). Neuropsychological profiles in bipolar affective disorder and complex partial seizure disorder. *Neuropsychology, 8,* 55–64.

Kagan, J., Reznick, J. S., & Snidman, N. (1988). Biological bases of childhood shyness. *Science, 240,* 167–171.

Kelley, W. M., Miezin, F. M., McDermott, K. B., Buckner, R. L., Raichle, M. E., Cohen, N. J., et al. (1998). Hemispheric specialization in human dorsal frontal cortex and medial temporal lobe for verbal and non-verbal memory encoding. *Neuron, 20,* 927–936.

Kerns, J. G., Cohen, J. D., MacDonald, A. W., 3rd, Cho, R. Y., Stenger, V. A., & Carter, C. S. (2004). Anterior cingulate conflict monitoring and adjustments in control. *Science, 303,* 1023–1026.

Kuhl, J., & Kazen, M. (1999). Volitional facilitation of difficult intentions: Joint activation of intention memory and positive affect removes Stroop interference. *Journal of Experimental Psychology: General, 128,* 382–399.

Lane, R. D., & Nadel, L. (Eds.). (2000). *Cognitive neuroscience of emotion.* New York: Oxford University Press.

Lang, P. J., Bradley, M. M., & Cuthbert, B. N. (1990). Emotion, attention, and the startle reflex. *Psychological Review, 97,* 377–395.

Larsen, R. J., & Ketelaar, E. (1991). Personality and susceptibility to positive and negative emotional states. *Journal of Personality and Social Psychology, 61,* 132–140.

Lazarus, R. S. (1991). Progress on a cognitive–motivational–relational theory of emotion. *American Psychologist, 46,* 819–834.

Leith, K. P., & Baumeister, R. F. (1996). Why do bad moods increase self-defeating behavior? Emotion, risk, and self-regulation. *Journal of Personality and Social Psychology, 71,* 1250–1267.

Lemelin, S., Baruch, P., Vincent, A., Everett, J., & Vincent, P. (1997). Distractibility and processing resource deficit in major depression. Evidence for two deficient attentional processing models. *Journal of Nervous and Mental Disease, 185,* 542–548.

Lemelin, S., Baruch, P., Vincent, A., Laplante, L., Everett, J., & Vincent, P. (1996). Attention disturbance in clinical depression: Deficient distractor inhibition or processing resource deficit? *Journal of Nervous and Mental Disease, 184,* 114–121.

Leon, M. R., & Revelle, W. (1985). Effects of anxiety on analogical reasoning: A test of three theoretical models. *Journal of Personality and Social Psychology, 49*(5), 1302–1315.

Lerner, J. S., Small, D. A., & Loewenstein, G. (2004). Heart strings and purse strings: Carryover effects of emotions on economic decisions. *Psychological Science, 15,* 337–341.

Lima, S. L., & Dill, L. M. (1990). Behavioral decisions made under risk of predation: A review and prospectus. *Canadian Journal of Zoology, 68,* 619–640.

Loewenstein, G. F., & Prelec, D. (1993). Preferences for sequences of outcomes. *Psychological Review, 100,* 91–108.

MacLeod, C. M. (1991). Half a century of research on the Stroop effect: An integrative review. *Psychological Bulletin, 109,* 163–203.

MacLeod, C. M., Mathews, A., & Tata, P. (1986). Attentional bias in emotional disorders. *Journal of Abnormal Psychology, 95,* 15–20.

Markham, R., & Darke, S. (1991). The effects of trait anxiety on verbal and spatial task performance. *Australian Journal of Psychology, 43,* 107–111.

Marr, D. (1982). *Vision.* New York: Freeman.

McNally, R. J. (1996). Cognitive bias in the anxiety disorders. *Nebraska Symposium on Motivation, 43,* 211–250.

McNally, R. J., Kaspi, S. P., Riemann, B. C., & Zeitlin, S. B. (1990). Selective processing of threat cues in post-traumatic stress disorder. *Journal of Abnormal Psychology, 99,* 398–402.

Metcalfe, J., & Mischel, W. (1999). A hot/cool-system analysis of delay of gratification: Dynamics of willpower. *Psychological Review, 106,* 3–19.

Miller, E. K., & Cohen, J. D. (2001). An integrative theory of prefrontal cortex function. *Annual Review of Neuroscience, 21,* 167–202.

Miller, N. E. (1944). Experimental studies of conflict. In J. McV. Hunt (Ed.), *Personality and the behavior disorders* (Vol. 1, pp. 431–465). New York: Ronald.

Mischel, W., Shoda, Y., & Rodriguez, M. L. (1989). Delay of gratification in children. *Science, 244,* 933–938.

Miyake, A., Friedman, N. P., Emerson, M. J., Witzki, A. H., Howerter, A., & Wager, T. D. (2000). The unity and diversity of executive functions and their contributions to complex "frontal lobe" tasks: A latent variable analysis. *Cognitive Psychology, 41,* 49–100.

Most, S. B., Scholl, B. J., Clifford, E., & Simons, D. J. (2005). What you see is what you set: Sustained inattentional blindness and the capture of awareness. *Psychological Review, 112,* 217–242.

Müller, H. J., & Rabbitt, P. M. A. (1989). Reflexive and voluntary orienting of visual attention: Time course of activation and resistance to interruption. *Journal of Experimental Psychology: Human Perception and Performance, 15,* 315–330.

Murphy, F. C., Sahakian, B. J., Rubinsztein, J. S., Michael, A., Rogers, R. D., Robbins, T. W., et al. (1999). Emotional bias and inhibitory control processes in mania and depression. *Psychological Medicine, 29*, 1307–1321.

Nakayama, K., & Mackeben, M. (1989). Sustained and transient components of focal visual attention. *Vision Research, 29*, 1631–1647.

Norman, D. A., & Shallice, T. (1986). Attention to action: Willed and automatic control of behavior. In R. J. Davidson, G. E. Schwartz, & D. Shapiro (Eds.), *Consciousness and self-regulation* (Vol. 4, pp. 1–18). New York: Plenum Press.

Oatley, K., & Johnson-Laird, P. N. (1987). Towards a cognitive theory of emotion. *Cognition and Emotion, 1*, 29–50.

Ochsner, K. N., Bunge, S. A., Gross, J. J., & Gabrieli, J. D. E. (2002). Rethinking feelings: An fMRI study of the cognitive regulation of emotion. *Journal of Cognitive Neuroscience, 14*, 1215–1229.

Öhman, A., Flykt, A., & Esteves, F. (2001). Emotion drives attention: Detecting the snake in the grass. *Journal of Experimental Psychology: General, 130*, 466–478.

Öhman, A., Lundqvist, D., & Esteves, F. (2001). The face in the crowd revisited: A threat advantage with schematic stimuli. *Journal of Personality and Social Psychology, 80*, 381–396.

Öhman, A., & Mineka, S. (2001). Fears, phobias, and preparedness: Toward an evolved module of fear and fear learning. *Psychological Review, 108*, 483–522.

Palfai, T. P., & Salovey, P. (1993). The influence of depressed and elated mood on deductive and inductive reasoning. *Imagination, Cognition, and Personality, 13*, 57–71.

Pardo, J. V., Fox, P. T., & Raichle, M. D. (1991). Localization of a human system for sustained attention by positron emission tomography. *Nature, 349*, 61–63.

Phillips, L. H., Bull, R., Adams, E., & Fraser, L. (2002). Positive mood and executive function: Evidence from Stroop and fluency tasks. *Emotion, 2*, 12–22.

Posner, M. I., & DiGirolamo, G. J. (1998). Executive attention: Conflict, target detection and cognitive control. In R. Parasuraman (Ed.), *The attentive brain* (pp. 401–423). Cambridge, MA: MIT Press.

Posner, M. I., & Petersen, S. E. (1990). The attention system of the human brain. *Annual Review of Neuroscience, 13*, 25–42.

Posner, M. I., & Snyder, C. R. R. (1975). Attention and cognitive control. In R. L. Solso (Ed.), *Information processing and cognition* (pp. 55–85). Hillsdale, NJ: Erlbaum.

Power, M., & Dalgleish, T. (1997). *Cognition and emotion: From order to disorder.* Hove, UK: Erlbaum.

Rilling, J., Gutman, D., Zeh, T., Pagnoni, G., Berns, G., & Kilts, C. (2002). A neural basis for social cooperation. *Neuron, 35*, 395–405.

Rosenberg, D. R., Dick, E. L., O'Hearn, K. M., & Sweeney, J. A. (1997). Response-inhibition deficits in obsessive–compulsive disorder: An indicator of dysfunction in frontostriatal circuits. *Journal of Psychiatry and Neuroscience, 22*, 29–38.

Rottenstreich, Y., & Hsee, C. K. (2001). Money, kisses, and electric shocks: On the affective psychology of risk. *Psychological Science, 12*, 185–190.

Russell, J. A., & Barrett, L. F. (1999). Core affect, prototypical emotional episodes, and other things called emotion: Dissecting the elephant. *Journal of Personality and Social Psychology, 76*, 805–819.

Salovey, P., Mayer, J. D., & Caruso, D. (2002). The positive psychology of emotional intelligence. In C. R. Snyder & S. J. Lopez (Eds.), *The handbook of positive psychology* (pp. 159–171). New York: Oxford University Press.

Savage, C. R., Baer, L., Keuthen, N. J., Brown, H. D., Rauch, S. L., & Jenike, M. A. (1999). Organizational strategies mediate nonverbal memory impairment in obsessive–compulsive disorder. *Biological Psychiatry, 45*, 905–916.

Savage, C. R., Deckersbach, T., Wilhelm, S., Rauch, S. L., Baer, L., Reid, T., et al. (2000). Strategic processing and episodic memory impairment in obsessive compulsive disorder. *Neuropsychology, 14*, 141–151.

Schaefer, A., Collette, F., Philippot, P., Vanderlinden, M., Laureys, S., Delfiore, G., et al. (2003). Neural correlates of "hot" and "cold" emotional processing: A multilevel approach to the functional anatomy of emotions. *Neuroimage, 18*, 938–949.

Scherer, K. R. (2001). Appraisal considered as a process of multilevel sequential checking. In K. R. Scherer, A. Schorr, & T. Johnstone (Eds.), *Appraisal processes in emotion: Theory, methods, research* (pp. 92–120). New York: Oxford University Press.

Shiffrin, R. M., & Schneider, W. (1977). Controlled and automatic human information processing: II. Perceptual learning automaticity, attending, and a general theory. *Psychological Review, 84*, 127–190.

Simon, H. A. (1967). Motivational and emotional controls of cognition. *Psychological Review, 74*(1), 29–39.

Smith, E. E., & Jonides, J. (1999). Storage and executive processes in the frontal lobes. *Science, 283*, 1657–1661.

Stein, M. B., Kennedy, C. M., & Twamley, E. W. (2002). Neuropsychological function in female victims of intimate partner violence with and without posttraumatic stress disorder. *Biological Psychiatry, 52*, 1079–1088.

Stroop, J. R. (1935). Studies of interference in serial verbal reactions. *Journal of Experimental Psychology, 18*, 643–662.

Sutton, S. K., & Davidson, R. J. (1997). Prefrontal brain asymmetry: A biological substrate of the behavioral approach and inhibition systems. *Psychological Science, 8*, 204–210.

Tomarken, A. J., & Keener, A. D. (1998). Frontal brain asymmetry and depression: A self-regulatory perspective. *Cognition and Emotion, 12*, 387–420.

Treisman, A., & Gelade, G. (1980). A feature-integration theory of attention. *Cognitive Psychology, 12*, 97–136.

Tucker, D. M., & Williamson, P. A. (1984). Asymmetric neural control systems in human self-regulation. *Psychological Review, 91*, 185–215.

Watkins, E., & Brown, R. G. (2002). Rumination and executive function in depression: An experimental study. *Journal of Neurology, Neurosurgery and Psychiatry, 72*, 400–402.

Williams, J. M. G., Mathews, A., & MacLeod, C. (1996). The emotional Stroop task and psychopathology. *Psychological Bulletin, 120*, 3–24.

Wood, J., Mathews, A., & Dalgleish, T. (2001). Anxiety and cognitive inhibition. *Emotion, 1,* 166–181.

Yantis, S., & Jonides, J. (1984). Abrupt visual onsets and selective attention: Evidence from visual search. *Journal of Experimental Psychology: Human Perception and Performance, 10,* 601–621.

Zacks, R. T., & Hasher, L. (1994). Directed ignoring: Inhibitory regulation of working memory. In D. Dagenbach & T. H. Carr (Eds.), *Inhibitory processes in attention, memory, and language* (pp. 241–264). San Diego: Academic Press.

PART II

Unconscious Emotional Processing
Perception of Visual Stimuli

CHAPTER 5

Caught by the Evil Eye

Nonconscious Information Processing, Emotion, and Attention to Facial Stimuli

DANIEL LUNDQVIST

ARNE ÖHMAN

A BIOLOGICAL PERSPECTIVE ON THE HUMAN FACE

The Face as an Evolved Structure

The mind's primary façade to the world, the face, is an amazingly complex biological structure. Functionally critical openings for breathing, ingestion of food and fluid, and emission of sounds, as well as more or less hidden sensory surfaces, are embedded in a multitude of muscles and richly wrinkled skin tissue. In spite of the constraints (two eyes placed above a nose, which is placed above the mouth, and so forth), there are nonetheless striking individual differences in the way we look. As a result, the face is the primary vehicle for visual recognition of individuals. In addition, it provides information about factors such as age, sex, attractiveness, and health (Bruce & Young, 1986; Cole, 1998). However, beyond these relatively static sources of information, the intricate musculature of the face provides rich dynamic information of primary psychological significance.

Facial Muscles and Their Neural Control

There are two layers of facial muscles (see, e.g., Fridlund, 1994, for a review). The inner layer contains very strong muscles of obvious biological significance, such as the masseter and the temporalis, which move the jaw-

1. *What is the scope of your proposed model? When you use the term* emotion, *how do you use it? What do you mean by terms such as* fear, anxiety, *or* happiness?

The account presented in this chapter addresses the face as an emotional stimulus. The basic premise is that humans are evolutionarily prepared to respond to and produce emotional facial gestures. This means that we respond automatically to emotional faces even if their expressions are masked from conscious recognition. Furthermore, threatening faces attract attention when presented among neutral or emotional distractor faces.

From the evolutionary perspective, emotions are viewed as dispositional states that give attentional priority to particular stimuli and prime responses that, in the long run, promote the transfer of genes between generations. A primary task of emotions is to evaluate which stimuli are good and bad in the sense that they should be approached or avoided. Emotions are action sets that prioritize particular classes of functional responses. They are complex responses incorporating diverse and partly independent components, such as expressive behavior (e.g., facial expressions), action tendencies (e.g., avoidance), attentional priorities, and autonomic responses (e.g., skin conductance, heart rate) that provide metabolic support for action and feelings (e.g., an urge to get out of the situation).

2. *Define your terms:* conscious, unconscious, awareness. *Or say why you do not use these terms.*

Un- (or non)conscious and conscious in this chapter simply mean nonreportable and reportable, respectively. To be aware of an event is to be able to report and comment on it.

3. *Does your model deal with what is conscious, what is unconscious, or their relationship? If you do not address this area specifically, can you speculate on the relationship between what is conscious and unconscious? Or if you do not like the conscious–unconscious distinction, or if you do not think this is a good question to ask, can you say why?*

The basic emotion systems are evolutionary old. Because they evolved in primitive brains, they rely on ancient systems deep in the human brain that are not readily available to more recently evolved structures such as the cerebral cortex. Therefore, emotions can be activated automatically and nonconsciously, independently of conscious access to the eliciting stimulus. The validity of this proposal is best documented for the emotion of fear. Because emotion is rapidly activated before the perceptual analysis of the emotional stimulus is complete, it is based on a crude sensory analysis likely to rely on critical features rather than on sophisticated configural analysis.

The rapid recruitment of subcortical emotional networks is consistent with a Jamesian view on emotion, according to which the feeling comes late and includes conscious appreciation of the bodily response in relation to the eliciting stimulus.

bone. In contrast, the function of the outer layer may appear somewhat obscure. It is composed of numerous small muscles that primarily move facial skin tissue rather than, like most other striped muscles, body limbs. The sphincter muscle encircling the eye, the orbicularis oculi, which mediates involuntary eyeblinks, and the corrugator supercilii, which lowers the medial part of the eyebrows, both serve obvious functions in protecting the eye. However, they are also used voluntarily in what appear to be biologically more arbitrary activities such as flirting or to emit "eyebrow flashes," a universal gesture of friendly greeting (Eibl-Eibesfeldt, 1970). Similarly, the zygomaticus major connects the corner of the mouth to the cheekbone, not to expose the canines but to produce the most universally recognized facial gesture, the smile (e.g., Russell, 1994).

The facial muscles are innervated from two quite distinct neural systems of different evolutionary origin. The evolutionarily older system originates in the striatum, the top level of what was once the reptilian brain, that controls reflexive behavior related to basic biological functions such as consumatory behavior, attack, and defense. This system exerts involuntary, symmetric, and bilateral control of the facial musculature (Fridlund, 1994). The other system, of much later evolutionary history, has the typical contralateral origin of voluntarily controlled muscles, with neurons starting in the face area of the motor cortex to provide fine-tuned control of muscles primarily around the mouth for sound articulation (Gazzaniga & Smylie, 1990). Its evolution was part of the emergence of the most human of all characteristics, language. However, the resulting fine-tuned control of the lower face not only benefited the repertoire of speech sounds but also supported voluntary facial actions that could be used for visual rather than vocal communication. Thus this control could override and partly conceal the facial responses evoked by the more reflexive older system originating in the striatum. Accordingly, intentional social smiles that do not necessarily mediate felt happiness primarily involves the mouth, whereas a felt "Duchenne smile" also incorporates the muscles around the eyes (e.g., Ekman, 2003).

Thus part of facial muscle control is likely to have coevolved with language, but the primary evolutionary contingencies for facial muscles derived from their role in social communication, as first recognized by Darwin (1872/1998). He pointed to similarities between human facial displays and those of other primates, and subsequent research has generated quite convincing evolutionary histories for some expressions, such as, for example, the smile (van Hooff, 1972). Indeed, modern evolutionary theory's emphasis on the importance of the social interaction in the shaping of humans (e.g., Alexander, 1974; Humphrey, 1983; Trivers, 1985; Wilson, 1976) gives the face a central role in human evolution.

The human face has a more complex facial musculature than that of other primates. It appears that the proliferation and diversification of facial muscles, as well as the enhanced versatility of their neural control, coincided with the rapid enlargement of the hominid brain volume during the past million years (Chevalier-Skolnikoff, 1973). Thus the capacity for complex facial displays is likely to have coevolved with enhanced potential for complex behavior and complex inner states (Cole, 1998).

The Role of the Face in Human Evolution

When exchanging life in the rain forest for that on the savanna, early hominids were exposed to new sets of survival contingencies. Such contingencies included not only an advantage for upright, two-legged locomotion, but also for living in larger, more stably organized groups. Living in large groups provided better protection from the big predators of the savanna and assisted group members in scavenging on their kills in competition with other scavengers. It also facilitated organized hunting of large prey. But living in large groups also posed its own set of critical selection contingencies. It necessitated the recognition of, and memory for, a large number of individuals and skillful navigation in a multitude of social relationships. Those successful in this endeavor had to be "natural psychologists" in order to understand, predict, and make use of fellow human beings to their own advantage (Humphrey, 1983). In short, "mind reading" was an important asset. For reading the minds of others, the face is a rich source of information because facial gestures convey clues to intentions as well as to emotional and motivational states. In the context of social interaction, skills in decoding the social signals emitted by another person are amplified when combined with some degree of volitional control of one's own signals. As every poker player knows, an expressionless face coupled with astute recognition of emotion in others is a key to success. But a gambler also knows that recognizing and trusting "gut feelings" are important preludes to managing one's own expressive behavior. As noted above, gaining voluntary control of facial muscles benefited both language articulation and control of facial gestures. Thus versatile control of the face muscles was a central component of the social intelligence that many theorists postulate as the critical driving force behind the rapid expansion of human brain size during the last few hundred thousand years (e.g., Dunbar, 1996; Humphrey, 1983). Often dubbed "Machiavellian intelligence" because the essence of this control was taken to be the ability to exploit social skills and insights in pursuing the interest of one's own genes (Whiten & Byrne, 1997), the possibility of concealing instinctive expression behind voluntarily controllable ones was a handy tool from this perspective.

Production and decoding of facial gestures are likely to have been shaped by mutually dependent evolutionary forces. The ability to produce distinctive displays (e.g., conveying threat) is clearly advantageous from an evolutionary perspective, whether the display communicates an aggressive intention or merely serves as a cue for impending negative consequences (Owren, Rendell, & Bachorowski, Chapter 8). But individuals who more efficiently read their opponents' threatening stance also have advantages in the next step of the interaction. In short, "displays co-evolve with vigilance for them" (Fridlund, 1997, p. 105). Thus social signaling and the understanding of social signals coevolve in a process where the "sender's" signal (signal meaning and signal behavior) and the "receiver's" neural responses to the signal influence each other to form an integrated social signaling system for the members of a species (e.g., Endler, 1992; Krebs, & Davies, 1993; Fridlund, 1997; Enquist & Arak, 1998; for an alternative view, see Owren et al., Chapter 8). Accordingly, research on human facial expression indicates that facial expressions comprise both stereotypic signals and signaling behavior (the looks and use of facial expressions of anger, happiness, fear, disgust, sorrow, and surprise; see, e.g., Ekman, 2003; for a critical view, see Barrett, Chapter 11), as well as specialized neural structures for recognition of facial emotion and facial identity.

Specialized Neural Structures for Facial Information

If this evolutionary scenario is valid, then one would expect there to be specific neural circuits in the human brain for recognizing the identity of a face as well as the emotions expressed by the face. This expectancy appears to receive support from the data. Processing of faces—in particular, processing of facial identity—has been found to involve the fusiform gyrus in the inferior temporal lobe, an area subsequently called the fusiform face area (FFA; e.g., Kanwisher, McDermott, & Chun, 1997; Bruce & Young, 1996; Bruce, Green, & Georgeson, 1996; Adolphs, 2002). Recognition of dynamic facial attributes such as gaze direction and emotional expression, on the other hand, is believed to rely mainly on structures in the superior temporal sulcus (STS)[1] (Haxby, Hoffman, & Gobbini, 2000), which has been proposed to constitute a system for social cognition in concert with the amygdala and the orbitofrontal cortex (Allison, Puce, & McCarthy, 2000). The notion that faces are processed by specific neural structures has also been supported by several reports of lost ability to recognize faces following brain damage. Thus damage to the ventromedial regions of the occipitotemporal cortex (including the FFA) typically cause prosopagnosia, a loss of face recognition ability (e.g., Sergent & Signoret, 1992; see also Marotta, Genovese, & Behrmann, 2001). Some patients with prosopagnosia, however, show unimpaired recognition of facial expressions of emotion (Tranel, Damasio, & Damasio, 1988), which supports the notion that facial identity and expression are processed in different areas.

Psychophysiological Responses to Facial Stimuli

Facial Muscle Responses

An evolutionary origin of facial signals implies that humans should possess efficient routines for automatically responding to facial signals. This hypothesis has been examined extensively by Dimberg (1982; see reviews by Dimberg, 1990; Dimberg & Öhman, 1996), who used electromyography (EMG) to record responses of facial muscles to facial stimuli. In this way, subtle responses from well-defined facial muscles, not necessarily detectable by the naked eye, could be accurately quantified. By measuring EMG from the corrugator and the zygomatic major muscles, Dimberg (1982) assessed activity in key muscles for displays of anger and happiness, respectively. The corrugator pulls the eyebrows together to produce the deep furrow in the forehead that signals discontent, anger, or threat, and the zygomatic major pulls the corner of the mouth toward the ear to help produce the universally recognized smile. Dimberg (1982) reported that research participants exposed to an angry face showed increased activity in the corrugator and little change in the zygomatic, whereas a happy face induced the opposite pattern: increased zygomatic activity, with little change in the corrugator. Thus these data suggested that emotional faces induced their mirror images in observers. A happy face activated key muscles in a happy display, and an angry face activated key muscles in an angry display. Lundquist and Dimberg (1995) extended this conclusion to a broader set of emotions (anger, happiness, fear, sadness, disgust, and surprise) by recording EMG from a larger set of muscles.

The responses in the corrugator and the zygomatic muscles to facial stimuli are rapid, demonstrating differential responses to angry and happy faces within 400 milliseconds after stimulus onset, and reaching peaks of activity within the first second of stimulation (Dimberg & Thunberg, 1998). The rapid activation in these facial muscles is consistent with the hypothesis that facial muscles respond automatically and nonconsciously to facial stimuli. This hypothesis was directly tested by Dimberg, Elmehed, and Thunberg (2000) using a backward masking technique (see Esteves & Öhman, 1993). Different groups of participants were exposed to briefly (30 milliseconds) presented angry, neutral, and happy faces that were immediately followed by a much longer (5 seconds) presentation of a neutral masking stimulus. With this arrangement of the stimuli, the participants could consciously perceive only the second, masking stimulus; they could not see the preceding target stimulus. Nevertheless, participants exposed to masked happy faces showed larger zygomatic responses than those exposed to masked neutral and angry faces, and those exposed to masked angry faces showed larger corrugator responses than those exposed to masked neutral and happy faces. In other words, the participants' facial muscles appeared to know more about the stimulus than what the participants were able to perceive consciously. This is a theoretically significant conclusion that is consistent with the facial feedback hypothesis of emotion (e.g., Izard, 1977). Thus, through fast feedback circuits to the brain, the automatically activated facial muscles could add a context that influences the interpretation of a stimulus as emotionally relevant (e.g., James, 1884/1976).

Autonomic Responses

Further support for the notion of automatic decoding of facial signals comes from experiments focusing on the emotional effect of angry faces. Öhman and Dimberg (1978) used facial expressions as stimuli in a Pavlovian conditioning experiment with humans, with skin conductance responses (SCRs) as their dependent variable. Different groups of subjects were trained to differentiate between two happy, two neutral, and two angry faces by having one of them followed by a mild electric shock to the fingers. All three groups acquired differential SCRs to the shock-associated and non-shock-associated face, but only those conditioned to angry faces showed lasting resistance to extinction when the shock was omitted. This basic finding, which has been replicated in several laboratories (see review by Dimberg & Öhman, 1996), has been taken as support for the hypothesis that evolution has prepared humans to persistently associate fear to evolutionarily relevant threat stimuli (Seligman, 1970; Öhman & Dimberg, 1984; Öhman & Mineka, 2001).

The Pavlovian face-conditioning paradigm has been exploited to analyze the nonconscious activation of autonomic responses. After undergoing conditioning to angry or happy faces presented in full view, research participants presented with masked versions of such stimuli continued to show elevated responses to conditioned angry faces, even though there was no sign of conscious recognition of the emotional expression of the stimulus (Esteves, Dimberg, & Öhman, 1994; Parra, Esteves, Flykt, & Öhman, 1997). Furthermore, Esteves, Parra, et al. (1994) demonstrated that enhanced SCRs can be conditioned to masked angry, but not to masked happy, faces. Thus not only can responses be elicited by emotionally provocative facial stimuli (with or without previous conditioning), but new responses can also be associated to masked, nonconsciously presented stimuli. Applied to face-to-face situations of social encounters, these data suggest that barely perceivable facial gestures can result in nonconsicous

Pavlovian conditioning of fear responses to a sender who induces aversive emotional states in the receiver.

Brain Responses to Masked Facial Stimuli

There is an extensive literature suggesting that the amygdala, a collection of neural nuclei in the anterior medial temporal lobe, is sensitive to visual information as it pertains to social interaction; a primary source for such information, of course, is the face (see reviews by, e.g., Adolphs, 2002; Öhman, 2002). Morris, Öhman, and Dolan (1998) examined amygdala responses to nonconsciously and consciously presented facial stimuli. They used a Pavlovian face-conditioning paradigm to induce enhanced emotional responding to an angry face by pairing it with an aversive noise. These conditioning trials were presented among other trials involving either of two neutral faces or another angry face, with none of these faces followed by the noise stimulus. Participants were then placed in a positron emission tomography (PET) scanner to assess regional changes in cerebral blood flow to facial stimuli presented under different conditions of awareness. The participants were exposed to scans involving repeated pair-wise presentations of the facial stimuli in different sequences. In different scans, the conditioned angry face was masked by one of the neutral faces, and the nonconditioned angry face was masked by the other neutral face. Participants could only perceive the neutral faces consciously and remained unaware of the preceding angry face. In this way, changes in regional cerebral blood flow could be contrasted between conditions involving two masked angry faces, one of which had been given enhanced emotional impact through conditioning.

Morris et al. (1998) reported reliable and specific activation of the right amygdala to the masked conditioned angry face, thus demonstrating that conscious perception of the emotional nature of the stimulus was not necessary for activation of the amygdala. Following up on these data, Morris, Öhman, and Dolan (1999) tried to delineate the network of structures that occasioned nonconscious activation of the amygdala to masked, emotionally provocative stimuli. They examined covariations between blood flow changes in the amygdala and changes in other brain areas. Morris et al. (1999) reported that two structures, the superior colliculus of the midbrain and the right pulvinar of the thalamus, were statistically tied to nonconscious activation of the right amygdala.

These results were replicated on a patient with blindsight (see Weiskrantz, 1985), who had blind areas in the visual field because of damage to the primary visual cortex (Morris, de Gelder, Weiskrantz & Dolan, 2001). The amygdala was activated by nonperceived faces presented in the blind areas of the visual field, and connectivity analyses tied this effect to the superior colliculi and the pulvinar. The superior colliculus and the pulvinar are closely linked to attentional systems of the brain that control eye movements and the selection of salient visual objects (Posner & Peterson, 1990; Robinson & Peterson, 1992; see also LaBerge, 1998; Wright, & Ward, 1998). These "magnocellular" pathways are served by large, rapidly conducting neurons that mediate low-frequency information and provide a rough outline of a scene, whereas more detailed high-frequency information is conveyed by a separate "parvocellular" system served by smaller neurons that provide information about color and objects. Vuilleumier, Armony, Driver, and Dolan (2003) filtered visual information to separately activate these two systems in response to facial stimuli. They showed that only low-frequency information activated the amygdala, supporting the hypothesis that the effect was mediated by the pathways that pass through the superior colliculi. Thus the results of Morris et al. (1998, 1999, 2001) and Vuilleumier et al. (2003) are consistent with LeDoux's (1996, 2000) model of fear activation, which proposes that the amygdala can be nonconsciously accessed from subcortical sites to rapidly redirect attention and to set emotion in progress, even before the eliciting stimulus has been registered in consciousness.

Conclusion: Biology and the Nonconscious Recognition of Emotional Facial Stimuli

The research reviewed in this section shows that faces presented under conditions that prevent their representation in conscious awareness nevertheless evoked psychophysiological responses that reflect nonspecific emotional activation. Furthermore, the data suggest that the perceptual processing required for these effects have a subcortical origin, relying on a network that includes the superior colliculi, the pulvinar, and the amygdala (for a similar view, see de Gelder, Chapter 6, and Atkinson & Adolphs, Chapter 7). This system is an evolutionarily ancient one (e.g., Allman, 1999), and the perceptual analysis it can accomplish is necessarily crude. It is temporally prior to the cortical processing of facial features (inferior occipital gyrus) and full faces (involving the FFA, the superior temporal sulcus, and the inferior temporal cortex). Because of the rich efferent connections between the amygdala and cortical areas involved in visual processing in primates (Amaral, Price, Pitkänen, & Carmichael, 1992), the subcortical system could serve to tune subsequent cortical processing of the stimuli.

The observations suggesting that threatening and friendly faces are segregated for differential processing at an early, subcortical level of visual processing could be taken to imply that the system is tuned to critical features in these faces that decide whether they should be interpreted as threatening or friendly. Because the superior colliculus provides the most advanced visual information in the brains of reptiles and birds, evolutionary considerations, as well as the previously reviewed data, suggest that functionally significant information can be extracted at this nonconscious level of information processing. Furthermore, the remaining vision that is seen in blindsight patients may be accounted for by the processing of visual information in the superior colliculus and the pulvinar nucleus in the thalamus (de Gelder, Chapter 6; Weiskrantz, 1985). However, it is unlikely that faces are recognized as faces at this preliminary level. As a result, individual features should have a greater impact on producing differential nonconscious effects on emotional activation. Finally, the functional advantage of this organization, which is presumably tuned to invariant features signaling one or the other facial emotion, is that the system can respond very quickly, alarming the amygdala to tune areas that perform further analysis of the input.

FACIAL FEATURES AND THEIR ROLE IN ATTENTION AND RECOGNITION

Critical Features for Recognition of Facial Emotion

Aronoff and coworkers (Aronoff, Barclay, & Stevenson, 1988; Aronoff, Woike, & Hyman, 1992) argued that there are general geometric properties in visual displays that carry critical information to determine the emotional valence of faces. For example, Aronoff et al. (1988) demonstrated that diagonal lines were perceived as more negative than horizontal or vertical lines, as were lines with sharp angles rather than smoothly curved shapes, and oval shapes were perceived as more energetic than circular ones. They also demonstrated that ceremonial masks that were regarded as threatening and evil in different cultures contained a multitude of features that were perceived as negative when presented in isolation.

Inspired by the results reported by Aronoff et al. (1988), Lundqvist, Esteves, and Öhman (1999, 2004) constructed schematic faces that were used to systematically examine the role of eyebrows, eyes, and mouths in conveying threatening and friendly impressions of faces. Participants rated their emotional impression of each stimulus face by means of 11 semantic differential scales that were factor analytically grouped into dimensions of evaluation (here, negative evaluation), potency, and activity before being subjected to analyses of variance (ANOVAs).

Eyebrows emerged as the most important and influential facial feature for conveying threat. Whether presented in isolation, in basic configurations with only a mouth, or in complete facial configurations that included eyes and mouth, the shape of the eyebrows had a strong impact on emotional impression. ∨-shaped eyebrows conveyed a negative and threatening impression, whereas ∧-shaped brows provided a positive, friendly impression. Data also showed that eyebrows presented outside a facial context *can* convey an emotional impression independent of a facial context (Lundqvist et al., 2004; cf. Aronoff et al., 1988, 1992). However, the effect of individual features was smaller when the feature was presented in isolation, and the effect of a feature was subordinate to the effect of the configuration. Thus eyebrows had basically no effect when placed under a mouth instead of above it. The upright basic eyebrows–mouth configurations (in the absence of eyes) conveyed threat as effectively as complete faces and predicted the emotional impression of complete faces.

Even though all examined facial features affected emotional impression to some degree, the weight of their effects differed. Eyebrows had the most profound effect on emotional impression, followed in order by mouth and eyes. Figure 5.1 illustrates these findings using a two-dimensional emotional space defined by *negative evaluation and activity*. This space was subdivided into areas of threat and nonthreat by the shape of the eyebrows. These areas, in turn, were segregated into "scheming" and friendly areas on the basis of the mouth, and these areas were further subdivided by the shape of the eyes. In this way, faces with consistently threatening or friendly features were placed at opposite poles of the emotional space. These results are consistent with face-processing theories that postulate a sequential, hierarchical processing of facial features (Marr, 1982; Bruce & Young, 1986; Haxby et al., 2000). Even though isolated features (especially ∨-shaped eyebrows and ∪-shaped mouth) have some ability to convey emotional impressions outside a facial context, the placement of features in a configuration with other features in a face-like structure is decisive both for the quality and strength of the emotional impression of the face. Conversely, placing features in a configuration deviating from normal faces (e.g., mouth above eyebrows) blocks the effect of the individual features.

The central role of ∨-shaped eyebrows in threatening faces and a ∪-shaped mouth in happy faces is further supported by data from image analyses of neutral, happy, and angry faces (Lundqvist, & Litton, 2004). Using the averaged Karolinska directed emotional faces (AKDEF; Lundqvist, & Litton, 1998) to analyze differences between emotional and neutral faces, the largest difference was found in the eyebrows/eyes area for angry faces, and in the mouth area for happy faces. Consistent with these image analyses, eye-tracking data from participants who freely viewed schematic threatening and friendly faces (unpublished data) showed that fixations were mainly directed to eyebrows and eyes for threatening faces, and to the mouth area for happy faces (see Figure 5.2).

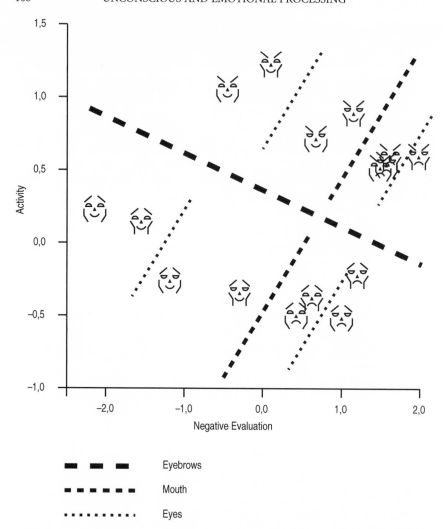

FIGURE 5.1. The two-dimensional plot over *activity* and *negative evaluation* for the ratings of schematic facial stimuli shows how the stimuli form a hierarchy of clusters around different facial features. First, faces are subdivided according to the different shapes of eyebrows. Second, faces form subclusters around the different shapes of mouth. Finally, within these subclusters, there are formations of faces around the different shapes of eyes.

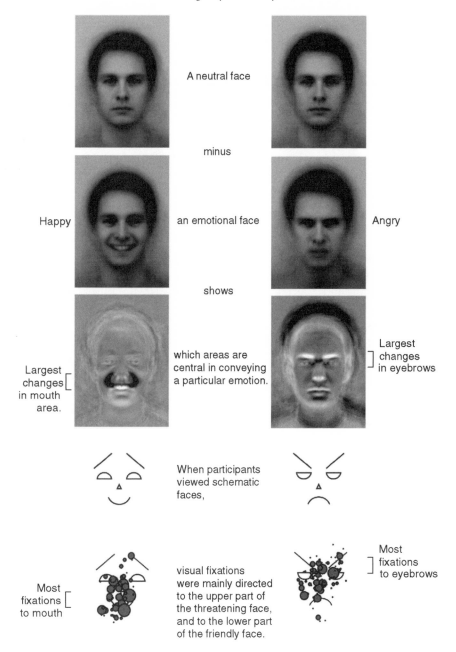

FIGURE 5.2. Image analysis of pictorial facial stimuli highlights the importance of eyebrows for threatening faces and the importance of mouth for friendly faces. Eye-tracking data show that visual attention is drawn to the eyebrow area on threatening faces, and to the mouth area on friendly faces.

Searching for Threat among Schematic Faces

Because threatening animal stimuli have been demonstrated to recruit attention very effectively in visual search tasks (Öhman, Flykt, & Esteves, 2001), visual search paradigms are good candidates for documenting behavioral effects of threat as conveyed by schematic faces. The first experiment used perceptually well-controlled schematic faces, based on the results reported by Lundqvist et al. (1999, 2004) to replicate a visual search experiment with real faces reported by Hansen and Hansen (1988; Öhman, Lundqvist, & Esteves, 2001). If a threat advantage could be demonstrated with these stimuli, the next aim would be to determine if the critical facial features for threat delineated in the rating studies (Lundqvist et al., 1999, 2004) also would be effective in recruiting attention (Lundqvist & Öhman, 2005). Thus Öhman, Lundqvist, et al. (2001) used schematic threatening, friendly, and neutral faces to test the hypothesis that humans preferentially orient their attention toward threat. The design of threatening and friendly faces incorporated the most threatening and the friendliest versions of the facial features (eyebrows, mouth, and eyes) into threatening and friendly faces, respectively, that were presented as targets among neutral or emotional (e.g., friendly faces for threatening targets) distractor faces (see Figure 5.3).

Across a number of experiments, threatening faces were detected reliably faster and more accurately than friendly faces, irrespective of whether the target faces were presented among neutral or emotional faces. However, when all faces in a matrix were identical, the time and accuracy to decide that a target stimulus was not present did not differ between matrices of threatening and friendly faces. The detection difference between threatening and friendly target faces was reliable across crowd sizes ranging from 4 to 25 faces (Öhman, Lundqvist, et al., 2001). Also, measurement of eye movements (Lundqvist & Öhman, 2004) showed that the eyes moved more directly, with shorter scan path and fewer fixations, toward a threatening than toward a friendly target among neutral distractors—which suggests that the former recruited attention more efficiently than the latter. Threatening angry faces were also detected faster and more accurately than other negative (scheming or sad) faces (Öhman, Lundqvist, et al., 2001), suggesting that the threat advantage can be attributed to the emotional impression of the face rather than to the differences in negative valence, uncommonness, or novelty among the different faces (cf. Whalen, 1998). The results show that, despite the basic physical–geometrical equality of schematic threatening and friendly faces, these facial stimuli affect attention differently. Whereas both types of faces were searched with equal efficiency in displays without a target, threatening faces guided attention faster and more accurately than friendly faces when they were presented as targets.

Typical pattern of results in the visual search experiments.

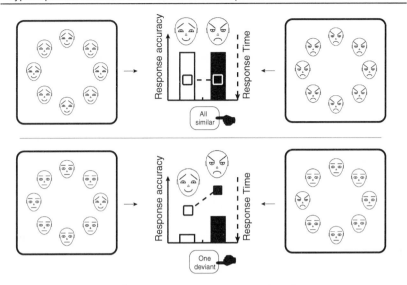

Results, Experiment 2, Öhman, Lundqvist, & Esteves (2001).

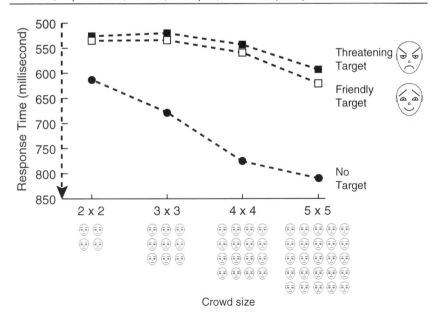

FIGURE 5.3. Visual search data reveal superior detection of a threatening target face, but equally efficient search of threatening and friendly crowds that are presented without any target.

The Relation between Facial Emotion and Visual Attention

Lundqvist and Öhman (2005) used visual search tasks to examine which emotional facial features and configurations were necessary and sufficient to produce the observed advantage in target detection. Participants were exposed to visual search tasks in which target faces had one, two, or three features (eyebrows, eyes, mouth) that provided differential emotional information (threatening, friendly) in relation to neutral background faces. After the visual search task, participants were asked to rate the stimuli as a way to examine the relationship between the emotional impression of a face and the visual search performance.

Somewhat surprisingly (particularly from the perspective of the rating data reported by Lundqvist et al., 2004), the results showed that emotional eyebrows alone (with neutral eyes and mouth) did not produce a consistent threat advantage with neutral distractors, but that the mouth alone (with neutral eyebrows and eyes) did (Lundqvist & Öhman, 2005, Experiments 3 and 4). However, for conditions in which the eyebrows varied (i.e., carried emotional information), the overall detection times were considerably shorter and the hit rate was close to ceiling, suggesting that eyebrows had processing priority. Perhaps because of floor (detection latency) and ceiling (hit rate) effects, the efficient performance when eyebrows varied tended to give smaller threat advantages. If a threatening target face could be discriminated from the distractors via eyebrows, it was detected very efficiently with short response latencies (mean 660 milliseconds for all conditions involving changes in eyebrows) and high hit rates (98%). When the mouth was used to discriminate between target and distractor faces, targets were detected less efficiently with intermediate detection latencies (803 milliseconds) and hit rates (91%). Finally, if the discrimination could be made only via the shape of the eyes, the detection of targets was comparatively inefficient, with slow detection latencies (839 milliseconds) and relatively low hit rates (86%).

Finally, a correlation analysis revealed a close relationship between emotion and attention measures. First, there were strong inverse relationships between detection latency and ratings of negative evaluation, activity, and potency for threatening, but not for friendly, facial configurations (Lundqvist & Öhman, 2005). Second, the attentional threat advantage (i.e., the difference in detection latency between threatening and friendly faces in a given stimulus pair) correlated closely with the contrast between these faces in emotion measures (see Figure 5.4). Thus a large difference in emotion scores for a contrasted pair of threatening and friendly faces was associated with a large difference between these faces in attention measures.

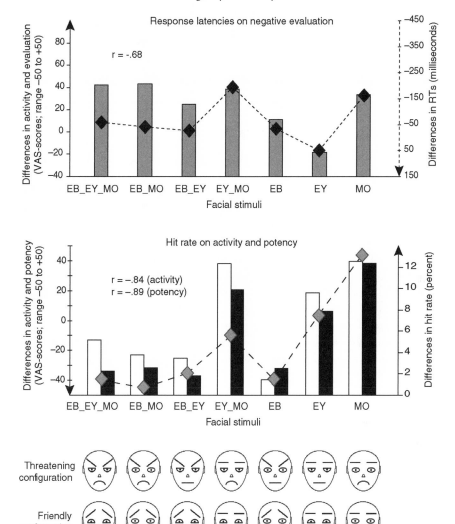

FIGURE 5.4. Differences between threatening and friendly faces on attention measures follow the differences in the same faces on emotion measures. The code under each set of stimuli signifies which feature(s) conveyed the facial emotion: EB, eyebrows; EY, eyes; MO, mouth. RTs, response latencies.

Taken together, the results from these experiments are consistent with the notion of a feature hierarchy that was initially observed in the rating studies. Furthermore, the results revealed a very close relation between emotion and attention measures, indicating that a threat advantage effect is closely linked to the emotional contrast between the compared stimuli.

The Role of Facial Features for Search of Faces

The apparent hierarchical relationship between eyebrows, mouth, and eyes may reflect the structural description (or feature detectors) underlying the recognition of facial emotion. In this case, the rank order effects of different features might be a consequence of the order with which features are matched to the specific structural description of a threatening/angry or friendly/happy face. Such an account would make a feature hierarchy an intrinsic part of the face-processing system. Alternatively, facial features might be differentially weighted according to how useful they are for discriminating emotions. Such a notion would locate the hierarchical feature effect in the stimulus itself. This notion was supported by the image analysis of pictorial emotional stimuli, which showed that the main change of information between a neutral and threatening face was found in the eyebrow region, and between a neutral and a friendly face in the mouth region (Figure 5.3). The priority of threatening faces would then result from the fact that a threatening face is more urgent to deal with than a friendly one.

The magnitude of the perceptual difference between an emotionally shaped feature (eyebrows, eyes, mouth) and the neutral control shape could be due to a nonemotional factor. However, even though target–distractor discriminability determines how faces are searched and discriminated (cf. Duncan & Humphrey, 1989), the close relation between attention and emotion suggests that the superior effect of threatening faces on attention is linked to the emotional rather than the perceptual properties of the facial stimuli.

Facial Emotion and Visual Attention: A Neural Model

The visual search data (Lundqvist & Öhman, 2005; Öhman, Lundqvist, et al., 2001) documented a strong association between emotional impression (e.g., high scores on negative evaluation) and efficient detection (short detection latencies and high hit rates). Moreover, the data indicated that the superior detection of threatening faces was closely related to the emotional contrast between the threatening and friendly configurations (Figure 5.4). These data indicate that the emotional impression of a facial stimulus regulates how that face affects attention. Such effects of emotion on visual attention imply that the facial emotion of the schematic stimuli was recognized preattentively (for a similar view see de Gelder, Chapter 6; Atkinson & Adolphs, Chapter 7), and that the recognized emotional properties of a particular face determined how attention was directed to that face.

The emotion literature contains related evidence showing clear relationships between the emotional significance of a stimulus and different psychophysiological response systems. Lang, Bradley, and Cuthbert (1997) showed that negative evaluation and activity reflect central motivational systems and signify a fundamental dimensionality that underlies human emotion. Their data showed strong positive relations between negative evaluation and EMG responses in the corrugator supercilii (the facial muscle mediating the eyebrow frown) and between negative evaluation and the magnitude of the startle reflex (measured by eye-blink responses to loud noises). Their data also revealed strong positive relations between activity (arousal) and skin conductance responses (Lang et al., 1997).

From this psychophysiological perspective, the more efficient attention to threatening compared to friendly configurations in our data (Lundqvist & Öhman, 2005; Öhman, Lundqvist, et al., 2001) may be interpreted as reflecting a similar modulation of neural activity as that shown by the data of Lang et al. (1997). In theory, the neural representation of each facial configuration would thus be nonconsciously modulated according to that face's emotional properties. Hence, a face conveying a threatening impression (e.g., high negative evaluation) would be modulated for enhanced processing and thereby stand out more from the background and be easier to detect. Conversely, a friendly configuration (e.g., low negative evaluation) would be modulated to a lower, possibly even inhibited, level and thus stand out comparatively less from background information.

Figure 5.5 illustrates how the neural representations of threatening and friendly faces may be modulated according to their emotional significance. The figure describes data from the visual search studies (Lundqvist & Öhman, 2005; Öhman, Lundqvist, et al., 2001) and is based on models of visual perception (e.g., Marr, 1982; Gegenfurtner & Sharpe, 1999), face processing (Bruce & Young, 1986; Haxby et al., 2000), and visual attention (Wright & Ward, 1998; LaBerge, 1998, 2002). According to the models of Bruce and Young (1986) and Haxby et al. (2000), face processing works sequentially, with increasing complexity over serial, modular levels. First, a basic component analysis of facial information is performed, the outcome of which is used for any subsequent specialized facial processes, such as identity and expression recognition. This core system then involves other neural structures, depending on task demands. Haxby et al. (2000) suggest that the basic, multipurpose extraction of facial information is carried out in the inferior occipital gyrus. The subsequent handling of facial emotional con-

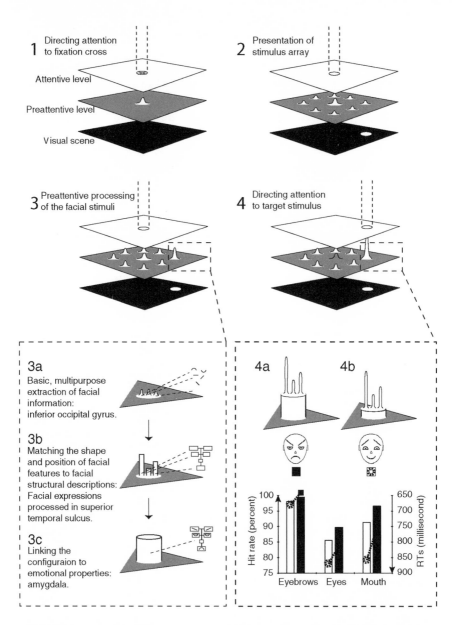

FIGURE 5.5. A model of how emotion modulates attention. The model illustrates how attention initially is directed to the pretrial fixation cross (1). When an array of faces is presented (2), the faces are processed sequentially (3). After a basic, multipurpose extraction of facial features and properties (3a), the shape and position of facial features is matched to facial structural descriptions (3b), the outcome of which links the configuration to its emotional properties (3c). Emotion modulates the neural firing rates, representing threatening and friendly configurations differently (4), resulting in quicker and more accurate detection of threatening configurations (4a) compared to friendly ones (4b).

figurations is performed in the superior temporal sulcus. Finally, connections between the superior temporal sulcus and the limbic system, foremost the amygdala, then link emotional properties to the facial configuration. However, the concept of a "low" subcortical route to the amygdala (LeDoux, 1996), the evidence for which was discussed earlier in this chapter (pp. 104–105), proposes that the amygdala is accessed even before, and can modulate initial processing in the visual cortex (this route is not illustrated in Figure 5.5).

The involvement of the amygdala in recognizing emotion in facial stimuli, such as the schematic faces used here, is also supported by an fMRI experiment by Wright, Martis, Shin, Fischer, and Rauch (2002). They exposed participants to blocks of threatening, friendly, and neutral schematic faces and reported a significant increase in the activation of the left amygdala for both threatening and friendly faces, compared to a neutral face. There was also a significant difference in activation in the left occipitotemporal cortex (OTC) for threatening and friendly faces. These data imply that the speculated activity modulation of threatening and friendly faces takes place in the inferior occipital cortex (IOC) in the OTC. The fact that the significant difference in activity is found in the OTC (Wright et al., 2002) does not necessarily mean that the difference in neural activity is caused by that area, only that it is expressed there.

CONCLUDING COMMENTS

Evolution has equipped humans with an expressive face that is useful for producing a versatile repertoire of social signals. The development of this repertoire is predicated on the ability of conspecifics to quickly recognize and react appropriately to each signal.

The data reviewed in this chapter argue quite persuasively that humans possess a highly efficient system for recognition of emotional faces. This system allows humans to recognize and react to facial stimuli without conscious experience of the stimuli and prior to a conscious awareness of the stimuli. In the first section of the chapter (A Biological Perspective on the Human Face), we reviewed data that illustrate how emotional facial stimuli can be decoded and responded to even during experimental conditions that bypass conscious awareness, because conscious recognition is blocked by backward masking. In the second section of the chapter (Facial Features and Their Role in Attention and Recognition), we reviewed data that suggest that the direction of visual attention to emotional facial stimuli is regulated by a preconscious recognition of the emotional properties of the faces.

These behavioral results can be accommodated by recent neural models of perception and attention, in which the amygdala is added as a central structure for emotional evaluations. The argument presented in this chapter provides a psychobiological starting point for understanding the processing of emotional information in the face. The existing data are largely limited to facial signals of threat. There are also some interesting results suggesting that happy faces can have nonconscious effects on motivation (Berridge & Winkielman, 2003; also see Winkielman, Berridge, & Wilbarger, Chapter 14), and that the recognition of happy faces is facilitated by a positive and impeded by a negative context, as provided by olfactory stimulation (Leppänen & Hietanen, 2003).

ACKNOWLEDGMENTS

This chapter is based on a doctoral dissertation (Lundqvist, 2003) presented to the Karolinska Institute by Daniel Lundqvist under supervision by Arne Öhman. The research was supported by grants from the Bank of Sweden Tercentennial Foundation to Arne Öhman.

NOTE

1. The differential involvement of the inferior temporal lobe and the STS in the processing of identity and expressions has also been demonstrated for the macaque monkey (see, e.g., Hasselmo, Rolls, & Baylis, 1989).

REFERENCES

Adolphs, R. (2002). Recognizing emotion from facial expressions: Psychological and neurological mechanisms. *Behavioural and Cognitive Neuroscience Reviews, 1,* 21–62.

Alexander, R. D. (1974). The evolution of social systems. *Annual Review of Ecology and Systematics, 5,* 325–383.

Allison, T., Puce, A., & McCarthy, G. (2000). Social perception from visual cues: Role of the STS region. *Trends in Cognitive Science, 4,* 267–278.

Allman, J. M. (1999). *Evolving brains.* New York: Scientific American Library.

Amaral, D. G., Price, J. L., Pitkänen, A., & Carmichael, T. S. (1992). Anatomical organization of the primate amygdaloid complex. In J. P. Aggleton (Ed.), *The amygdala: Neurobiological aspects of emotion, memory, and mental dysfunction* (pp. 1–66). New York: Wiley-Liss.

Aronoff, J., Barclay, A. M., & Stevenson, L. A. (1988). The recognition of threatening facial stimuli. *Journal of Personality and Social Psychology, 54,* 647–655.

Aronoff, J., Woike, B. A., & Hyman, L. M. (1992). Which are the stimuli in facial displays of anger and happiness? Configurational bases of emotion recognition. *Journal of Personality and Social Psychology, 62*, 1050–1066.

Berridge, K. C., & Winkielman, P. (2003). What is an unconscious emotion?: The case for unconscious "liking." *Cognition and Emotion, 17*, 181–212.

Bruce, V., Green, P. R., & Georgeson, M. A. (1996). *Visual perception: Physiology, psychology, and ecology* (3rd ed.). Hove, East Sussex, UK: Psychology Press.

Bruce, V., & Young, A. W. (1986). Understanding face recognition. *British Journal of Psychology, 77*, 305–327.

Bruce, V., & Young, A. W. (1996). *In the eye of the beholder: The science of face perception.* New York: Oxford University Press.

Chevalier-Skolnikoff, S. (1973). Facial expression of emotion in nonhuman primates. In P. Ekman (Ed.), *Darwin and facial expression: A century of research in review* (pp. 11–83). New York: Academic Press.

Cole, J. (1998). *About face.* Cambridge, MA: MIT Press.

Darwin, C. (1998). *The expression of emotions in man and animal.* New York: Oxford University Press. (Original work published 1872)

Dimberg, U. (1982). Facial reactions to facial expressions. *Psychophysiology, 19*, 643–647.

Dimberg, U. (1990). Facial electromyography and emotional reactions. *Psychophysiology, 27*, 481–494.

Dimberg, U., Elmehed, K., & Thunberg, M. (2000). Facial reactions to masked stimuli: Unconsciously evoked emotional responses. *Psychological Science, 11*, 86–89.

Dimberg, U., & Öhman, A. (1996). Behold the wrath: Psychophysiological responses to facial stimuli. *Motivation and Emotion, 20*, 149–182.

Dimberg, U., & Thunberg, M. (1998). Rapid facial reactions to different emotionally relevant stimuli. *Scandinavian Journal of Psychology, 39*, 39–45.

Duncan, J., & Humphreys, G. W. (1989). Visual search and stimulus similarity. *Psychological Review, 96*, 433–458.

Dunbar, R. I. M. (1996). *Grooming, gossip, and the evolution of language.* London: Faber & Faber.

Eibl-Eibesfeldt, I. (1970). *Ethology: The biology of behavior.* New York: Holt, Rinehart & Winston.

Ekman, P. (2003). *Emotions revealed: Recognizing faces and feelings to improve communication and emotional life.* New York: Times Books.

Endler, J. A. (1992). Signals, signal conditions and the direction of evolution. *American Naturalist, 139*(Suppl.), 125–153.

Enquist, M., & Arak, A. (1998). Neural representation and the evolution of signal form. In R. Dukas (Ed.), *Cognitive ecology: The evolutionary ecology of information processing and decision making* (pp. 21–87). Chicago: University of Chicago Press.

Esteves, F., & Öhman, A. (1993). Masking the face: Recognition of emotional facial expressions as a function of the parameters of backward masking. *Scandinavian Journal of Psychology, 34*, 1–18.

Esteves, F., Dimberg, U., & Öhman, A. (1994). Automatically elicited fear: Conditioned skin conductance responses to masked facial expressions. *Cognition and Emotion, 8,* 393–413.

Esteves, F., Parra, C., Dimberg, U., & Öhman, A. (1994). Nonconscious associative learning: Pavlovian conditioning of skin conductance responses to masked fear-relevant stimuli. *Psychophysiology, 31,* 375–385.

Fridlund, A. J. (1994). *Human facial expressions: An evolutionary view.* New York: Academic Press.

Fridlund, A. J. (1997). The new ethology of human facial expression. In J. A. Russell & J. M. Fernández-Dols (Eds.), *The psychology of facial expression* (pp. 103–129). Cambridge, UK: Cambridge University Press.

Gazzaniga, M. S., & Smylie, C.S. (1990). Hemispheric mechanisms controlling voluntary and spontaneous facial expressions. *Journal of Cognitive Neuroscience, 2,* 239–245.

Gegenfurtner, K. R., & Sharpe, L. T. (1999). *Color vision: From genes to perception.* New York: Cambridge University Press.

Hansen, C., & Hansen, R. (1988). Finding the face in the crowd: An anger superiority effect. *Journal of Personality and Social Psychology, 54,* 917–924.

Hasselmo, M. E., Rolls, E. T., & Baylis, G. C. (1989). The role of expression and identity in the face selective responses of neurons in the temporal visual cortex of the monkey. *Behavioural Brain Research, 32,* 203–218.

Haxby, J. V., Hoffman, E. A., & Gobbini, M. I. (2000). The distributed human neural system for face perception. *Trends in Cognitive Sciences, 4,* 223–233.

Humphrey, N. (1983). *Consciousness regained.* Oxford, UK: Oxford University Press.

Izard, C. (1977). *Human emotions.* New York: Plenum Press.

James, W. (1884). What is an emotion? *Mind, 9,* 188–205.

Kanwisher, N., McDermott, J., & Chun, M. M. (1997). The fusiform face area: A module in human extrastriate cortex specialized for face perception. *The Journal of Neouroscience, 17,* 4302–4311.

Krebs, J. R., & Davies, N. B. (1993). *An introduction to behavioral ecology* (3rd ed.). Oxford, UK: Blackwell.

LaBerge, D. (1998). Attentional emphasis in visual orienting and resolving. In R. D. Wright (Ed.), *Visual attention* (pp. 417–454). New York: Oxford University Press.

LaBerge, D. (2002). Attentional control: Brief and prolonged. *Psychological Research, 66,* 220–233.

Lang, P., Bradley, M., & Cuthbert, M. (1997). Motivated attention: Affect, activation and action. In P. Lang, R. Simons, & M. Balaban (Eds.), *Attention and orienting: Sensory and motivational processes* (pp. 97–136). Hillsdale, NJ: Erlbaum.

LeDoux, J. E. (1996). *The emotional brain.* New York: Simon & Schuster.

LeDoux, J. E. (2000). Emotion circuits in the brain. *Annual Review of Neuroscience, 23,* 155–184.

Leppänen, J.M., & Hietanen, J. K. (2003). Affect and face perception: Odors modulate the recognition advantage of happy faces. *Emotion, 3,* 315–326.

Lundquist, L.-O., & Dimberg, U. (1995). Facial expressions are contagious. *Journal of Psychophysiology, 9*, 203–211.

Lundqvist, D. (2003). *The face of wrath: How facial emotion captures visual attention.* Stockholm: Karolinska University Press.

Lundqvist, D., Esteves, F., & Öhman, A. (1999). The face of wrath: Critical features for conveying facial threat. *Cognition and Emotion, 13*, 691–711.

Lundqvist, D., Esteves, F., & Öhman, A. (2004). The face of wrath: The role of features and configurations in conveying social threat. *Cognition and Emotion, 18*, 161–182.

Lundqvist, D., & Litton, J. E. (1998). *The averaged Karolinska directed emotional faces—AKDEF.* CD ROM from Department of Clinical Neuroscience, psychology section, Karolinska Institutet, ISBN 91–630–7164–9.

Lundqvist, D., & Litton, J. E. (2004). *The essence of human facial emotions: Image analysis of information changes between neutral and emotional faces.* Manuscript in preparation.

Lundqvist, D., & Öhman, A. (2004). *Eye movements during visual search for emotional faces.* Manuscript in preparation.

Lundqvist, D., & Öhman, A. (2005). Emotion regulates attention: Relation between facial configurations, facial emotion and visual attention. *Visual Cognition, 12*, 51–84.

Marotta, J. J., Genovese, C. R., & Behrmann, M. (2001). A functional MRI study of face recognition in patients with prosopagnosia. *Cognitive Neuroscience, 12*, 1–7.

Marr, D. (1982). *Vision: A computational investigation into the human representation and processing of visual information.* San Francisco: Freeman.

Morris, J. S., de Gelder, B., Weiskrantz, L., & Dolan, R. J. (2001). Differential extrageniculostriate and amygdala responses to presentation of emotional faces in a cortically blind field. *Brain, 124*, 1241–1252.

Morris, J. S., Öhman, A., & Dolan, R. J. (1998). Conscious and unconscious emotional learning in the human amygdala. *Nature, 393*, 467–470.

Morris, J. S., Öhman, A., & Dolan, R. J. (1999). A subcortical pathway to the right amygdala mediating "unseen" fear. *Proceedings of the National Academy of Sciences, 96*, 1680–1685.

Öhman, A. (2002). Automaticity and the amygdala: Nonconscious responses to emotional faces. *Current Directions in Psychological Science, 11*, 62–66.

Öhman, A., & Dimberg, U. (1978). Facial expressions as conditioned stimuli for electrodermal responses: A case of "preparedness"? *Journal of Personality and Social Psychology, 36*, 1251–1258.

Öhman, A., & Dimberg, U. (1984). An evolutionary perspective on human social behavior. In W. M. Waid (Ed.), *Sociophysiology* (pp. 47–86). New York: Springer-Verlag.

Öhman, A., Flykt, A., & Esteves, F. (2001). Emotion drives attention: Detecting the snake in the grass. *Journal of Experimental Psychology: General, 130*, 466–478.

Öhman, A., Lundqvist, D., & Esteves, F. (2001). The face in the crowd revisited: A threat advantage with schematic stimuli. *Journal of Personality and Social Psychology, 80*, 381–396.

Öhman, A., & Mineka, S. (2001). Fears, phobias, and preparedness: Toward an evolved module of fear and fear learning. *Psychological Review, 108,* 483–522.

Parra, C., Esteves, F., Flykt, A., & Öhman, A. (1997). Pavlovian conditioning to social stimuli: Backward masking and the dissociation of implicit and explicit cognitive processes. *European Psychologist, 2,* 106–117.

Posner, M. I., & Peterson, S. E. (1990). The attention system of the human brain. *Annual Review of Neuroscience, 13,* 25–42.

Robinson, D. L., & Peterson, S. E. (1992). The pulvinar and visual salience. *Trends in Neuroscience, 15,* 127–132.

Russell, J. A. (1994). Is there universal recognition of emotion from facial expression? *Psychological Bulletin, 115,* 102–141.

Seligman, M. E. P. (1970). On the generality of the laws of learning. *Psychological Review, 77,* 406–418.

Sergent, J., & Signoret, J. L. (1992). Functional and anatomical decomposition of face processing: Evidence from prosopagnosia and PET study of normal subjects. *Philosophical Transactions of the Royal Society of London, B, 335,* 55–62.

Tranel, D., Damasio, A. R., & Damasio, H. (1988). Intact recognition of facial expression, gender and age in patients with impaired recognition of face identity. *Neurology, 38,* 690–696.

Trivers, R. (1985). *Social evolution.* Menlo Park, CA: Benjamin/Cummings.

van Hooff, J. A. R. A. M. (1972). A comparative approach to the phylogeny of laughter and smiling. In R. A. Hinde (Ed.), *Non-verbal communication* (pp. 209–243). Cambridge, UK: Cambridge University Press.

Vuilleumier, P., Armony, J. L., Driver, J., & Dolan, R. J. (2003). Distinct spatial frequency sensitivities for processing faces and emotional expressions. *Nature Neuroscience, 6,* 624–631.

Weiskrantz, L. (1985). *Blindsight: A case study and implications.* Oxford, UK: Oxford University Press.

Whalen, P. J. (1998). Fear, vigilance and ambiguity: Initial neuroimaging studies of the human amygdala. *Current Directions in Psychological Science, 7,* 177–188.

Whiten, A., & Byrne, R. W. (Eds.). (1997). *Machiavellian intelligence II: Extensions and evaluations.* Cambridge, UK: Cambridge University Press.

Wilson, E. O. (1976). *Sociobiology: The new synthesis.* Cambridge, MA: Harvard University Press.

Wright, C. H., Martis, B., Shin, L. M., Fischer, H., & Rauch, S. L. (2002). Enhanced amygdala responses to emotional versus neutral schematic facial expressions. *Neuroreport, 13,* 785–790.

Wright, R. D., & Ward, L. M. (1998). The control of visual attention. In R. D. Wright (Ed.), *Visual attention* (pp. 132–186). New York: Oxford University Press.

CHAPTER 6

Nonconscious Emotions

New Findings and Perspectives on Nonconscious Facial Expression Recognition and Its Voice and Whole-Body Contexts

BEATRICE DE GELDER

In the early days of scientific psychology, the notion of unconscious information processing was much debated and controversial. The idea that our thoughts result from deliberations we are not aware of is no longer provocative. But emotional information processing may still occupy a special niche in this changed and broadened intellectual landscape. The notion that our brain processes crucial *emotional* information outside of awareness seems to present a challenge for traditional Western notions of autonomy, the self, and free will. Not only are emotions even more personal and related to first-person authority than are cognitions, but emotion also has a special link with adaptive behavior and action. As a consequence, the very idea of unconscious emotional information leading straight to action may be a cause for concern.

The last decade has seen significant progress in the scientific understanding of how emotional information is processed. By far, most research has focused on the recognition of facial expressions. There is now a growing consensus that facial expressions of emotion can be processed outside awareness. There is also increasing insight into the neural underpinnings of conscious and nonconscious recognition of facial expressions. Functional neuroimaging studies in both healthy subjects and brain-damaged patients

1. *What is the scope of your proposed model? When you use the term* emotion, *how do you use it? What do you mean by terms such as* fear, anxiety, *or* happiness?

All the research reported and discussed in the chapter deals with perceptual processes, whether conscious or unconscious.

2. *Define your terms:* conscious, unconscious, awareness. *Or say why you do not use these terms.*

In distinguishing conscious and nonconscious emotions, we usually adopt a methodological criterion that defines what counts as purely perceptual process. This distinction between conscious and nonconscious is not important. Whether or not the observer is aware of the stimulus does not matter for the stage of processing in which we are interested. The obvious exception is, of course, affective blindsight. But this phenomenon is important because it has the power to reveal alternative processing routes.

3. *Does your model deal with what is conscious, what is unconscious, or their relationship? If you do not address this area specifically, can you speculate on the relationship between what is conscious and unconscious? Or if you do not like the conscious–unconscious distinction, or if you do not think this is a good question to ask, can you say why?*

From the methodological perspective just described, this distinction is not critical. What counts is whether or not a perceptual process leads automatically and in a mandatory way to a representation. Subsequent perceptual elaboration often depends on consciousness, but our research is not about those later postperceptual cognitive processes.

converge to indicate that amygdala and orbitofrontal areas are activated by emotional faces, independently of voluntary attention and even without any awareness of the stimuli presented (Adolphs, 2002b; Breiter et al., 1996; Morris et al., 1996). Presumably, this primitive emotion system operates independently of awareness and higher cognition; indeed, it is often referred to as the fast and automatic emotional processing route. The amygdala plays a central role in this basic emotional system. In addition to receiving input from various sensory systems, the amygdala may directly modulate the fusiform cortex to enhance the processing of salient face stimuli. A more controversial and challenging idea is that amygdala responses to emotional stimuli could be driven by subcortical inputs that are independent of preliminary analysis in the striate cortex and more anterior visual areas (Morris, Friston, et al., 1998; de Gelder, 1999). This "low" route (as it is sometimes called) conveys rather crude information based on a coarse parsing of a face stimulus; this crude information, in itself, is sufficient to trigger an emotional response. If conscious and unconscious processes have their own neural networks (LeDoux, 1992, 2000; see Edelman & Tononi, 2000, for a review), then it is theoretically possible that both routes interact and that conflicts can arise between conscious and unconscious processes. Such conflicts, in turn, can be seen against the background of the larger question regarding the role nonconscious emotional processes play in daily life.

The first part of this chapter reviews recent research on nonconscious recognition of facial expressions and discusses the most far-reaching conception of nonconscious emotion perception and its neural underpinnings. The second half is devoted to research that moves beyond the face and concentrates on two contexts in which faces routinely appear in everyday life: the voice (expressions of emotion in the tone of voice) and the whole body (bodily expressions of emotion). This extended perspective draws attention to synergies between different emotional subsystems, with one subsystem specific for fear. It moves scientists away from a picture of nonconscious emotion as dominated solely by vision toward a more embodied notion of emotion processing and cognition, which could be integrated with the research on emotional experience, not discussed here. In this sense, my final conclusions about the importance of action and simulation in emotion processing are consistent with those suggested by several contributors to this volume (e.g., Niedenthal, Barsalou, Ric, & Krauth-Gruber, Chapter 2; Barrett, Chapter 11; Prinz, Chapter 15).

Within the limits of the chapter we cannot address fundamental questions on the nature of emotion and consciousness. When relevant, specific implications of the research for the big issues of emotion and consciousness will be noted. Instead, I will build a case for the hypothesis that emotional information, like any other kind of information that impinges on the sensory systems, is processed at the perceptual level in an automatic and mandatory way. In this chapter I do not use the term *emotion* to refer to a specific type of response, such as a behavior or a coordinated packet of behaviors, feeling, facial movements, physiology, etc., as in traditional definitions of emotion (de Gelder & Bertelson, 2003; see also Barrett, Chapter 11). Instead, the research discussed mainly focuses on automatic perceptual processing of emotional signals. Within this perspective of the research on perception of emotional signals presented here, there is no compelling reason for making a distinction between absence of consciousness and absence of awareness. I therefore use these two notions interchangeably.

NONCONSCIOUS RECOGNITION
OF FACIAL EXPRESSIONS

Facial expressions are, by far, the most prominent emotional objects studied in the emotion literature. This state of affairs is related as much to the widespread use of the stimulus set provided by Ekman and Friesen as it is to the prominence of facial expressions in social communication. Among the facial expressions that have been studied thus far, researchers have targeted fear. During the past decade there has been an avalanche of neurobiological studies linking the amygdala to the processing of facial expressions of fear (see Zald, 2003). To date, the link between the amygdala and fearful faces has guided the cognitive neuroscience agenda for conducting research on emotion. A number of studies has tackled the question of the role of the amygdala in nonconscious recognition of fearful facial expressions, following the first reports (Breiter et al., 1996; Morris et al., 1996).

Over the last decade, two different sets of results have converged on the notion that emotional information, in general (and fear expressions, in particular) may be processed without awareness (see also Lundqvist & Öhman, Chapter 5; Atkinson & Adolphs, Chapter 7). One set belongs to the tradition of defining the conscious versus nonconscious distinction in terms of attention. The other set of results examines noncortically based visual abilities. For the sake of clarity, I refer to these two different meanings of nonconscious emotions and the underlying differences in scope and explanation as *unattended* versus *unseen*. In the final sections I relate this distinction to the contrast I propose between visual emotion perception and visual emotion cognition.

Facial Expressions Processed without Attention

Over the last decade studies using various methods such as priming, pop out, inattentional blindness, redundant target presentation, and masking have provided evidence for nonconscious face recognition. The majority of studies are linked in some way to theories of attention, either directly, as when a specific model of attention is tested, or indirectly, as when specific attentional deficits (e.g., hemi-neglect—not paying attention to stimuli in the visual field contralateral to the lesion—or extinction) are investigated. Models of attention come in many varieties, but for the present purpose they all have in common the idea that nonconscious perception is related to availability of processing resources. When no attention is allocated to a stimulus, the information is not processed, or at least not processed sufficiently to sustain object recognition (Lavie, 1995; Treisman & Gelade, 1980). Patients suffering from hemi-neglect (i.e., a condition predominantly following damage to the right parietal cortex, whereby the patient no longer pays attention to his or her left visual field) or extinction (a condition with an etiology similar to neglect, whereby the patient attends to left-hemispace stimuli in the absence of right-hemispace stimuli but ignores the stimulus to the left when the right stimuli is presented simultaneously) provide an interesting opportunity for assessing the role of attention in the processing of facial expressions (Vuilleumier, 2000). As predicted, the emotional significance of faces does influence spatial attention during visual processing, thereby reducing neglect in brain-damaged patients with unilateral inattention. Faces may capture attention and overcome extinction, in part, because of their special biological status as well because of the highly automatized perceptual processing that is activated.

Research on nonconscious perception that manipulates attention suffers from the problem that attention is a relative notion, making the conclusive interpretation of results somewhat difficult. It is difficult to find a task that objectively measures the degree to which a stimulus occupies the observers' attention, because attention is difficult to quantify. An upper or a lower limit cannot be fixed in absolute terms. For example, based on their own results using functional magnetic resonance imaging (fMRI) in normal controls, some researchers have argued that, consistent with observations in animals, unattended stimuli do not produce a neural response (Pessoa, McKenna, Gutierrez, & Ungerleider, 2002), suggesting that they are not processed at all. Yet this area is a matter of hot debate. Recent studies have shown selective fluctuations in the network of attention (e.g., subcortical vs. cortical components), wherein some components are sensitive to attentional fluctuations, and others are not. These findings suggest that the arousal aspect of a face, in addition to its intrinsic valence, may also influence how it is processed (although see Charland, Chapter 10, on the idea of intrinsic valence).

To try and avoid the problems associated with manipulating attention, research on the nonconscious recognition of emotion has used visual masking techniques to block stimulus awareness (i.e., the faces of interest are unseen by the participants, who only consciously register the mask). Masking not only ensures that the face of interest is not consciously perceived, but it also interferes with the normal processing of that face in the visual cortex. Backward masking is thought to interfere with the specific role played by the primary visual cortex in the elaboration of a percept after initial stimulus encoding (Bullier, 2001). Studies using this technique have shown that when confronted with a backwardly masked, hence unseen, angry face, the observer nevertheless gives a reliable skin conductance response (Esteves, Dimberg, & Öhman, 1994). Facial expressions of fear increase the activation level of the amygdala, an effect that is lateralized as a function of whether or not the observer can perceive the faces consciously: right amygdala for unseen, left for seen masked presentation (Morris, Öhman, & Dolan, 1998). Faces displaying fear expressions followed by a backward mask lead to increased activities among the right amygdala, pulvinar, and superior colliculus (although see Atkinson & Adolphs, Chapter 7, on the consistency of this lateralization effect). This result and subsequent ones clearly suggest the existence of a primitive processing route for fear faces that functions independently of stimulus awareness.

It has been argued that presenting backwardly masked stimuli creates in normal viewers a situation that is functionally equivalent to that which exists in patients with a lesion in the primary visual cortex or hemianopia (Macknik & Livingstone, 1998). An important difference between backward masking and striate cortex lesion is that in the latter case, the primary visual cortex is no longer able to receive initial input whatsoever. Because subcortical structures are normally intact in these patients, they present a unique opportunity for assessing residual visual abilities when the primary visual cortex is destroyed. These patients can discriminate some elementary visual stimulus attributes of visual stimuli projected to their blind field, a phenomenon called *blindsight* (Weiskrantz, 1986, 1997). Residual vision for emotional stimuli such as facial expressions is referred to as *affective blindsight* (de Gelder, Vroomen, Pourtois, & Weiskrantz, 1999). In studies of affective blindsight, patients are instructed to make guesses about a stimulus because they are not able to see that there is a stimulus present. This method provides researchers with a clearer instance of unconscious perception (when compared to studies that simply manipulate attention) because patients are literally not able to see that there is a stimulus present (Weiskrantz, 2001). Although absence of awareness makes for a comparable experience in neglect and blindsight patients, intact sensory processes in the former, but not in the latter, make their situation very different. As a result, studies of blindsight patients are extremely useful in understanding the role of nonconscious perception of facial expressions.

Affective Blindsight: Radical Nonconsciousness of Facial Expressions

Research on blindsight patients confirms that the primary visual cortex is not essential in processing visual emotional signals or in combining unseen emotional signals with auditory ones. My collaborators and I have shown that patients with lesions in the striate cortex had residual nonconscious vision for facial expressions and were able to discriminate between facial expressions they could not see and were not aware of (de Gelder, Vroomen, et al., 1999; de Gelder, Vroomen, Pourtois, & Weiskrantz, 2000). More recently, Hamm and collaborators (Hamm et al., 2003) classically conditioned a person with bilateral loss of the striate cortex to a visual stimulus. The subject was completely blind (both behaviorally and experientially), yet responded to a visual stimulus that had been paired with an electric shock. These results are consistent with the notion that masked facial expressions are processed in normal subjects via a subcortical pathway involving the right amygdala, pulvinar, and superior colliculus. In contrast, processing of consciously seen faces increases connectivity between fusiform and orbitofrontal cortices (Morris, de Gelder, Weiskrantz, & Dolan, 2001).

The findings of blindsight have been controversial. Some older objections to the phenomenon are now irrelevant, thanks in part to the use of new technologies. First, the possibility that the remarkable visual abilities of cortically blind patients were due to an island of intact striate cortex or to light scattering has been definitively laid to rest by findings from brain imaging: Structural scans show that there is no intact striate cortex in these patients (Barbur, Watson, Frackowiak, & Zeki, 1993; Cowey & Stoerig, 2004).

The interesting questions are: How effective is blindsight, and what visual functions do these different pathways sustain? We know from studies in both monkey and human blindsight patients that residual discrimination of color and movement is possible, but both forms of discrimination are quantitatively and qualitatively different from the normal situation. For example, one may argue that facial expressions are too subtle and complex to survive striate cortex damage. But it is clear from recent research that subcortical structures play a crucial role in the processing of unseen faces (whether due to lesions in the striate cortex or to backward masking). Information from the retina is sent, via the superior colliculus, to the thalamic pulvinar nucleus and on to the amygdala, where the visual information is coded for its emotional significance. This action occurs in the absence of cortical activity (for a similar argument, see Atkinson & Adolphs, Chapter 7). Research on residual vision of facial expressions of fear provides support for the model that, in animals, fear reactions to auditory stimuli can be accounted for by two separate pathways (LeDoux, 1992). This dual-route approach has gained acceptance among emotion researchers as a general model of emotion processing (e.g., Adolphs, 2002b).Yet many details about its anatomical and functional implementation are still lacking. Although there is clear evidence from animal research of a noncortical route in auditory processing (LeDoux, 1992), clear-cut anatomical evidence of the corresponding situation for visual processes in humans is still lacking. Nevertheless, there are several reasons to assume that this route exists.

First, facial expressions should be among the most likely candidates for non-striate-based perception. Many types of information provided by the face are indeed rather subtle, such as age, gender, trustworthiness, attractiveness, and, most obviously, personal identity. These sources of information are processed with contributions from multiple cortical brain areas. Yet facial expressions of emotion can be recognized even when stimuli are much degraded. For example, using images with spatial frequencies below 8 cycles filtered out, the emotional expression on a face (but not the person's identity) can still be recognized almost faultlessly (Morrison & Schyns, 2001; Vuilleumier, Armony, Driver, & Dolan, 2003). This range of spatial frequencies corresponds to the range within which patients with a striate cortex lesion can still discriminate visual patterns, indicating that processing facial expression is within the range of the visual abilities sustained by a subcortical route.

Second, the subcortical route is comparatively faster than processing in the occipitotemporal cortex. And facial expressions of emotion can be processed, at least at some level, very quickly. Evidence for this speed comes from recordings of event-related potentials (ERPs), magnetoencelography (MEG), and to some extent, single-unit recordings. Facial expressions of emotion begin to be distinguished at 80–110 milliseconds poststimulus, with the signal located in the midline occipital cortex (Halgren, Raij, Marinkovic, Jousmaki, & Hari, 2000; Pizzagalli, Regard, & Lehmann, 1999; Streit et al., 1999). Activity at around 160 milliseconds is seen in the fusiform gyrus and superior temporal sulcus and corresponds to the time window of the N170, a negative wave form occurring at around 170 milliseconds and associated with the structural encoding of faces (but also bodies; Stekelenburg & de Gelder, 2004). We observed that the emotional content of faces affected the left N170, the occipitoparietal P2, and the frontocentral N2 (Stekelenburg & de Gelder, 2004). So far, all these studies concern cortical sources of activity and, as such, do not provide support for a subcortical route in emotion face processing. Recordings from the amygdala in animals and in humans suggest that the earliest activity is around 220 milliseconds (Streit et al., 1999), which is later than the occipital signal. But, interestingly, one study using single-unit recording in a patient reported discrimination between faces and scenes expressing fear or happiness in the orbitiofrontal cortex after only 120 milliseconds (Kawasaki et al., 2001). This latency is suggestive of a direct subcortical route from the amygdala to the orbitofrontal cortex. More recently, significant differences were found between emotion and neutral face conditions for peak amplitudes and latencies throughout the whole network of brain structures involved in emotion. The earliest peak of activation located in the calcarine sulcus (or primary visual cortex) appeared around 90 milliseconds and showed specificity to upright faces, which cannot be attributed to the low-level features of the stimulus (Meeren, Hadjikhani, Ahlfors, & de Gelder, 2005). The second peak of activation was stronger for meaningful stimuli, in general, but faces, in particular, elicited the strongest amount of activation. These findings suggest that the early visual areas do not merely process the physical features of the stimuli but are an intricate part of the face recognition network. The most interesting suggestion comes from the various time-course data that include evidence for biphasic face activity and current models of conscious and nonconscious cortically based and noncortically based processing routes. Unfortunately, the methods that provide highly specific information about time-course, such as ERP and MEG, do not allow direct inferences about subcortical structures.

In summary, at present the evidence for a functional role of a direct subcortical route for visual emotion signals in humans is still mostly indirect, with the strongest arguments provided by studies of blindsight, the points raised above, and the behavioral and brain-imaging data from unseen faces.

Reciprocal interactions between the visual system, other sensory systems, and the motor system open the possibility that visual deficits in the primary visual projections to the striate cortex may be compensated for not only by alternative visual pathways but also by links between these alternative visual pathways and, for example, the motor system. A relevant example is provided by the superior colliculus–putamen link that sustains orientation behavior. An important role of the superior colliculus in emotional perception may be directly related to its functional anatomical properties. The superficial layers of the superior colliculus consist of neurons that have predominantly visual properties, whereas the deep layers contain sensorimotor neurons. Superficial to deep-layer projections provide spatially ordered visual signals directly to the superior colliculus neurons that are involved in coordinating sensory inputs with motor outputs (Doubell, Skaliora, Baron, & King, 2003).

Visual perception can be achieved by the standard visual route, based on the lateral geniculate nucleus and projections to the primary visual cortex. However, it may or may not involve conceptual knowledge of the stimulus, memory, and influence from context (e.g., see Niedenthal et al., Chapter 2; Atkinson & Adolphs, Chapter 7; Barrett, Chapter 11; Prinz, Chapter 15). Yet even the enriched visual perception system does not operate in isolation. The visual system has direct links with the motor system, as shown by studies on action representation, of which the observations of mirror neurons are the most widely known (Grèzes & Decety, 2001). Our own research (de Gelder et al., 2004) has shown that a three-way modulation of the visual areas of the brain, the structures that comprise the emotional system of the brain, and the motor systems is the most noticeable when subjects watch fearful, as contrasted with happy or neutral, body movements, as I discuss below.

It has also been noted that dim visual abilities may be enriched in other ways than through contributions that improve the visual signal. There is increasing evidence that other phenomena accompanying visual perception without awareness may be more important in nonconscious visual perception. During testing, patients with blindsight sometimes report *feeling* that a stimulus is present without having any visual experience (Weiskrantz, 2001). This report is consistent with the notion that processing of emotional signals is associated with changes in bodily states during the early stages of emotion processing (Damasio, 1999), perhaps producing something like a primitive core affective state (see Barrett, Chapter 11) Affective blindsight may be related, in part, to a patient's interoceptive access to his or her bodily reactions to unseen stimuli. I have considered this possibility previously (de Gelder, Vroomen, et al., 2000). Other mechanisms, such as sensorimotor correlates of mandatory eye movements toward a target in the blind field, may help explain the puzzling finding that G.Y. (a patient with a unilateral hemianopia) performed above chance in a gender-decision task (Morris et al., 2001). In keeping with the limited range of spatial frequencies within which the superior colliculus–putamen pathway is functional, purely visually based gender discrimination, in itself, seems to less likely, although male and female faces might have different reward functions, and reward mechanisms may, in turn, supplement poor subcortical visual discrimination abilities.

Emotional Conflict Situations without Awareness of Conflict

The notion of partly independent processing streams for consciously and nonconsciously perceived emotional stimuli allows for the possibility of interactions between the two. Patients with unilateral visual cortex damage provide a unique occasion to explore this intriguing processing conflict, because it is possible to present simultaneously two stimuli (left and right of central fixation) under circumstances where there is no visual awareness of one or the other stimulus. Interhemispheric cooperation or conflict can be manipulated by manipulating whether the two stimuli carry the same or different emotional significance (de Gelder, Pourtois, van Raamsdonk, Vroomen, & Weiskrantz, 2001). One experiment used chimeric faces (consisting of two half-faces presented to each visual half-field). A second experiment simultaneously presented two full faces to the right and left visual fields. The stimulus presented in the contralesional field was perceived in patients with striate cortex damage, yet we also obtained clear evidence that the stimulus presented in the blind field influenced the emotional categorization of the stimulus seen in the intact field, as shown by lower performance in the emotion–face categorization of faces presented in the good field that were accompanied by an incongruent facial expression presented to the blind field.

Imaging studies contribute to our understanding of the neural architecture underlying the interactions between processing seen and unseen faces. Interhemispheric congruence effects between seen and unseen facial expressions modulate brain activity in the medial prefrontal cortex, superior colliculus, amygdala, and fusiform cortex (de Gelder, Morris, & Dolan, 2005). First, the overall congruency effects reflected in the medial prefrontal cortex indicate that there is an interaction between overt, conscious and covert, unconscious processing. The increase in activity for congruent, as opposed to incongruent, pairs in the medial prefrontal cortex is consistent with the role of this area in behavioral regulation (Bechara, Damasio, Damasio, & Anderson, 1994) more than in specific emotion-related information processing. The prefrontal cortex has been shown to govern the top-down control of behavior, executive functioning, higher-level emotional processing, and conscious behavioral control (Dolan et al., 1996; Dolan, Fletcher, McKenna, Friston, & Frith, 1999; Miller, 2000; Miller & Cohen, 2001). In particular, the ventral medial prefrontal cortex receives sensory information from the body and the external environment via the orbitofrontal cortex and is connected with the amygdala and the ventral striatum (Bechara et al., 1994), suggesting its role in the integration of emotional and cognitive processes (by incorporating visceromotor signals into decision-making processes). By presenting facial expressions simultaneously to the two visual fields, neural processes in subcortical structures related to an interaction between conscious and nonconsiously recognized images can be investigated. The presence of unseen fear faces has an influence on how consciously recognized fear or happy faces and fear or happy voices are perceived. Our results indicate that here also emotional congruency between visual and auditory stimulation led to enhancement in amygdala and superior colliculus activity for blind relative to intact field presentations. By comparing voice–face and voice–scene pairs, we were able to assess that the effect of unseen visual information on emotional voices is specific to faces and not with affective pictures. Our findings indicate that processing fear in the human face is mandatory and independent of awareness and that it remains robust even in the light of concurrent incongruent emotional information whether provided by a facial expression or an emotional voice of which the observer is aware. At the functional level, this asymmetry suggests that the integration between perception and behavior may be different as a function of whether the organism is engaged in automatic-reflexive or in controlled-reflective fear behavior. This asymmetry may mirror psychological reality: Our unconscious desires, anxieties, etc., influence our conscious thoughts and actions, but we cannot simply "think away" or remove our unconscious fears.

BEYOND THE FACE: EMOTIONAL CUES FROM VOICES AND BODY MOVEMENTS

Laboratory investigations of affective processes in humans tend to focus on one sensory system at a time—and most often, the visual system. The majority of studies focuses on affective information that can be gleaned from the face. In daily life, however, visual emotional signals from the face are usually accompanied by other information. Context influences how we see a facial expression (for a discussion, see Barrett, Chapter 11). The natural scene context in which a face appears has some influence on how it is perceived and how well it is remembered afterward. We investigated the role of natural scenes with affective meaning on the N170 (an electroencephalographic [EEG] wave selectively sensitive to faces, presumably reflecting the initial stage of face encoding and related to activity in fusiform cortex). We predicted that embedding facial expressions in an affective picture context would significantly modulate the N170, because viewing faces in the context of emotional scenes would trigger amygdala activation, which in turn would lead to increased activation of the fusiform cortex. Indeed, the results indicated that face expression and affective meaning of the scene interacted to generate the highest N170 amplitudes for the combination of fearful faces and fear-inspiring scenes (Righart & de Gelder, 2005). Our preliminary data also indicate an effect of natural scenes on memory for faces with a detrimental effect of fear-inspiring scenes on subsequent recognition of person identity.

In daily life, visual perception of the face is usually accompanied by signals from other sensory modalities. Multisensory emotion integration is particularly relevant for the issue of nonconscious emotional processing, because it is an automatic, mandatory process. People integrate information from multiply sensory channels even when they are unaware of the inputs or devote little conscious attention to integrating them. An increasing number of studies provide evidence that integration of information across different sensory modalities is a powerful mechanism for increasing adaptive responses (de Gelder & Bertelson, 2003). In the next section we discuss research that has expanded beyond face recognition research to consider expressions of emotion in the voice and whole body.

Emotional Voices

In contrast to the wealth of studies that explore the processing of facial expressions, there have been relatively few attempts at identifying the specific neural sites for processing emotions in the voice (see Buck, 2000, for a review; George et al., 1996; Scherer, 1995). Some studies have investigated common processing resources and overlapping brain structures for face and voice expressions (Borod, Tabert, Santschi, & Strauss, 2000; Royet et al., 2000). Insights into the neurobiological basis of voice processing are also based on neuropsychological findings (Adolphs, Damasio, & Tranel, 2002). For example, impaired recognition of emotional prosody is associated mostly with damage in the right frontal cortex, but also suggests a role of the temporal pole. The issue of common brain structures for processing emotional signals provided by different sensory systems has mainly been addressed by looking for correlations between emotional processing in different sensory channels. For example, parallel impairments were observed in recognition of fear in the face and in the voice in patients with amygdalectomy (Scott et al., 1997; but see Anderson & Phelps, 1998). Right-brain-damaged patients were impaired in tasks of emotional perception that involved facial, prosodic, and lexical stimuli. Yet to understand fully how the brain combines multiple sources of affective information, it is not sufficient to combine results obtained in studies that have investigated visual and auditory emotion perception separately. The issue of multisensory integration is altogether a different one from that of merely looking for common processing resources, because it concerns the online integration of the two sensory sources.

Perceiving Emotion in Face and Voice

Facial expressions of fear, anger, or sadness naturally go together with specific properties of the voice (for an alternative view, see Owren, Rendall, & Bachorowski, Chapter 8). People are quite confident that the shrieking voice they hear emanates from a face expressing fear rather than from one exhibiting a smile, as any parent watching children in a playground can testify. The ability to associate the emotional expression of a voice with accompanying visual information from the face seems to occur effortlessly and to be largely automatic. We have investigated a number of multisensory situations involving perception of emotional signals and argued for automatic binding of fear expressed in a face with fear present in a voice (for an overview, see de Gelder, Vroomen, & Pourtois, 2004).

Patients suffering from visual agnosia, which sometimes also includes an inability to recognize facial expressions of emotion, present a good opportunity for investigating the cross-modal processing of emotional information in faces and voices. We studied patient A.D., who has visual agnosia with severe face recognition problems due to bilateral occipito-temporal damage (de Gelder, Pourtois, Vroomen, & Bachoud-Levi, 2000). Her recognition of facial expressions of emotion is almost completely lost, whereas her recognition of emotions in the voice is intact. This combination allowed us to examine her perceptual abilities within a cross-modal bias paradigm. In the critical experiment she was asked to rate the emotion expressed in short spoken fragments while watching the facial expressions appearing on the screen. The evidence clearly indicated that the presentation of facial expression stimuli significantly influenced A.D.'s recognition of emotions in the voice, suggesting that she was able to process the facial expressions at a covert level that contributed to her ability to recognize emotion in vocal stimuli (de Gelder, Pourtois et al., 2000).

In other studies, the time-course of the integration between an affective tone of voice and facial expression was examined using ERP signals that track the processing of unexpected changes in the properties of auditory stimuli (whether in intensity, duration, or location). In the majority of trials, subjects were simultaneously presented with congruent facial (e.g., fearful) and vocal expressions. In the deviant trials, however, the voice was accompanied by an incongruent facial expression (e.g., a fearful voice and happy face). As predicted, we found a change in the auditory ERP as a function of a change in the visual component of the stimulus pair, indicating that the perceptual system was sensitive to the combination of these inputs rather than to the auditory one alone. We replicated this finding in a subsequent study, by showing that congruent facial/vocal stimuli (e.g., a sentence fragment spoken in an emotional tone of voice paired with a facial expression) gave rise to an increase in the amplitude of auditory evoked potentials (Pourtois, de Gelder, Vroomen, Rossion, & Crommelinck, 2000). A third study (Pourtois, Debatisse, Despland, & de Gelder, 2002) suggested that the processing of affective prosody is delayed when there is an incongruent facial expression present. Source localization indicated activation in the anterior cingulate cortex, an area selectively implicated in processing congruency or conflict between stimuli (Cabeza & Nyberg, 2000; MacLeod & MacDonald, 2000). The anterior cingulate cortex is not normally considered a multisensory processing area, but it is one of the areas associated with the processing of human motivational and emotional cues and with detection of error (Mesulam, 1998). Results indicated that adding visual affective information to the voice translates as an ERP amplitude increase of early auditory evoked potentials, an effect that obtains for both naturalistic (voice–face) and semantic (voice–affective picture) pairings in the intact field, but is only observed for the naturalistic pairings in the blind field (de Gelder, Pourtois, & Weiskrantz, 2002). Taken together, these four studies converge toward the conclusion that when emotional cues from the face and the voice are present, they influence each other rapidly and automatically. This conclusion does not imply that each stimulus is consciously perceived, that the observer is aware of their congruence, or that their integration proceeds in a deliberate manner.

The study of cortically blind patients allows the possibility of investigating intersensory integration of affective information with seen and unseen faces. We investigated the neural correlates of audiovisual integration when subjects categorize a facial expression while listening to an emotional voice (Dolan, Morris, & de Gelder, 2001). Participants were scanned while hearing a happy- or a fearful-sounding voice paired with either a congruent or an incongruent facial expression. Their task was to judge the facial emotion. When a fearful face was accompanied by a fearful voice, activation level in the amygdala and the fusiform gyrus increased. No such effect was observed when the voice and the face expressed conflicting emotions or when both expressed happiness. Interestingly, in contrast to our behavioral studies in which we observed that this cross-modal influence occurred equally for both "fearful" and "happy" pairs, no such increase in activation was observed for the latter. Further research is required to establish whether this reflects the different ecological importance of happy and fearful emotions.

Expressions of Emotion through Body Movements

At present, we know much less about how the human voice conveys emotion when compared to the human face. Even less is known about the emotional signals provided by the human body. Historically, body movements have frequently been analyzed as potent emotional signals. In his treatise on physiognomics, Aristotle remarked that the body as a whole signaled a person's emotional states and that facial expressions and intonations of the voice were part of a whole organism. In the 19th century German and Dutch expression physiologists and psychologists promoted the study of body expressions. Continuing initial explorations by Bell, Gratiolet, and Duchène de Boulogne, Darwin (1872/1998) described in detail the body expressions associated with emotions in animals and humans and proposed principles underlying the organization of these expressions. In his view, the expression of an emotional state by movements of the whole body is to be viewed as a simulation of the action normally associated with the emotion expressed. In view of the current usage of the term *mental simulation* (e.g., Niedenthal et al., Chapter 2), it should be noted that Darwin's view did not postulate a mentalist stage at which this simulation is initiated (as compared with James's ideomotor theory; James, 1890).

In general, there have been few scientific studies of emotion perception based on the bodily movements in others. The few occasional reports assessed recognition of body emotions in normal adults (Ekman & Friesen, 1976). Developmental data suggest that observation of bodily behavior is a better indicator of reaction to surprise than is facial expression (Camras et al., 2002). For a discussion of these findings and others, see Atkinson & Adolphs (Chapter 7).

Recently my colleagues and I initiated research on the functional and neural basis of whole-body expressions of emotion. Our findings indicate some similarities to the way that posed facial expressions are processed. First, we found that perceptions of whole-body expressions are processed configurally (as are emotion expressions on the face) and showed the familiar inversion effect and context effects (Stekelenburg & de Gelder, 2004). These results are consistent with configural perception of neutral body postures (Reed, Stone, Bozova, & Tanaka, 2003) as well as with studies of biological motion indicating that the global structure of whole-body movement is perceived, and that perception is not interrupted by anomalies in local relations (Berthental & Pinto, 1994; Grèzes & Decety, 2001; Grèzes et al., 2001).

Second, we found that perceptions of whole-body expressions produced neural activations that are similar to those seen in face perception. Exposure to body expressions of fear, compared to neutral body postures, activates the fusiform gyrus and the amygdala bilaterally (de Gelder, Snyder, et al., 2004). In the emotion literature these two areas have predominantly been associated with face processing (Adolphs, 2002a, 2002b; Kanwisher, McDermott, & Chun, 1997; Morris, Friston et al., 1998). These findings are consistent with those from studies of biological motion that used dance-like movements represented by point-light displays contrasted with randomly moving dots. The biological movement patterns were experienced as pleasant and activated subcortical structures, including the amygdala (Bonda, Petrides, Ostry, & Evans, 1996), consistent with results indicating that the role of the amygdala in recognizing emotion is not restricted to faces. A further finding of related interest is that visual perception of biological motion activates two areas in the occipital and fusiform cortices (Grossman & Blake, 2002). This result goes in the same direction as the preceding one, in the sense that it indicates that areas hitherto best known for processing faces are also involved in processing properties associated with human bodies.

Subjects were presented with short blocks of body expressions of fear alternating with blocks of images of emotionally neutral but meaningful body gestures. The face was blurred in all images to avoid confounds due to the facial expression. The results indicated that although the processing of emotional information from faces and bodies is somewhat similar, emotional bodies generate activity in a whole network of areas more comprehensive than the visual system (de Gelder, Snyder, et al., 2004). The major finding of this study is the existence of condition-specific activity associated with seeing fearful bodily expressions, as compared to neutral but meaningful body actions. A similar comparison for happy bodily expressions did not yield a result that was anywhere comparable. Foci of activity were located in areas involved in *stimulus detection and orientation* (e.g., in the superior colliculus), in *visual* areas so far mostly associated with the processing of fearful face expressions (e.g., amygdala and fusiform cortex). Passive viewing of still images of bodily expressions activates areas in the occipito-parietal pathway, predominantly the supplememtary motor area, cingulate gyrus, and middle frontal gyrus, which have been observed in studies of voluntary imitation (Decety et al., 1997; Passingham, 1996) and suggests that passive viewing can initiate motor preparation. This finding would seem particularly important in view of the Darwinian notion that the role of emotions is to facilitate adaptive action.

In the same study we also observed activity in the putamen and caudate nucleus in subjects viewing bodily expressions of fear. Both the caudate nucleus and putamen are predominantly known for their involvement in motor tasks but have also been associated with motivational–emotional task components. The caudate and putamen are damaged in Huntington's and Parkinson's diseases, which are both characterized by motor as well as emotion deficits. Although the nature of the relation between the emotional and the motor disorders is not yet fully understood, preliminary data indicate that these patients have a significant impairment in recognition of whole-body expressions of emotion (de Gelder, van den Stock, de Diego Balaguer & Bachoud-Levi, 2005).

Taken together, the available evidence suggests that the integrated activity in processing bodily expressions of fear may constitute a mechanism for fear contagion. This possibility is consistent with the view that simulating an emotion may be the basis upon which emotion is perceived (see Niedenthal et al., Chapter 2; Atkinson & Adolphs, Chapter 7; Barrett, Chapter 11; Prinz, Chapter 15). Most importantly, the preparation for action in response to fear seems to operate in a direct, automatic, and noninferential fashion in fear perception.

Emotional Synergies: Combining Faces and Bodies

In natural situations, a particular body expression is most likely to be accompanied by a congruent face expression. It is also well known from animal research that information from body expressions can play a role in reducing the ambiguity of facial expression (van Hoof, 1962). Moreover, it has been shown that observers' judgments of infants' emotional states depend on whole-body behavior more than on facial expressions alone (Camras et al., 2002). My colleagues and I have begun to explore the issue of synergies between facial expressions and bodily expressions of emotion using behavioral methods and EEG measurements. In one study we used a paradigm of categorical perception (reminiscent of the cross-modal studies in which we explored the influence of an emotional voice expression on a face) to assess how emotionally congruent or incongruent bodily expression influences the accuracy and speed of face categorization (Meeren, van Heynsberger, & de Gelder, 2005). The results of this experiment were very consistent with those found in studies of face–voice interactions: The way in which observers rated the facial expression was clearly influenced by the emotion expressed in the body, to which they were not paying attention.

CONCLUSIONS

For many years emotion researchers have been occupied with crucial issues regarding what emotions are, how they are perceived, how the sender intends them, and whether or not there are basic emotions. For the present-day cognitive psychologist, there is nothing shocking about the idea that unconscious processing assists our conscious mind from behind the curtains of awareness. It is generally agreed that unconscious mental machinery allows the conscious mind to operate more efficiently, without overloading it with irrelevant details. In line with this understanding, subjective reports are no longer viewed as the stumbling block for a science of the mind. Instead subjective reports may be viewed as the output of a complex but presumably lawful mental machinery (Dennett, 1991). A crucial question for emotion researchers is whether or not nonconscious emotional processes can be viewed within the information-processing paradigm that has characterized mainstream cognitive psychology for several decades. The general consensus seems to be yes (see also Scherer, Chapter 13; Winkielman et al., Chapter 14; for a different view see Clore, Storbeck, Robinson, & Centerbar, Chapter 16). This assumption yields several insights about emotion processing, more generally.

Levels of Processing, Qualitative Differences

Conscious and nonconscious emotional processes obey different principles and may ultimately require quite different research methods. For example, a major argument against basic, culture-independent emotions has been that studies of facial and vocal expressions of emotion have failed to produce convincing results (see Russell, Bachorowski, & Fernandez-Dols, 2003, for overview and discussion). It may be the case, however, that the majority of studies has been designed to measure conscious derivatives of emotion; therefore these data really do not speak to the possibility of basic unconscious emotion mechanisms.

Thus, when investigating how the organism specifically processes emotional information at the perceptual level, as contrasted with higher levels of cognition (e.g., thinking and decision making), it is important to exert proper methodological caution such that processing levels are not confounded. Without such empirical control, it is difficult to avoid the interpretation that the observed results reflect task demands and subjective coping strategies. When the experimental subject is aware of the goals and the design of the study, the experimental situation is transparent, and deliberate response strategies may contaminate the findings (Bertelson & de Gelder, 2004; de Gelder & Bertelson, 2003; Weiskrantz, 2001). If control is fully achieved, participants are neither aware of a stimulus nor of its properties, and the results are not contaminated by response strategies.

Awareness, Seeing, and Attending

As noted in the first part of this chapter, two kinds of neurological deficits have dominated research on nonconscious processes in the last decade: deficits of attention (e.g., visual neglect) and deficits of vision (e.g., blindsight). Similarities and differences between neglect versus blindsight have been compared in the past (Driver & Vuilleumier, 2001). In human research, affective blindsight probably offers the clearest and most radical instance of emotional perception without awareness. Unlike inattentional recognition of emotional objects in neglect patients, blindsight is not modulated by degree of attention or by the fact that attentional resources are otherwise engaged. This finding is consistent with the view that attention and awareness can be manipulated independently (Kentridge, Heywood, & Weiskrantz, 1999), and that the cognitive processes involved in attention and alerting are spared in blindsight (Kentridge & Heywood, 2001).

Findings from studies of patients with blindsight suggest that visual awareness deficits are relatively independent from cognitive awareness deficits. Furthermore, although the networks involved in each are not well understood, it does seem to be the case that they contribute separately to the nonconscious processing of emotion. For example, the means by which the amygdala plays its role in alerting the organism to fear signals and modulates visual processes may be different in the two cases. In both cases fear signals are often processed automatically. But automaticity on its own does not count as a touchstone for absence of awareness. Many daily activities are performed in an automatic fashion, but we are still aware of them taking place.

Perception and Recognition

A longstanding intuition is reflected in the association of perception with intermediate vision (linked with nonconscious processing) and recognition with conscious cognition, although more recently the boundary between perception and recognition has become blurred (e.g., meaningful but nonconscious processes are often termed *nonconscious recognition*). The central issue in this distinction is the role of concepts in providing a firm

ground for empirical knowledge. The traditional association between recognition and consciousness stems from the longstanding epistemological
claim that knowledge (as involved in recognition and contrasted with perception) requires concepts, and that concepts belong to the realm of the
thinking mind, not that of sensory perception. The epistemological roots
are reflected in 19th- and early 20th-century psychological theories of
visual perception and continue to influence our thinking, including our cat-
egorizations of patients' experiences. For example, the contrast between
perception and cognition (previously called *apperception*) is at the basis of
the classical distinction between apperceptive and associative agnosia
(Lissauer, 1890).

The perception–cognition distinction also owns its persistence to the
fact that it maps easily onto a traditional hierarchical model of the visual
system. Yet recent findings make it increasingly doubtful that perception
(sensory, visual) and recognition (cognitive, conceptual) are sequentially
organized (for a similar point, see Niedenthal et al., Chapter 2; Barrett,
Chapter 11). For example, findings about recurrent networks and feedback
loops from frontal areas back to temporo-occipetal areas (Bullier, 2001)
challenge a strictly hierarchical organization of visual perception and cognition. The notion that recognition requires concepts is also challenged by
the discovery of new ways in which an organism can instantiate a concept
outside conscious control (e.g., via perceptual categorization through automatic mimicry, imitation, action representation, and the "most cognitive"
variant, theory of mind). When recognition involves activity in structures
devoted to action representation and in motor structures, as shown for
observation of object-directed actions (Grèzes & Decety, 2001) and emotional body movements (de Gelder, 2004), then the meaning of perception
is extended to include perceptual abilities rooted in systems that involve
broadly distributed abilities related to bodily implementation and embodiment of emotion.

In view of these developments, there is no compelling reason to distinguish between perception and recognition, at least not along the traditional
sensory–cognitive or nonconscious–conscious divide. A similar comment
applies, albeit for different reasons, to partly overlapping contrasts between
implicit–explicit and attended–unattended processes. Each of these distinctions is built upon a mix of intuitions, behavioral findings, and experimental evidence obtained with widely different methodologies, experiential reports, and neuroanatomical facts whose interconnections we do not
clearly envisage at present. As far as studies of the perception of emotions
are concerned, in the conscious versus unconscious debate, we have sal-
vaged one reasonably circumscribed and clear dimension that is linked to
perceptual and postperceptual processes. In cases where the methodology

used allows for applying it, conscious and nonconscious processes can be distinguished.

Seeing Is Feeling: A Thorny Issue

Traditionally, emotion researchers have focused on facial expressions of emotion, and this focus may help explain why visual perception of aspects of emotional behavior have received the most attention. This focus may have some advantages for disentangling conscious from nonconscious perception, however, because the methods to do so are much more advanced in the visual domain than in any other sensory domain . Facial expressions, affective pictures, vocalizations, emotional tone of voice in language, and whole-body movements are viewed as the observable consequences of internal emotional states intended by a sender and decoded by a receiver. Yet many emotional displays function in a way that transcends the relatively complex notion of making internal states visible or even of communicating them. Action-based perception models consider visual perception and communication from a richer and more evolutionary inspired perspective that is potentially more appropriate for emotions (de Waal, 2002). Emotional communication is more direct than envisaged in traditional models; the first data now available clearly indicate that seeing fear "contaminates" motor structures for the sake of preparing for action (de Gelder, 2004).

Interesting findings about emotional mimicry from Dimberg and collaborators (Dimberg, 2000) are sometimes used in support of the role of mirror neurons in social communication. The activations observed in our study (de Gelder, 2004) in premotor, parietal, and inferior frontal gyri are consistent with a role for mirror neurons somewhere along the line, yet it is unknown at present just what this role may be (di Pellegrino, Fadiga, Fogassi, Gallese, & Rizzolatti, 1992). Future research is needed to disentangle the role of the different components in the fear contagion system. As we suggested, this is likely to be a complex system with multipurpose components that acquire significance for emotion only in the context of the whole. This complex system suggests a limitation for accounts of social communication based only on imitation implemented by neural mechanisms that model observed behavior. For example, several studies inspired by the reports on mirror neurons recently reported deficits in imitation in autistic individuals, suggesting a failure of this imitation-mirror mechanism in autism. We recently tested the hypothesis that facial expression mimicry may be impaired in autism. But our observations clearly indicated that there is no difference in EMG activity in response to facial expressions of anger or joy in autistic participants with clear deficits in recognition of facial expressions and social communication (Magnee, Stekelenburg, de Gelder, Van Engeland, & Kemner, 2005). Given that the communicative disorders of populations with autism are well documented, this result suggests that caution should be exercised in jumping from a reflex-like activity in facial muscles to a conclusion regarding mirror-neuron-based imitation and ultimately to the presence of social cognition and empathy in these individuals. At present no single approach and, *a fortiori*, no single cause seems to be able to render the different dimensions of perceiving, producing, and experiencing emotion.

ACKNOWLEDGMENTS

Many thanks to the editors for fruitful comments on earlier drafts, to W. A. C. van de Riet for assistance with the manuscript, and to the collaborators of the various studies summarized here.

REFERENCES

Adolphs, R. (2002a). Neural systems for recognizing emotion. *Current Opinion in Neurobiology, 12*(2), 169–177.

Adolphs, R. (2002b). Recognizing emotion from facial expressions: Psychological and neurological mechanisms. *Behavioral and Cognitive Neuroscience Review, 1*, 21–61.

Adolphs, R., Damasio, H., & Tranel, D. (2002). Neural systems for recognition of emotional prosody: A 3-D lesion study. *Emotion, 2*(1), 23–51.

Anderson, A. K., & Phelps, E. A. (1998). Intact recognition of vocal expressions of fear following bilateral lesions of the human amygdala. *NeuroReport, 9*(16), 3607–3613.

Barbur, J. L., Watson, J. D., Frackowiak, R. S., & Zeki, S. (1993). Conscious visual perception without V1. *Brain, 116*(Pt. 6), 1293–1302.

Bechara, A., Damasio, A. R., Damasio, H., & Anderson, S. W. (1994). Insensitivity to future consequences following damage to human prefrontal cortex. *Cognition, 50*(1–3), 7–15.

Bertelson, P., & de Gelder, B. (2004). The psychology of multimodal perception. In C. Spence & J. Driver (Eds.), *Crossmodal space and crossmodal attention* (pp. 151–177). Oxford, UK: Oxford University Press.

Berthental, B. I., & Pinto, J. (1994). Global processing of biological motion. *Psychological Science, 5*, 221–225.

Bonda, E., Petrides, M., Ostry, D., & Evans, A. (1996). Specific involvement of human parietal systems and the amygdala in the perception of biological motion. *Journal of Neuroscience, 16*(11), 3737–3744.

Borod, J., Tabert, M., Santschi, C., & Strauss, E. (2000). Neuropsychological assessment of emotional processing in brain-damaged patients. In J. Borod (Ed.), *The neuropsychology of emotion* New York: Oxford University Press.

Breiter, H. C., Etcoff, N. L., Whalen, P. J., Kennedy, W. A., Rauch, S. L., Buckner, R. L., et al. (1996). Response and habituation of the human amygdala during visual processing of facial expression. *Neuron, 17*(5), 875–887.

Buck, R. (2000). The epistemology of reason and affect. In J. Borod (Ed.), *The neuropsychology of emotion* (pp. 31–55). Oxford, UK: Oxford University Press.

Bullier, J. (2001). Feedback connections and conscious vision. *Trends in Cognitive Sciences, 5*(9), 369–370.

Cabeza, R., & Nyberg, L. (2000). Imaging cognition II: An empirical review of 275 PET and fMRI studies. *Journal of Cognitive Neuroscience, 12*(1), 1–47.

Camras, L. A., Meng, Z., Ujiie, T., Dharamsi, S., Miyake, K., Oster, H., et al. (2002). Observing emotion in infants: Facial expression, body behavior, and rater judgments of responses to an expectancy-violating event. *Emotion, 2*(2), 179–193.

Cowey, A., & Stoerig, P. (2004). Stimulus cueing in blindsight. *Progress in Brain Research, 144*, 261–277.

Damasio, A. R. (1999). *The feeling of what happens*. New York: Harcourt Brace.

Darwin, C. (1998). *The expresion of the emotions in man and animals*. New York: Oxford University Press. (Original work published 1872)

Decety, J., Grèzes, J., Costes, N., Perani, D., Jeannerod, M., Procyk, E., et al. (1997). Brain activity during observation of actions: Influence of action content and subject's strategy. *Brain, 120*(Pt. 10), 1763–1777.

de Gelder, B. (1999). Recognizing emotions by ear and by eye. In R. Lane & L. Nadel (Eds.), *Cognitive neuroscience of emotions* (pp. 84–105). Oxford, UK: Oxford University Press.

de Gelder, B., & Bertelson, P. (2003). Multisensory integration, perception and ecological validity. *Trends in Cognitive Sciences, 7*(10), 460–467.

de Gelder, B., Morris, J. S., & Dolan, R. J. (2005). *Two emotions in one brain: The influence of nonconsciously processed facial expression on consciously recognized faces and voices*. Manuscript submitted for publication.

de Gelder, B., Pourtois, G., van Raamsdonk, M., Vroomen, J., & Weiskrantz, L. (2001). Unseen stimuli modulate conscious visual experience: Evidence from inter-hemispheric summation. *NeuroReport, 12*(2), 385–391.

de Gelder, B., Pourtois, G., Vroomen, J., & Bachoud-Levi, A. C. (2000). Covert processing of faces in prosopagnosia is restricted to facial expressions: Evidence from cross-modal bias. *Brain and Cognition, 44*(3), 425–444.

de Gelder, B., Pourtois, G., & Weiskrantz, L. (2002). Fear recognition in the voice is modulated by unconsciously recognized facial expressions but not by unconsciously recognized affective pictures. *Proceedings of the National Academy of Sciences USA, 99*(6), 4121–4126.

de Gelder, B., Snyder, J., Greve, D., Gerard, G., & Hadjikhani, N. (2004). Fear fosters flight: A mechanism for fear contagion when perceiving emotion expressed by a whole body. *Proceedings of the National Academy of Sciences USA, 101*, 16701–16706.

de Gelder, B., van den Stock, J., de Diego Balaguer, R., & Bachoud-Levi, A.-C. (2005). *Impaired recognition of facial expressions, instrumental and body actions in Huntington's disease*. Manuscript in preparation.

de Gelder, B., Vroomen, J., & Pourtois, G. (2004). Multisensory perception of affect, its time course and its neural basis. In G. Calvert, C. Spence, & B. E. Stein (Eds.), *Handbook of multisensory processes* (pp. 581–596). Cambridge, MA: MIT Press.

de Gelder, B., Vroomen, J., Pourtois, G., & Weiskrantz, L. (1999). Non-conscious recognition of affect in the absence of striate cortex. *NeuroReport, 10*(18), 3759–3763.

de Gelder, B., Vroomen, J., Pourtois, G., & Weiskrantz, L. (2000). Affective blindsight: Are we blindly led by emotions?: Response to Heywood and Kentridge (2000). *Trends in Cognitive Sciences, 4*(4), 126–127.

Dennett, D. C. (1991). *Consciousness explained.* Boston: Little, Brown.

di Pellegrino, G., Fadiga, L., Fogassi, L., Gallese, V., & Rizzolatti, G. (1992). Understanding motor events: A neurophysiological study. *Experimemtal Brain Research, 91*, 176–180.

Dolan, R. J., Fletcher, P. C., McKenna, P., Friston, K. J., & Frith, C. D. (1999). Abnormal neural integration related to cognition in schizophrenia. *Acta Psychiatrica Scandinavica Supplement, 395*, 58–67.

Dolan, R. J., Fletcher, P., Morris, J., Kapur, N., Deakin, J. F., & Frith, C. D. (1996). Neural activation during covert processing of positive emotional facial expressions. *NeuroImage, 4*(3, Pt. 1), 194–200.

Dolan, R. J., Morris, J. S., & de Gelder, B. (2001). Crossmodal binding of fear in voice and face. *Proceedings of the National Academy of Sciences USA, 98*(17), 10006–10010.

Doubell, T. P., Skaliora, I., Baron, J., & King, A. J. (2003). Functional connectivity between the superficial and deeper layers of the superior colliculus: An anatomical substrate for sensorimotor integration. *Journal of Neuroscience, 23*(16), 6596–6607.

Driver, J., & Vuilleumier, P. (2001). Unconscious processing in neglect and extinction. In B. de Gelder, E. H. F. de Haan, & C. A. Heywood (Eds.), *Out of mind: Varieties of unconscious processes* (pp. 107–139). Oxford, UK: Oxford University Press.

Edelman, G. M., & Tononi, G. (2000). *A universe of consciousness.* New York: Basic Books.

Ekman, P., & Friesen, W. V. (1976). *Pictures of facial affects.* Palo Alto, CA: Consulting Psychologists Press.

Esteves, F., Dimberg, U., & Öhman, A. (1994). Automatically elicited fear: Conditioned skin conductance responses to masked facial expressions. *Cognition and Emotion, 9*, 99–108.

George, J. S., Schmidt, D. M., Mosher, J. C., Aine, C. J., Ranken, D. M., Wood, C. C., et al. (1996, February). *Dynamic neuroimaging by MEG, constrained by MRI and fMRI.* Paper presented at the Tenth International Conference on Biomagnetism, Santa Fe, NM.

Grèzes, J., & Decety, J. (2001). Functional anatomy of execution, mental simulation, observation, and verb generation of actions: A meta-analysis. *Human Brain Mapping, 12*(1), 1–19.

Grèzes, J., Fonlupt, P., Bertenthal, B., Delon-Martin, C., Segebarth, C., & Decety, J.

(2001). Does perception of biological motion rely on specific brain regions? *NeuroImage, 13*(5), 775–785.

Grossman, E. D., & Blake, R. (2002). Brain areas active during visual perception of biological motion. *Neuron, 35*(6), 1167–1175.

Halgren, E., Raij, T., Marinkovic, K., Jousmaki, V., & Hari, R. (2000). Cognitive response profile of the human fusiform face area as determined by MEG. *Cerebral Cortex, 10*(1), 69–81.

Hamm, A. O., Weike, A. I., Schupp, H. T., Treig, T., Dressel, A., & Kessler, C. (2003). Affective blindsight: Intact fear conditioning to a visual cue in a cortically blind patient. *Brain, 126*(Pt. 2), 267–275.

James, W. (1890). *Principles of psychology.* New York: Holt.

Kanwisher, N., McDermott, J., & Chun, M. M. (1997). The fusiform face area: A module in human extrastriate cortex specialized for face perception. *Journal of Neuroscience, 17*(11), 4302–4311.

Kawasaki, H., Kaufman, O., Damasio, H., Damasio, A. R., Granner, M., Bakken, H., et al. (2001). Single-neuron responses to emotional visual stimuli recorded in human ventral prefrontal cortex. *Nature Neuroscience, 4*(1), 15–16.

Kentridge, R. W., & Heywood, C. A. (2001). In B. de Gelder, E. H. F. de Haan, & C. A. Haywood (Eds.), *Out of mind: Varieties of unconscious processes* (pp. 163–184). Oxford, UK: Oxford University Press.

Kentridge, R. W., Heywood, C. A., & Weiskrantz, L. (1999). Attention without awareness in blindsight. *Proceedings of the Royal Society of London B: Biological Sciences, 266*(1430), 1805–1811.

LaBar, K. S., Crupain, M. J., Voyvodic, J. T., & McCarthy, G. (2003). Dynamic perception of facial affect and identity in the human brain. *Cereb Cortex, 13*(10), 1023–1033.

Lavie, N. (1995). Perceptual load as a necessary condition for selective attention. *Journal of Experimental Psychology: Human Perception and Performance, 21*(3), 451–468.

LeDoux, J. E. (1992). Brain mechanisms of emotion and emotional learning. *Current Opinion in Neurobiology, 2*(2), 191–197.

LeDoux, J.E. (2000). Emotion circuits in the brain. *Annual Review of Neuroscience, 23,* 155–184.

Lissauer, H. (1890). *Ein Fall von Seelenblindheit nebst einem Beitrage zur Theorie derselben* [A case of visual agnosia with a contribution to theory]. *Archiv für Psychiatrie und Nervenkrankheiten, 21,* 222–270.

Macknik, S. L., & Livingstone, M. S. (1998). Neuronal correlates of visibility and invisibility in the primate visual system. *Nature Reviews Neuroscience, 1*(2), 144–149.

MacLeod, C. M., & MacDonald, P. A. (2000). Interdimensional interference in the Stroop effect: Uncovering the cognitive and neural anatomy of attention. *Trends in Cognitive Sciences, 4*(10), 383–391.

Magnee, M. J. C. M., Stecklenburg, J. J., de Gelder, B., Van Engeland, H., & Kemner, C. (2005). *Facial EMG and affect processing in autism.* Manuscript in preparation.

Meeren, H., Hadjikhani, N., Ahlfors, S., & de Gelder, B. (2004). *MEG source analy-*

sis of early visual responses during face perception: Anatomically-constraint noise-normalized minimum norm estimates. Manuscript in preparation.

Meeren, H., van Heynsberger, C., & de Gelder, B. (2005). Rapid integration of facial expressions and whole body emotions. Manuscript in preparation.

Mesulam, M. M. (1998). From sensation to cognition. Brain, 121(Pt. 6), 1013–1052.

Miller, E. K. (2000). The prefrontal cortex and cognitive control. Nature Reviews Neuroscience, 1(1), 59–65.

Miller, E. K., & Cohen, J. D. (2001). An integrative theory of prefrontal cortex function. Annual Review of Neuroscience, 24, 167–202.

Morris, J. S., de Gelder, B., Weiskrantz, L., & Dolan, R. J. (2001). Differential extrageniculostriate and amygdala responses to presentation of emotional faces in a cortically blind field. Brain, 124(Pt. 6), 1241–1252.

Morris, J. S., Friston, K. J., Buchel, C., Frith, C. D., Young, A. W., Calder, A. J., et al. (1998). A neuromodulatory role for the human amygdala in processing emotional facial expressions. Brain, 121(Pt. 1), 47–57.

Morris, J. S., Frith, C. D., Perrett, D. I., Rowland, D., Young, A. W., Calder, A. J., et al. (1996). A differential neural response in the human amygdala to fearful and happy facial expressions. Nature, 383(6603), 812–815.

Morris, J. S., Öhman, A., & Dolan, R. J. (1998). Conscious and unconscious emotional learning in the human amygdala. Nature, 393(6684), 467–470.

Morrison, D. J., & Schyns, P. G. (2001). Usage of spatial scales for the categorization of faces, objects, and scenes. Psychonomic Bulletin and Review, 8(3), 454–469.

Passingham, R. E. (1996). Attention to action. Philosophical Transactions of the Royal Society of London B: Biological Sciences, 351(1346), 1473–1479.

Pessoa, L., McKenna, M., Gutierrez, E., & Ungerleider, L. G. (2002). Neural processing of emotional faces requires attention. Proceedings of the National Academy of Sciences USA, 99(17), 11458–11463.

Pizzagalli, D., Regard, M., & Lehmann, D. (1999). Rapid emotional face processing in the human right and left brain hemispheres: An ERP study. NeuroReport, 10(13), 2691–2698.

Pourtois, G., de Gelder, B., Vroomen, J., Rossion, B., & Crommelinck, M. (2000). The time-course of intermodal binding between seeing and hearing affective information. NeuroReport, 11(6), 1329–1333.

Pourtois, G., Debatisse, D., Despland, P. A., & de Gelder, B. (2002). Facial expressions modulate the time course of long latency auditory brain potentials. Brain Research, Cognitive Brain Research, 14(1), 99–105.

Reed, C. L., Stone, V., Bozova, S., & Tanaka, J. (2003). The body inversion effect. Psychological Science, 14, 302–308.

Righart, R., & de Gelder, B. (2005). Context influences early perceptual analysis of faces: An electrophysiological study. Manuscript in preparation.

Royet, J. P., Zald, D., Versace, R., Costes, N., Lavenne, F., Koenig, O., et al. (2000). Emotional responses to pleasant and unpleasant olfactory, visual, and auditory stimuli: A positron emission tomography study. Journal of Neuroscience, 20(20), 7752–7759.

Russell, J. A., Bachorowski, J. A., & Fernandez-Dols, J. M. (2003). Facial and vocal expressions of emotion. Annual Review of Psychology, 54, 329–349.

Scherer, K. R. (1995). Expression of emotion in voice and music. *Journal of Voice, 9*(3), 235–248.

Scott, S. K., Young, A. W., Calder, A. J., Hellawell, D. J., Aggleton, J. P., & Johnson, M. (1997). Impaired auditory recognition of fear and anger following bilateral amygdala lesions. *Nature, 385*(6613), 254–257.

Simpson, J. R., Ongur, D., Akbudak, E., Conturo, T. E., Ollinger, J. M., Snyder, A. Z., et al. (2000). The emotional modulation of cognitive processing: An fMRI study. *Journal of Cognitive Neuroscience, 12*(Suppl. 2), 157–170.

Stekelenburg, J. J., & de Gelder, B. (2004). The neural correlates of perceiving human bodies: An ERP study on the body-inversion effect. *NeuroReport, 15*(5), 777–780.

Streit, M., Ioannides, A. A., Liu, L., Wolwer, W., Dammers, J., Gross, J., et al. (1999). Neurophysiological correlates of the recognition of facial expressions of emotion as revealed by magnetoencephalography. *Brain Research, Cognitive Brain Research, 7*(4), 481–491.

Treisman, A. M., & Gelade, G. (1980). A feature-integration theory of attention. *Cognitive Psychology, 12*(1), 97–136.

van Hooff, J. A. (1962). Facial expressions in higher primates. *Symposium of the Zoological Society of London, 8*, 97–125.

Vuilleumier, P. (2000). Faces call for attention: Evidence from patients with visual extinction. *Neuropsychologia, 38*(5), 693–700.

Vuilleumier, P., Armony, J. L., Driver, J., & Dolan, R. J. (2003). Distinct spatial frequency sensitivities for processing faces and emotional expressions. *Nature Neuroscience, 6*(6), 624–631.

Weiskrantz, L. (1986). *Blindsight: A case study and implications.* Oxford, UK: Clarendon Press.

Weiskrantz, L. (1997). *Consciousness lost and found.* Oxford, UK: Oxford University Press.

Weiskrantz, L. (2001). Blindsight—putting beta on the back burner. In B. de Gelder, E. H. F. de Haan, & C. A. Heywood (Eds.), *Out of mind: Varieties of unconscious processes* (pp. 20–31). Oxford, UK: Oxford University Press.

Zald, D. H. (2003). The human amygdala and the emotional evaluation of sensory stimuli. *Brain Research, Brain Research Reviews, 41*(1), 88–123.

CHAPTER 7

Visual Emotion Perception

Mechanisms and Processes

ANTHONY P. ATKINSON

RALPH ADOLPHS

Perceiving and interpreting other people's emotional states is essential for effective social interaction. Its very importance is likely to have resulted in the evolution of complex mechanisms that underlie it. A basic capacity to attach emotional significance to stimuli and respond to them appropriately, without any conscious experience, is likely to have evolved under different selection pressures and considerably earlier than the capacity for conscious emotional responses—a hypothesis that now enjoys considerable empirical support (LeDoux, 1998). Emotion perception is similarly bifurcated in this way. At times emotion perception is automatic and fast (and thus, typically, unconscious), and at other times deliberate, slow, and effortful (and thus, typically, conscious). Recent evidence indicates that this distinction at the behavioral level reflects a division in the underlying cognitive processes and neural substrate (for a similar view, see Winkielman, Berridge, & Wilbarger, Chapter 14).

The focus of this chapter is the perception of emotion from visual cues. In the first section we highlight some of the conceptual issues surrounding the distinction between conscious and unconscious emotion perception, and the different methods used to probe these capacities. Then, in the second section, we outline the neural substrate of emotion perception from facial expressions, weighing the evidence for a degree of emotion-specific func-

1. *What is emotion?*

From an evolutionary perspective, emotions are central states shaped by natural selection that enable animals to cope with threats and opportunities presented to them by their physical and social environments. Emotions achieve these effects by coordinating a large number of changes in brain, body, and behavior. Most or all of the so-called basic emotions (Ekman, 1992)—fear, disgust, anger, joy, sadness, surprise—can be thought of as packages of response coordination sculpted by evolution to meet particular environmental challenges, such as avoiding physical harm (fear) and contaminants (disgust). Somewhat more controversially, some of the more complex social emotions, such as jealousy, guilt, and embarrassment, can be analyzed in this way as well (e.g., Cosmides & Tooby, 2000). Such an adaptationist perspective encompasses both the production and perception of emotion signals—capacities that many have argued coevolved (e.g., Darwin, 1872/1998; Plutchik, 1980; although see Owren, Rendall, & Bachorowski, Chapter 8; Owren & Bachorowski, 2001, for an account of why the evolution of emotion signaling and perception might be decoupled in some cases). Emotion signals can be considered as aspects of coordinated systems of emotional response, as outward expressions of internal emotional states, or as communicative acts that can be causally divorced from the emotional states that they usually signal. We do not make these distinctions in this chapter, and refer to all three types of emotion signal as emotional expressions.

Consonant with this view of emotions as solutions to distinct adaptive problems is an expectation that the underlying neural systems will be organized in a modular fashion, to some degree. Both the requirement for speed and the need to trigger a particular class of behaviors may make specialized systems advantageous, and may have resulted in neural mechanisms that are relatively specialized to process certain emotionally relevant information. Some theories of emotion, in fact, categorize emotions according to the neural systems that implement ecological packages of behavioral mechanisms (Panksepp, 1998). The main purpose of this initial processing is to provide a crude assessment of the value of the stimulus (good/bad, harmful/pleasant) and thus to motivate behavior (e.g., approach–avoid). In addition to this very fast, automatic, and coarse processing, the presentation of an emotional stimulus also typically initiates more detailed perceptual and recognition processing, which is likely to be less classically modular (e.g., slower, less automatic, and less encapsulated), and can include more complex attributions and rationalizations of the causes of an emotion and regulation of its expression.

Roughly, we view feeling (the awareness of one's emotional state and what it is like to be in that state) and behavior (emotional response) as only dispositionally linked to emotion, as such. Measurements of feelings (via subjective report) or behavior (via facial expression or autonomic response) can be taken as evidence for an emotional state, but are not themselves constitutive of that state. That is, although we use evidence of what people say and do to infer

(continued)

their emotional states, those emotional states are not to be identified with any one particular piece of that evidence (behavior, vouched feeling), nor, indeed, with that evidence in the round. This view differs from many other emotion theories. It may be closest in spirit to Russell's notion of "core affect" (Russell, 2003), although we do not share all his views. In particular, we agree that people are often unaware of the causal networks linking stimuli, emotions, feelings, and behavior. In attributing an emotion to someone, or even to oneself, one might be unaware of the actual causal networks because one's causal attribution is mistaken, only partial, or both, or because one has failed to attribute any causes at all (see also Winkielman, Berridge, & Wilbarger, Chapter 14). In our view, emotions are theoretical central states that are assigned to an organism on the basis of our observations of its interaction with its environment, its somatic response, and (for humans) its verbal report of feelings. In this sense, we believe emotions to be implemented neurologically. Although there are particular words to describe emotions, and although we use the basic emotion labels in this chapter, we fully acknowledge that emotions are continuous states that accompany all of our waking lives, not just discrete, strongly emotional episodes—an idea consonant with the theoretical frameworks of Russell (2003), Damasio (1994, 1999), and others.

2. *How does one measure conscious versus unconscious perception?*

Implicit or covert abilities are typically measured by performance on indirect tests, whereas explicit or overt abilities are typically measured by performance on direct tests. In a *direct* test of a perceptual ability, subjects are given explicit instructions to perform a perceptual task, and performance on that task is the measure of interest for the experimenter. Direct tests of emotion perception include tasks that require (1) matching emotional expressions across two or more identities, (2) distinguishing between varying degrees of emotional intensity, (3) forced-choice emotion labeling, (4) rating viewed faces as to how much of each of a given number of emotions they contain, and (5) identifying the expressed emotion in a free-response procedure. By contrast, in an *indirect* test of a perceptual ability, performance on the task specified in the instructions is not the measure of interest but nevertheless involves the to-be-measured perceptual ability. (Indirect tests thus typically involve both direct and indirect measures.) No reference is made to the perceptual ability or measure of interest in the instructions given to the subjects. One of several examples of indirect tests of emotion perception discussed in the main text involves recording changes in the skin conductance response (SCR) in the absence of reported awareness of the very briefly presented masked expressions (Esteves, Parra, Dimberg, & Öhman, 1994); another involves measuring changes in facial electromyographic (EMG) response.

The terms *direct* and *indirect* are used to describe different types of empirical measures (performances on tasks), whereas the terms *explicit* or *overt*

(continued)

and *implicit* or *covert* refer to types of knowledge or information processes and, in particular, describe the degree of participants' awareness of their abilities (Reingold & Merikle, 1988). Direct measures are often accompanied by explicit knowledge, and indirect measures by implicit knowledge, but not always: For instance, it is possible for certain brain-damaged patients to generate implicit knowledge on direct tests, such as when blindsight patients successfully discriminate stimuli presented in their blind fields in a direct, forced-choice task (Weiskrantz, 1990), even though they lack visual awareness of those stimuli.

3. *What are the stimuli for the study of biological motion perception?*

In order to assess our ability to make various judgments on the basis of face and body movements (biological motion), including the ability to discriminate and identify emotional expressions, it is important to be able to study the contribution of movement information in the absence of all other cues that might contribute to those judgments, especially static-form information. Johansson (1973) devised a technique for studying the perception of biological motion that minimizes or eliminates static-form information from the stimulus but retains motion information. In these point-light or patch-light displays, the moving figure, such as a face or body, is represented by a small number of illuminated dots or patches, positioned so as to highlight the motion of the facial muscles or body parts. Video clips are made in which the only visible elements are these bright points. When static, the display gives the impression of a relatively meaningless configuration of points, but when moving, this meaningless configuration is transformed into a striking impression of a moving face or body. Researchers have shown that people recognize not just types of locomotive movement from point-light biological motion stimuli, but also gender from the actor's gait (Kozlowski & Cutting, 1977), the identity of familiar people from their gait (Cutting & Kozlowski, 1977) or arm movement (Hill & Pollick, 2000), traits such as vulnerability (Gunns, Johnston, & Hudson, 2002), and emotional states from facial movement (Bassili 1978) and whole-body (Dittrich et al., 1996) or arm (Pollick et al., 2001) movement. Even young infants are sensitive to biological motion in point-light displays (Fox & McDaniel, 1982). In sum, people's ability to derive socially relevant information from such impoverished cues is striking: Facial and body movement are clearly useful sources of information about others' states and traits.

tional organization in these neural mechanisms, and arguing the need for further research using dynamic portrayals of emotion. In the third section we consider the evidence that a subcortical pathway from the retina to amygdala, bypassing the primary visual cortex, subserves unconscious emotion perception. In the fourth section we explore whether the neural structures involved in emotion perception from faces might also subserve emotion perception from other visual cues, especially body posture and movement.

A variety of evidence suggests an intimate link between emotion perception and emotional experience (see also Barrett, Chapter 11; Prinz, Chapter 15), and between the neural mechanisms subserving these capacities. One idea, elaborated in the fifth section, is that we come to know or recognize the emotional state of others via our perception of an emotional response within ourselves (see also Niedenthal, Barsalou, Ric, & Krauth-Gruber, Chapter 2). The importance of the dynamic aspect of emotional expressions shows itself here, for if, as we suggest, emotion understanding occurs via mimicry or simulation, then it is plausible to suppose that what is mimicked or simulated is the dynamic production of an expression, rather than some snapshot at, or near, the emotional peak.

CONSCIOUS VERSUS UNCONSCIOUS EMOTION PERCEPTION

As we illustrate below, it is possible to perceive another's emotional expression without the observer being consciously aware of perceiving the posture or movement of the other person's face or body, or, indeed, without being aware of the face or body at all. At the other end of the spectrum, the observer might consciously perceive another's face or body, its features and their configuration, and its emotional expression. In between these two extremes lie other possible degrees or levels of awareness, such as consciously perceiving a face or body, its posture and movement, and its affective quality (e.g., as having a positive or negative valence) without being aware of what specific emotion it conveys, without recognizing or otherwise *knowing that* it is an expression of fear, for example (technically, a form of fear agnosia). At work in these cases is a distinction known to philosophers as that between the *perception of things* and the *perception of facts*, or nonepistemic versus epistemic perception (Dretske, 1969). Perceiving an object or event, such as a fearful facial expression, does not require that the object or event be recognized or interpreted in any particular way; it does not require that we associate what we perceive with any additional knowledge about what it means. Perceiving a fact, on the other hand, means grasping the fact and entails coming to know that it *is* a fact. Epistemically seeing an expression of fear, for example, involves recognizing or coming to know this fact via the visual modality.

In psychology, the term *perception* is often used to cover both nonepistemic and epistemic perception; unless otherwise noted, this is how we use the term in this chapter. Nonetheless, the two types of perception still mark a useful distinction that corresponds to discrete types or stages of processing. *Perception of things* refers to processes that occur very soon after the onset of the stimulus, and are presumed to rely largely on early sensory cortices. These processes make explicit the distinct features of stimuli and their geometric configurations to allow discrimination among different stimuli on the basis of their appearance. In contrast, *perception of facts* refers to processes that require additional knowledge that could not be obtained solely from an inspection of the features of the stimulus. The latter set of processes is quite heterogeneous. For instance, recognition of fear from a facial expression may occur by linking the perceptual properties of the facial stimulus to various knowledge-based processes. These include the knowledge components of the concept of fear, the lexical label *fear*, and the perception of the emotional fear response (or a central representation thereof) that the stimulus triggers in the observer. Although a common conception is that higher-level cognitive abilities such as these are grounded in knowledge-based processes that do not involve sensory cortices and are thus amodal, an alternative viewpoint, which we endorse, is that these abilities are, in fact, grounded in sensory–motor representations, but at a more abstract or higher level (e.g., Barsalou, Simmons, Barbey, & Wilson, 2003; Damasio, 1999; Niedenthal et al., Chapter 2).

It may be tempting to identify early perceptual processing (perception of things) with unconscious perception, and later perceptual and recognition processing (perception of facts) with conscious perception. Later perceptual and recognition processing need not be conscious, however, as evidenced by the various ways in which conceptual knowledge can shape perception without awareness (see Barrett, Chapter 11; Smith & Neumann, Chapter 12). Indeed, it may even be that emotionally and socially relevant conceptual knowledge is particularly adept at shaping perception with or without awareness, that recognition of emotional and other social information is, in some sense, obligatory and colors our perception of the social world, even when that perception is unconscious. If true, then early visual processing is not sufficient for unconscious emotion perception.

There are several ways of measuring unconscious emotion perception (see "A Subcortical Pathway . . . " and "Emotion Recognition . . . "; see also Lundqvist & Öhman, Chapter 5; de Gelder, Chapter 6), but it remains unclear as to exactly what the informational content is of the representations produced by such unconscious processing. For example, one current controversy that we explore below concerns the role of a subcortical pathway from the retina to amygdala, which some investigators argue subserves unconscious emotion perception. Does activity of this pathway, in response to faces of which the subject is unaware, reflect that pathway's ability to distinguish between certain specific facial emotions (e.g., fearful from happy and sad), or threatening from nonthreatening faces, or more simply, emotional from nonemotional faces? Bound up with this issue is the additional question of whether this subcortical pathway subserves unconscious emotion perception on its own, or whether its activation reflects some involvement of cortical processing.

THE NEURAL SUBSTRATE OF EMOTION PERCEPTION FROM FACIAL EXPRESSIONS

Some of the most important neural structures underpinning emotion perception from the face are the occipital and temporal cortices, amygdala, orbitofrontal cortex (including its ventromedial aspect), right inferior parietal cortices, especially somatosensory cortex, and basal ganglia (see Figures 7.1 and 7.2). These structures are engaged in multiple processes and at various points in time, making it difficult to assign a single function to a structure. (For a more detailed review, see Adolphs, 2002.) Early visual processing of facial emotion, up to 150–180 milliseconds poststimulus onset, proceeds along two parallel routes that later interact: a subcortical pathway to the amygdala via the superior colliculus and pulvinar, for the fast processing of highly salient, especially threatening, stimuli; and a slower cortical route, via thalamus and striate cortices, to regions of inferior and superior temporal cortices. Later, more detailed processing of emotional faces, occurring after about 180 milliseconds poststimulus onset, appears to involve interactions between the amygdala and several cortical regions, especially fusiform, superior temporal, and orbitofrontal cortices. This claim is consistent with the findings of projections between the amygdala and orbitofrontal cortex, and projections from those two structures to the superior temporal and fusiform cortices (e.g., Carmichael & Price, 1995), and is supported by direct evidence of correlations between amygdala activity and activity in these cortical regions in response to static facial expressions (e.g., Iidaka et al., 2001; Morris, Öhman, & Dolan, 1998). Direct, causal evidence in humans that amygdala activity modulates the processing of emotional stimuli in cortical regions was, until very recently, lacking. By combining functional imaging and lesion data, Vuilleumier, Richardson, Armony, Driver, and Dolan (2004) found that amygdala activity enhances sensory processing in occipital as well as fusiform visual areas, when participants were viewing fearful, as compared to emotionally neutral, faces.

Along with the orbitofrontal cortex, especially its ventromedial sector, and the amygdala, the insular and parietal somatosensory cortices are involved in the modulation of emotional reactions involving the body via connections to brainstem structures (Damasio, 1994, 1999; LeDoux, 1998). This function of the insular and parietal somatosensory cortices may under-

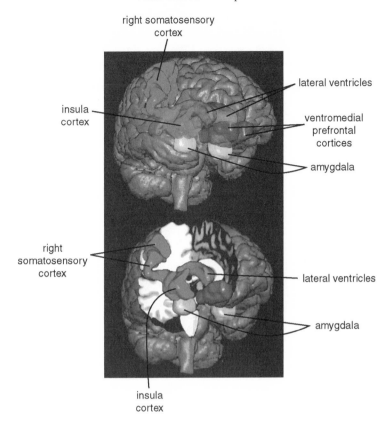

FIGURE 7.1. Neuroanatomy of some of the key structures implicated in recognition of facial emotion. Three-dimensional renderings of the amygdala, ventromedial prefrontal cortex, right somatosensory cortices (SI, SII, and insula), and, for orientation, the lateral ventricles were obtained from segmentation of these structures from serial magnetic resonance images of a normal human brain. The structures were corendered with a three-dimensional reconstruction of the entire brain (top) and a reconstruction of the brain with the anterior right quarter removed to clearly show location of the internal structures (bottom). From Adolphs (2002). Copyright 2002 by Ralph Adolphs. Reprinted by permission.

lie their important role in emotion perception (Adolphs, Damasio, Tranel, Cooper, & Damasio, 2000; Heberlein, Adolphs, Tranel, & Damasio, 2004; Winston, O'Doherty, & Dolan, 2003), which is likely to involve the activation of conceptual knowledge associated with the emotion signaled by the viewed face, perhaps via their connections with the orbitofrontal cortex and superior temporal cortex. As we discuss in the section "Emotion Recognition via Contagion . . . ," the processes that engage parietal somatosensory

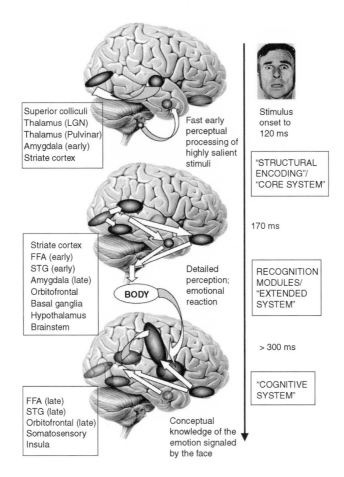

FIGURE 7.2. The time-course of emotion processing and the associated neural structures. The time-course is represented from the onset of the stimulus at the top, through perception, to final recognition of the emotion at the bottom. FFA, fusiform face area; STG, superior temporal gyrus. Many of the mechanisms outlined here may be shared when recognizing emotion from other classes of stimuli, such as body movement and prosody. From Adolphs (2002). Copyright 2002 by Ralph Adolphs. Reprinted by permission.

and insular cortices may involve simulating the viewed emotional state via the generation of a somatosensory image of the associated body state.

It is clear that the perception of any given facial configuration depends on a complex interaction of multiple brain regions and that many distinct brain regions are multifunctional, participating in a range of psychological processes. Nonetheless, neuropsychological and neurophysiological research suggests that distinct brain regions are disproportionately involved in the perception of certain facially expressed basic emotions (for a review, see Calder, Lawrence, & Young, 2001). Patients with bilateral amygdala damage have particular difficulty recognizing fearful and, in some cases, angry facial expressions in static images, but have relatively little difficulty recognizing other emotions expressed in the face, such as disgust, happiness, and sadness (e.g., Adolphs, Tranel, Damasio, & Damasio, 1994; Calder et al., 1996). In contrast, people with damage to the anterior insula and surrounding tissue have particular difficulty recognizing facial expressions of disgust, but are not so impaired at recognizing other facial expressions, including fear and anger (e.g., Calder, Keane, Manes, Antoun, & Young, 2000b; Sprengelmeyer et al., 1997). More recently, a selective impairment in the recognition of anger from facial expressions has been demonstrated in patients with damage to a region of the subcortical basal ganglia known as the ventral striatum (Calder, Keane, Lawrence, & Manes, 2004), as well as in healthy participants who are administered sulpride, an antipsychotic drug that reduces aggression and operates by blocking dopamine receptors (Lawrence, Calder, McGowan, & Grasby, 2002). Although this lesion evidence is persuasive, it is important to note that there is some criticism and evidence to the contrary (e.g., Rapcsak et al., 2000). Moreover, that amygdala damage can sometimes impair anger as well as fear perception suggests a deficit in arousal responses to signals of threat, rather than a deficit in recognizing a specific basic emotion. This interpretation is supported by the finding that bilateral amygdala damage can impair the ability to judge the level of arousal (but not the valence) in facial expressions and spoken words and sentences that depict unpleasant emotions, especially those relating to fear and anger (Adolphs, Russell, & Tranel, 1999).

One problem cited in regard to many of the older studies in the literature that reported emotion-specific impairments is that they did not adequately control for effects of differential difficulty between emotions (Rapcsak et al., 2000). Functional imaging studies with static facial expressions, however, do not appear to be subject to the possible confounds of difficulty that may be present in some of the lesion studies. Although functional imaging techniques support only correlational rather than causal claims about brain function, studies that make use of them nevertheless corroborate the inference from human lesion studies of a degree of emotion-specific functional organization in the neural substrate of emotion perception (see Murphy, Nimmo-Smith & Lawrence, 2003, and Phan, Wager, Taylor, & Liberzon, 2002, for meta-analyses of imaging studies, but see also Winston et al., 2003, for some recent counterevidence). In particular, static facial expressions of fear are associated with bilateral amygdala functioning, especially in the left hemisphere (e.g., Breiter et al., 1996; Morris et al., 1998), whereas static facial expressions of disgust are associated with functioning of the anterior insula, especially in the left hemisphere, and striatum in the right hemisphere, especially the globus pallidus and caudate nucleus (e.g., Phillips et al., 1997; Sprengelmeyer, Rausch, Eysel, & Przuntek, 1998). A recent study, however, suggests that this selective activity for expressions of fear and disgust may be restricted to conditions of conscious perception (Phillips et al., 2004). It is noteworthy that the occasional reports of amygdala activation for happy faces may well be due to the fact that those studies did not control sufficiently for personality, because the amygdala's response to happy faces, but not to expressions of fear or other basic emotions, has been positively correlated with degree of extraversion (Canli, Sivers, Whitfield, Gotlib, & Gabrieli, 2002). The few studies that have examined neural responses specifically to angry facial expressions have tended to find relatively widespread activation for anger compared to expressions of other basic emotions, yet the lateral orbitofrontal cortex appears to be a region of common overlap (Murphy et al., 2003).

In contrast to the current state of knowledge about the perception of basic emotions and its neural substrate, much less is known about the social and moral emotions, such as shame, embarrassment, pride, and guilt. What little research there is has focused on the amygdala. Baron-Cohen, Wheelwright, and Joliffe (1997) explored the recognition of complex mental and emotional states, including social emotions, from the face. Their findings were threefold: (1) such complex mental states are recognized disproportionately by information from the region of the eyes in the face (Baron-Cohen et al., 1997; Baron-Cohen, Wheelwright, Hull, Raste, & Plumb, 2001); (2) when making judgments about such states from images of the eye region of the face, normal subjects showed activation of the amygdala in functional imaging studies (Baron-Cohen et al., 1999); and (3) this amygdala activation was not found in individuals diagnosed with autism (Baron-Cohen et al., 1999), who are impaired in their ability to recognize complex mental states from the eyes. These findings, together with many others, have suggested that the severe impairments in everyday social behavior exhibited by people with autism may be attributable, in part, to dysfunction in circuits that include the amygdala (Baron-Cohen et al., 2000). Indeed, a lesion study (Adolphs, Baron-Cohen, & Tranel, 2002) found that amygdala damage resulted in a disproportionate impairment in perceiving social emotions from facial expressions, notably from the eye region of the face. Furthermore, there was some indication that, in fact, subjects with amygdala damage may be more impaired in their perception and judgments of social emotions than of basic emotions. Although preliminary, those findings are consistent with the possibility that the amygdala might be relatively specialized to process emotional information that is socially relevant—a function that may be particular to the human amygdala (Adolphs, 2003).

Although studies using static face stimuli are valuable (Lundqvist & Öhman, Chapter 5) and have yielded a good deal of knowledge about visual emotion perception and its neural substrate (Adolphs, 2002), they will not provide a complete account of emotion perception and its neural basis. For one thing, postures and movement of the body or its parts can make a substantial contribution to emotional and other nonverbal communication. For another, it is clear that dynamic portrayals of emotional expressions have greater ecological validity than static portrayals, because faces and bodies move a great deal in social interactions, especially when we are emotional, whereas emotions portrayed in static images correspond only to identifiable peaks or intermediate stages of socially meaningful movements. It is also evident that dynamic properties of emotional expressions, such as their time-course and vigor, influence recognition performance and ratings of emotional intensity (Atkinson, Dittrich, Gemmell, & Young, 2004; Kamachi et al., 2001; Pollick, Paterson, Bruderlin, & Sanford, 2001; Pollick, Hill, Calder, & Paterson, 2003). Moreover, there is now considerable evidence for the existence of a neural system, critically involving the superior temporal sulcus, dedicated to the perception of high-level motion stimuli, especially facial and body movements (for reviews, see Allison, Puce, & McCarthy, 2000; Puce & Perrett, 2003), with the suggestion that it might also play an important role in the perception of emotional expressions (Narumoto, Okada, Sadato, Fukui, & Yonekura, 2001).

It remains to be confirmed whether the circumscribed deficits in recognizing facial expressions of fear, disgust, and anger encompass both dynamic as well as static expressions, or whether the patients might derive some benefit from facial (or body) movement—or indeed, whether the patients still show a relative deficit in recognizing expressions of fear, disgust, or anger, despite deriving some benefit from movement. An early report of a patient with bilateral amygdala damage indicated that she was no better at identifying basic emotions in dynamic than static full-light facial expressions (Young, Hellawell, Van De Wal, & Johnson, 1996). As we discussed above, further studies with this and other patients with amygdala lesions have shown that the recognition deficit is most evident for expressions of fear in static faces, but the apparent lack of facilitation for facial movement has not been pursued. More recently, there has been a report of a patient with brain damage encompassing the insula in both hemispheres, whose recognition performance was significantly better for dynamic than for static facial expressions, except in the case of disgust (Adolphs, Tranel, & Damasio, 2003).

Any facilitation of emotion perception provided by dynamic compared to static expressions may well depend on a combination of the tasks and stimuli. Wehrle, Kaiser, Schmidt, and Scherer (2000) found that dynamic presentations of synthetic facial expressions increased overall recognition

accuracy and reduced confusions between unrelated emotions, compared
to static presentations of those faces, in neurologically healthy participants.
However, participants in Kamachi et al.'s (2001) study were no better at
recognizing dynamic compared to static facial expressions of sadness, happiness, surprise, and anger (where the dynamic stimuli were generated by
morphing between still images of a neutral face and an emotional expression for a given actor). Nevertheless, the speed and time-course of the facial
movements influenced forced-choice recognition accuracy: Happiness, and
to a lesser extent, surprise, were more accurately identified from faster
movements, whereas sadness was more accurately identified from slower
movements, and anger from movements of medium pace. The same pattern
of recognition accuracy was obtained in an emotion-rating task. Moreover,
Kamachi et al. found that ratings of emotional intensity tended to be higher
for the dynamic than the static expressions, when the dynamic expressions
were played at the speed that produced the best recognition performance.

Emotional intensity ratings of happy and angry facial expressions did
not differ between static and dynamic presentations in Kilts, Egan, Gideon,
Ely, and Hoffman's (2003) study. Thornton and Kourtzi (2002) found that
the time to match the emotion of a static target face (frowning or smiling)
with that of a briefly presented (540 milliseconds) prime face was essentially similar whether the prime was dynamic (from neutral to emotional
expression) or static. The same dynamic primes did, however, facilitate
reaction times for matching the identity of the same faces, compared to the
static primes. Facial movement as represented in point-light displays has
been shown to facilitate judgments of emotional expression and gender, relative to judgments from static, fully illuminated faces, in a patient with
bilateral damage to the occipital lobes who has severe visual object and
face recognition impairments (Humphreys, Donnelly, & Riddoch, 1993).
Yet patients with schizophrenia have shown impairment in recognizing
dynamic as well as static facial expressions of emotion, although movement
information does improve their ability to match the identity of unfamiliar
faces and to recognize the identity of familiar faces (Archer, Hay, & Young,
1994).

To date, only a handful of functional imaging studies has examined the
perception of dynamic facial expressions of emotion, and these studies have
used full-light but not point-light displays. Nevertheless, these studies provide further evidence for the disproportionate involvement of certain neural structures in processing signals of specific emotions. Most notably, the
amygdala was found to respond preferentially to fearful compared to
happy and angry expressions, with greater activation for dynamic face
morphs compared to static expressions and dynamic control stimuli (LaBar,
Crupain, Voyrodic, & McCarthy, 2003; Sato, Kochiyama, Yoshikawa, Naito,

& Matsumura, 2004). Furthermore, the anterior insula, and to a lesser extent, the anterior cingulate cortex, but not the amygdala, were selectively activated by dynamic facial expressions of disgust, relative to dynamic displays of emotionally neutral face movements (Wicker et al., 2003). The superior temporal sulcus was strongly implicated in the processing of facial expressions of emotion, especially dynamic portrayals, in all four of these studies, consonant with previous findings of STS involvement in the perception of biological motion, mentioned earlier. However, whereas this differential activation of the superior temporal sulcus by dynamic compared to static expressions was found for angry faces in Kilts et al.'s study and for fearful faces in Sato et al.'s study, both studies reported that it was activity in the middle temporal cortex that better differentiated dynamic from static happy faces. Note that Kilts et al.'s participants were required to make explicit judgments of emotional expression for the angry and happy faces, but judged the spatial orientation of the neutral faces. Thus it is possible that the observed differential brain activations might reflect, in part, that difference in tasks. Indeed, it is known that different tasks can differentially modulate neural responses to facial expressions (e.g., Lange et al., 2003; Phillips et al., 1997).

A SUBCORTICAL PATHWAY FOR THE UNCONSCIOUS PERCEPTION OF EMOTION?

The subcortical pathway appears to underpin the processing of information about others' emotional states, without any involvement of the visual cortex, and even, as some investigators have suggested, without any involvement of conscious awareness. One line of evidence comes from reports of patient G.Y., who has blindsight—that is, a lack of conscious visual experience for stimuli presented in part of his visual field as a result of damage to the striate cortex (V1), yet a spared ability to discriminate and localize simple visual stimuli presented in that blind field (see also de Gelder, Chapter 6). This residual vision in the blind field is thought to rely on subcortical pathways from the retina to extrastriate cortex, via the pulvinar and superior colliculus, which bypass V1 (Cowey & Stoerig, 1991). G.Y. showed significantly above-chance forced-choice discrimination of happy, sad, fearful, and angry facial expressions presented in his blind field, and he was more accurate discriminating happy and sad than angry and fearful expressions, yet he was not aware of the faces to which he responded (de Gelder, Vroomen, Pourtois, & Weiskrantz, 1999). G.Y.'s performance was considerably better for short-duration dynamic displays than for static images, with which he had only very limited success. In a later study, his performance was at chance level for nonconscious discrimination between fearful and happy static facial expressions, though interestingly, another blindsight patient, D.B., was significantly above chance at this task, and both patients successfully discriminated between fearful and happy complex static scenes presented in their blind fields (de Gelder, Pourtois, & Weiskrantz, 2002). Covert perception of the emotional content of faces appears to have consequences over and above covert perception of the emotional content of scenes in these patients, however. Event-related potentials to words spoken in fearful or happy tones were modulated by the emotional congruency of fearful and happy faces as well as scenes when presented in D.B.'s and G.Y.'s good visual fields, but only by the emotional congruency of the faces when presented in their blind fields (de Gelder et al., 2002). Static faces elicited early extrastriate occipital activity when presented either in G.Y.'s good or blind hemifields, beginning at about 120 milliseconds poststimulus onset for his good field and at about 140 milliseconds for his blind field, demonstrating that V1 activity is not necessary for an extrastriate response to these static images (Rossion, de Gelder, Pourtois, Guerit, & Weiskrantz, 2000). When scanned using functional magnetic resonance imaging (fMRI), differential amygdala activity was observed in G.Y. to fearful versus happy static faces presented either to his blind or seeing hemifield, whereas striate, fusiform, and prefrontal activation was observed only for faces presented to his seeing hemifield (Morris, de Gelder, Weiskrantz, & Dolan, 2001). Although this is tantalizing evidence that the subcortical route to the amygdala subserves covert emotion perception, it is not conclusive, because the relatively poor temporal resolution of fMRI does not allow an alternative explanation to be ruled out, namely, that the amygdala activity to emotional faces is due to feedback to the amygdala from extrastriate cortices.

A second line of evidence that the subcortical pathway can subserve covert emotion perception comes from functional imaging studies with healthy volunteers. Morris, Öhman, and Dolan (1999) found that aversively conditioned static angry expressions enhanced the activity of the right amygdala when the faces were presented very briefly and backward masked, such that they were not consciously seen, whereas these faces enhanced activity of the left amygdala only when they were unmasked and thus consciously seen, replicating these authors' earlier findings (Morris et al., 1998). Importantly, the responses of the pulvinar and superior colliculus were positively correlated, whereas the responses of the fusiform and orbitofrontal cortices were negatively correlated, with the right amygdala response to the masked angry ("unseen") faces. Even without aversive conditioning, backward-masked presentations of fearful expressions can increase, whereas happy expressions decrease amygdala activity relative to neutral expressions (Whalen et al., 1998). However, in a more recent study,

Phillips et al. (2004) did not find significant amygdala activation to sublimi-nally presented masked fearful faces. Killgore and Yurgelun-Todd (2004) reported significant bilateral amygdala and anterior cingulate activation to subliminally presented masked happy faces, and left anterior cingulate but no amygdala activation to masked sad facial expressions—which, they argue, is not consistent with the subcortical pathway account of covert emotion perception.

Although most of these studies support the idea that a subcortical pathway from the retina to amygdala subserves covert emotion percep-tion, that interpretation is not watertight for two reasons, at least. First, the reported amygdala activity in response to emotional expressions in the absence of awareness might, in fact, reflect the amygdala's involve-ment in degraded but intact processing in cortical systems that subserve face and emotion perception (e.g., Pessoa, Kastner, & Ungerleider, 2002; Rolls, 1999). Second, the data may be subject to criterion effects. That is, subjects could be reporting that they were unaware of the stimulus or of the particular emotion when they were not completely sure about their response. Two recent studies attempted to address these problems and together strengthen the claim that the subcortical pathway to the amyg-dala is a neural substrate of unconscious emotion perception. Pasley, Mayes, and Schultz (2004) used fMRI in conjunction with binocular rivalry to investigate the subcortical discrimination of fearful faces versus non-face objects when these stimuli were not consciously perceived. Bin-ocular rivalry occurs when different monocular stimuli (such as a face and a chair) are presented independently to the two eyes. After a few seconds of apparently monocular perception, the dominant image is replaced by the other completely monocular image. This procedure allows the experi-menter to determine the effect of a visual stimulus that we can be more confident the participant does not consciously perceive (e.g., Crick, 1996). Pasley et al. found left amygdala but not inferotemporal cortex activation to unperceived or suppressed fearful static faces, compared to a non-face object, consonant with the proposition of a subcortical route to the amygdala that subserves unconscious emotion perception. The activation of the amygdala via this subcortical route does not appear to be limited to expressions of fear, however. Also using fMRI, Williams, Morris, McGlone, Abbott, and Mattingley (2004) found increased amygdala activity to both fearful and happy, compared to neutral, static faces when the faces were suppressed (bilateral for fear; right hemisphere for happy), but only to fearful faces when they were consciously perceived (right amygdala). This finding suggests that the activity of a subregion of the amygdala (primar-ily in the right hemisphere) does not differentiate between threatening and nonthreatening facial expressions, at least when the subcortical route is selectively engaged.

PERCEIVING EMOTIONS FROM BODY EXPRESSIONS AND OTHER DYNAMIC VISUAL STIMULI

Body posture and movement stimuli have rarely been used in investigations of emotion perception in patient populations or in functional imaging studies. Yet characteristic body postures and movements indicate specific emotional states (e.g., Wallbott, 1998), and distinct expressions of at least the basic emotions are readily recognized in the absence of facial and vocal cues when portrayed by static body postures (e.g., Atkinson et al., 2004) and by whole-body movement (e.g., Atkinson et al., 2004; Dittrich, Troscianko, Lea, & Morgan, 1996). The neural substrate of emotion perception from body expressions is beginning to be revealed. Three brain regions have been implicated so far, all of which are also involved in the processing of facially expressed emotion: the amygdala and the fusiform and somatosensory cortices.

Sprengelmeyer et al. (1999) reported a patient with bilateral amygdala damage who has a deficit in recognizing fear from static body postures as well as from static faces. However, the amygdala's role in processing emotional information from bodies may be less important than its role in processing emotional information from faces. Adolphs and Tranel (2003) showed that bilateral amygdala damage reduces the ability to recognize emotions from static images of complex social scenes when subjects utilize information from facial expressions, but not for negative emotions when the faces are obscured, such that participants have to rely on other cues such as body posture, hand gestures, and interpersonal stances. Remarkably, patients with bilateral amygdala damage were, in fact, more accurate in recognizing anger from scenes with faces erased than with faces present—a response that Adolphs and Tranel (2003) attribute, in part, to their particular impairment in recognizing anger from faces shown in isolation. The amygdala has also been implicated as a key structure in the processing of static, fearful body expressions, along with several cortical regions, including the fusiform cortex, in two fMRI studies (de Gelder, Snyder, Greve, Gerard, & Hadjikhani, 2004; Hadjikhani & de Gelder, 2003).

Further studies are required that employ dynamic as well as static body stimuli, along with expressions of other emotions. Heberlein et al.'s (2004) study is step in this direction. These researchers found that impairments in judging emotions from point-light walkers were associated with damage to several components of a network of neural structures, in which the most reliable region of lesion overlap associated with this impairment was in the right somatosensory cortices. In contrast, impairments in judging personality traits from point-light walkers were associated with damage to the left frontal operculum. The involvement of right somatosensory cortices in emotion perception from these dynamic stimuli parallels the role of these structures in emotion perception from static facial expressions, as demonstrated by a study involving over 100 patients with focal brain damage, which also found that impaired emotion perception correlated best with right somatosensory cortex lesions (Adolphs et al., 2000).

As mentioned above, the superior temporal cortex appears to be selectively involved in processing body (as well as facial) movement, as opposed to nonbiological motion and static body (and facial) form (e.g., Grossman et al., 2000). Activity in the lingual gyrus, especially at the cuneus border (Servos, Osu, Santi, & Kawato, 2002; Vaina, Solomon, Chowdhury, Sinha, & Belliveau, 2001), and in the occipital and fusiform face areas (Grossman & Blake, 2002) also distinguishes biological from nonbiological motion. But very little is yet known about the roles these areas play in processing body expressions of emotion—for example, whether their contribution is simply in the processing of biological motion, regardless of emotional content, or whether some part of these areas might be specialized for processing the emotional meaning of body (and perhaps also facial) movement.

Another interesting class of pure visual motion stimuli that conveys emotional and social information consists of displays in which social interactions are depicted by relative visual motion between multiple objects. One such stimulus shows simple geometric shapes moving on a plain white background (Figure 7.3). Solely on the basis of the movements of these shapes, normal subjects attribute social and emotional states to the objects (Heider & Simmel, 1944). The reliable, automatic, and obligatory emotional and social perception triggered by this visual motion stimulus has been confirmed in numerous studies (Berry, Misovich, Kean, & Baron, 1992). Intriguingly, such simple geometric shapes can, in virtue of their motion, activate the fusiform face area in humans (Schultz et al., 2003); furthermore, people with autism (Klin, 2000) or bilateral amygdala damage (Heberlein & Adolphs, 2004) fail to perceive this stimulus in emotional–social terms. This impairment was most striking in a rare subject with bilat-

FIGURE 7.3. A representation of a frame from a version of the Heider and Simmel (1944) video.

eral amygdala damage, who perceived the geometric motion of the stimuli entirely accurately, but completely failed to see any emotional or social meaning in those movements.

EMOTION RECOGNITION VIA CONTAGION OR SIMULATION

How do we come to associate particular postures and movements of another's face and body with specific emotional states? Several closely related proposals, which are examples of the "embodied cognition" concept (e.g., Niedenthal et al., in press), center on the idea that processes of emotional contagion or simulation (or both) provide the means by which we come to know what others are feeling. Here we provide a brief summary of this class of proposals and the experimental findings that support them; the proposals are delineated in more detail elsewhere (Atkinson, in preparation; Goldman & Sripada, 2005; see also Niedenthal et al., Chapter 2).

The idea that emotional contagion underpins emotion recognition is the view that a visual representation of another's expression leads us to experience what that person is feeling, which then allows us to infer that person's emotional state. Current versions of this idea say little, if anything, about the latter, inferential process, but all state or assume that the grounds for inferring the viewed person's emotional state is knowledge from the "inside," that experiencing the emotion for oneself (even in an attenuated or unconscious form) is an important, perhaps necessary, step to making accurate inferences about others' emotions. This perspective suggests a close connection between the neural substrates of emotion perception and emotional experience. The perceptual mechanisms might relay information to separate mechanisms underlying emotional experience, either directly or via facial mimicry, or the perceptual mechanisms might also subserve emotional experience (see also Barrett, Chapter 11; Prinz, Chapter 15). A different but conceivably compatible idea is that coming to know what another is feeling involves simulating the viewed emotional state via the generation of a somatosensory image of the associated body state, or simulating the motor programs for producing the viewed expression.

There is direct evidence that at least some of the neural systems involved in emotion perception mediate emotional experience as well. For example, somatosensory and cingulate cortices were prominent among those structures engaged by the recall of personal episodes of happiness, sadness, anger, and fear (Damasio et al., 2000), and the medial prefrontal cortex was engaged during episodes of positive and negative emotion, and by more specific experience of happiness, sadness, and disgust, as induced by emotional films, pictures, and recall (Lane, Reiman, Ahern, Schwartz, & Davidson, 1997; Lane, Reiman, Bradley, et al., 1997). Moreover, several studies support a degree of emotion-specific processing consonant with the emotion perception literature. For example, procaine-induced feelings of intense fear were associated with significant left amygdala activity, compared to euphoric feelings, in a study by Ketter et al. (1996), and direct electrical stimulation within the medial temporal lobe, primarily of the amygdala and hippocampus, evoked unpleasant feelings that were predominantly reported as fear or anxiety (Halgren, Walter, Cherlow, & Crandall, 1978). Direct stimulation of insula neurons can generate reports of unpleasant sensations in the throat, spreading up to the mouth, lips, and nose (Krolak-Salmon et al., 2003), responses related more to disgust than to other emotions, though so can stimulation of the amygdala and hippocampus, which can also elicit sensations in the stomach that are typically described as nausea (Halgren et al., 1978). More recently, Wicker et al. (2003) found anterior insula activation when participants felt disgusted as well as when they saw someone else produce genuine expressions of disgust.

A large degree of overlap or close connection between the neural substrates of emotion perception and emotional experience is also suggested by the finding that patients who have circumscribed emotion perception deficits may also have a corresponding circumscribed deficit in their phenomenal experience of the same emotions (e.g., Calder, Keane, Manes, et al., 2000; Sprengelmeyer et al., 1997). However, not all such patients appear to have abnormal emotional experience. For example, amygdala lesions do not necessarily impair emotional experience, either as assessed by a questionnaire asking about the typicality of experienced positive and negative emotions, or by a daily diary record of experienced positive and negative emotions (Anderson & Phelps, 2002). Thus whereas emotion perception may engage processes that are also involved in emotional experience, either their engagement is not necessary for emotion perception, or, if those processes are necessarily engaged, then their operation may not necessarily produce the relevant emotional experience. Nevertheless, we should record a caveat here: Given the difficulty of obtaining accurate and reliable online measures of specific emotions (for a review, see Barrett, Chapter 11), and that such measures have rarely been used in the patient studies, the possibility is left open that any processes of emotional contagion or mental simulation underpinning emotion perception may involve, at least as a by-product, subjects' experience of the emotion they are viewing in another as they are viewing it.

Further evidence that contagion or simulation, or both, may also play a role in recognition of the actions that comprise emotional facial expressions comes from disparate experiments. The experience and expression of emotion can be correlated (Rosenberg & Ekman, 1994; although they need not be—see Cacioppo, Berntson, Larsen, Poehlmann, & Ito, 2000) and offer an intriguing causal relationship: Production of emotional facial expressions (Adelmann & Zajonc, 1989) and other somatovisceral responses (Cacioppo, Berntson, & Klein, 1992) can lead to changes in emotional experience. Producing a facial expression to command influences the feeling and autonomic correlates of the emotional state (Levenson, Ekman, & Friesen, 1990) as well as its electroencephalographic (EEG) correlates (Ekman & Davidson, 1993). Viewing facial expressions results in expressions on one's own face that may not be readily visible but that can be measured with facial electromyography (EMG; Dimberg, 1982) and that mimic the expression shown in the stimulus (Hess & Blairy, 2001), even in the absence of conscious recognition of the stimulus (Dimberg, Thunberg, & Elmehed, 2000; see also Lundqvist & Öhman, Chapter 5). Viewing facial expressions can also elicit autonomic correlates indicative of a change in emotional state, such as the skin conductance response (Dimberg, 1982), even during unconscious stimulus presentations (Williams et al., 2004) and changes in feeling (Schneider, Gur, Gur, & Muenz, 1994; Wild, Erb, & Bartels, 2001).

We have already mentioned the finding that lesions involving right somatosensory cortices (including SI, SII, and the insular cortex) are associated with a general impairment in the recognition of emotion from facial (Adolphs et al., 2000) and body (Heberlein et al., 2004) expressions. These findings suggest that emotion recognition may involve simulating the viewed emotional state via the generation of a somatosensory image of the associated body state. Indeed, Adolphs et al. (2000) also found a correlation between impaired perception of emotion from facial expressions and impaired somatic touch sensation in the viewer! What is not yet clear, however, is exactly how somatosensory cortices contribute to emotion perception. If, for example, emotion recognition involves the unintentional mimicry of the viewed expression, then one might expect the activity of the facial muscles to be reflected in the face regions of primary and secondary somatosensory cortices, which raises the question of whether it is such proprioceptive activity that plays a role in emotion recognition, either directly or by inducing the corresponding emotional state. The possibility has also been raised of a more direct connection between the visual processing of emotional expressions and activity in the primary and secondary somatosensory cortices, which does not involve mimicry of the other's expressions: namely, that observing another's facial emotion directly elicits the proprioceptive activity in the observer appropriate to the viewed expression, as if the observer were making the movements him- or herself (what Goldman & Sripada, 2004, call "reverse simulation with 'as if' loop").

(In the case of observing emotional body postures and movements, one might also expect activity in regions representing proprioceptive information about the corresponding parts of the observer's body.) Another possibility is that primary and secondary somatosensory cortex activity in emotion perception arises as a consequence of the offline simulation of another's facial (or body) movements, either as a by-product of that simulation process or as a causal link in the chain leading eventually to emotion recognition and attribution.

Both lesion and imaging studies indicate a more general role for the insula cortex in emotion perception, in addition to the role its anterior portion seems to play in the perception and experience of disgust. The insula's role in emotional experience is likely linked to its function in representing visceral and other interoceptive, rather than proprioceptive, information (Craig, 2003), suggesting several possibilities for which one would expect insula involvement in emotion perception. One is that viewing an emotional expression induces that same emotion in the observer, either directly or via some mediating process such as motor mimicry. Another possibility is that visual representations of the emotional expression directly modulate interoceptive structures that generate the feeling, without causing actual bodily changes—that is, the offline simulation of an emotional state (akin to Damasio's, 1994, 1999, "as-if" loop). That this simulation proposal requires the possibility of such a direct, central mechanism is borne out by the finding that patients with congenital facial paralysis are able nonetheless to recognize facial emotion (Calder, Keane, Cole, et al., 2000).

If emotion perception involves mimicking the viewed expression or executing its motor program offline, then we might expect to find neural mechanisms common to both the perception and production of facial expressions. Evidence of such a common neural substrate comes from work on mirror neurons. Neurons in the premotor cortex of monkeys respond not only when the monkey prepares to perform an action itself, but also when the monkey observes the same visually presented action performed by another individual (monkey or human, e.g., Rizzolatti, Fadiga, Gallese, & Fogassi, 1996). Various supportive findings have also been obtained in humans. Observing another's actions results in desynchronization in the motor cortex, as measured with magnetoencephalography (Hari et al., 1998), and lowers the threshold for producing motor responses when transcranial magnetic stimulation is used to activate the motor cortex (Strafella & Paus, 2000). Imitating another's actions via observation activates the premotor cortex in functional imaging studies (Iacoboni et al., 1999); moreover, such activation is somatotopic with regard to the body part that is observed to perform the action, even in the absence of any overt action on the part of the subject (Buccino et al., 2001). There may also be

mirror neurons for emotional facial actions: A largely similar neural network is activated when subjects either passively view or deliberately imitate static facial expressions of basic emotions (Carr, Iacoboni, Dubeau,
Maziotta, & Lenzi, 2003) and dynamic smiling and frowning expressions
(Leslie, Johnson-Frey, & Grafton, 2004). Premotor areas, especially the
inferior prefrontal area responsible for face movement, are prominent in
this network. Imitation elicited greater and more bilateral activation of
these areas than passive viewing, corresponding to an additive effect of
expression observation and execution. Other regions implicated in this network include the superior temporal cortex (in both studies), insula, and
amygdala (in Carr et al.'s study).

The findings discussed so far suggest that viewing dynamic expressions may facilitate simulation, compared to static expressions. However,
the results of one study were taken by its authors to suggest the opposite,
namely, that emotion perception in dynamic facial expressions relies less on
motor simulation. Kilts et al. (2003) found that judging the emotional intensity of static, but not dynamic angry and happy, compared to neutral, faces
activated cortical motor-related regions, including primary motor and
premotor cortices, and the left somatosensory cortex. Presumably the idea
is that the brain, in implementing a simulation process, has to try harder or
do more to decipher the emotion in static compared to dynamic images.
Clearly, though, this interpretation is in stark contrast to our earlier suggestion that the dynamic production of an expression is more likely to be simulated than some snapshot at or near the emotional peak. A decision
between these alternatives awaits further research, using facial and body
expressions.

CLOSING REMARKS

Regions of the visual cortex and certain other structures, including the
amygdala and insula, appear to be relatively specialized to process emotionally and socially relevant information. Some of this processing occurs
very early in time, subsequent to the onset of an emotionally salient visual
stimulus, with latencies around 100–300 milliseconds. It is likely that much
of this early processing is driven by feed-forward connections between
lower visual areas and higher regions, including the amygdala. Yet, as we
noted, the amygdala also receives emotional information via a subcortical
pathway involving the superior colliculus and pulvinar; this pathway might
underpin the processing of information about others' emotional states without the involvement of the visual cortex—and even without any conscious
awareness. There are at least three reasons to suspect that this early cortical

and subcortical processing does not contribute directly to the contents of our conscious perceptual experience of the emotional expression (Prinz, Chapter 15; Clore, Storbeck, Robinson, & Centerbar, Chapter 16). First, it happens too quickly, apparently permitting insufficient time for a window within which integrated neural activity could generate a conscious percept (cf. Libet, 1981). Indeed, the early phase of emotional information processing can occur with stimuli that are either backward masked or suppressed under binocular rivalry, and especially in the latter case we can be sure that the emotional expression cannot be consciously perceived. A second reason to doubt that the informational contents of such early processing constitute the contents of our conscious perception of the emotional expression is that the representation of the stimulus or of the emotional response that the stimulus produces is somewhat impoverished or lacking in detail, relative to the properties of the visual world represented in experience. That is, the information that is represented by such early processing looks to be of a much coarser grain than our conscious experience. For example, the subcortical route to the amygdala carries only low-spatial-frequency information that is nevertheless sufficient to activate the amygdala in response to fearful faces (Vuilleumier, Armony, Driver, & Dolan, 2003), yet we experience the stimulus with much richer perceptual and emotional content. Hence it is prima facie doubtful that the contents of this early processing are directly related to the contents of conscious perception. (Nevertheless, they could be related indirectly, insofar as the informational contents of this early processing might contribute to, or be necessary precursors of, the informational contents that constitute the contents of experience.) A third reason is more empirical: Recent findings argue strongly that feedback projections from higher processing stages back to lower ones are necessary in order for conscious experience to occur (e.g., Pascual-Leone & Walsh, 2001).

Nonetheless, research (Pascual-Leone & Walsh, 2001) has also shown that conscious experience depends on lower-processing regions, anatomically—just at a later point in time. So, although conscious processing requires temporally later stages, it draws upon anatomical regions that are both "higher" and "lower" in a processing hierarchy. Occipital visual cortices, the amygdala, and other structures that are engaged very early in processing do indeed contribute directly to conscious experience, but they do so during a later iteration of processing, when the activity driven by the external stimulus can be compared with activity driven by feedback from higher regions. Thus it is fallacious to assign conscious perception to any particular anatomical regions: Both anatomy and time are critical. Certain sets of structures, engaged at certain points in time, are the subvenience base for conscious experience.

Having said this much, an obvious next question is: What is the content of the conscious experiences so generated? Suppose we see an emotional facial expression. Our argument has been that perception of the emotion can include at least the following components. We perceive the structural features of the visual stimulus (i.e., the features of the face and their configuration). We also perceive the emotion shown in the face, and, we have argued, one mechanism whereby we do that is by perceiving our own emotional response to the face shown. This latter component depends on first triggering an emotional response to the face, via structures such as the amygdala, and second, neurally representing that emotional response, via structures such as the somatosensory cortices and insula. Finally, the way we actually perceive the emotional face in our conscious awareness is not merely as a combination of these different components, but as the face imbued with the emotion that we attribute to it. A key open question concerns exactly how this process occurs. From what we have said so far, we might expect that the viewer would simply perceive a face, and perceive his or her own emotional state. But that is not what happens—the emotional state is attributed to the face, not to oneself as the viewer. Clearly, there must be mechanisms in place that automatically prevent such misattribution and permit the emotion to be linked to the stimulus in the right way. The sense of self—and thus the ability to distinguish between self and others when attributing emotions, thoughts, and actions—develops as a consequence of interpersonal interactions and a capacity to imitate, and may well be implemented by a system involving the inferior parietal cortex in conjunction with the prefrontal cortex (Decety & Chaminade, 2003).

ACKNOWLEDGMENTS

The writing of this chapter was aided by a conference travel grant awarded to Anthony P. Atkinson by the British Academy. Ralph Adolphs's work reported here was funded by grants from the U.S. National Institutes of Health and the James S. McDonnell Foundation. We are grateful to Lisa Feldman Barrett and Piotr Winkielman for helpful comments on an earlier version of the chapter.

REFERENCES

Adelmann, P. K., & Zajonc, R. B. (1989). Facial efference and the experience of emotion. *Annual Review of Psychology, 40,* 249–280.
Adolphs, R. (2002). Recognizing emotion from facial expressions: Psychological and neurological mechanisms. *Behavioral and Cognitive Neuroscience Reviews, 1,* 21–62.

Adolphs, R. (2003). Is the human amygdala specialized for social cognition? *Annals of the New York Academy of Sciences, 985,* 326–340.

Adolphs, R., Baron-Cohen, S., & Tranel, D. (2002). Impaired recognition of social emotions following amygdala damage. *Journal of Cognitive Neuroscience, 14,* 1264–1274.

Adolphs, R., Damasio, H., Tranel, D., Cooper, G., & Damasio, A. R. (2000). A role for somatosensory cortices in the visual recognition of emotion as revealed by 3–D lesion mapping. *Journal of Neuroscience, 20,* 2683–2690.

Adolphs, R., Russell, J. A., & Tranel, D. (1999). A role for the human amygdala in recognizing emotional arousal from unpleasant stimuli. *Psychological Science, 10,* 167–171.

Adolphs, R., & Tranel, D. (2003). Amygdala damage impairs emotion recognition from scenes only when they contain facial expressions. *Neuropsychologia, 41,* 1281–1289.

Adolphs, R., Tranel, D., & Damasio, A. R. (2003). Dissociable neural systems for recognizing emotions. *Brain and Cognition, 52,* 61–69.

Adolphs, R., Tranel, D., Damasio, H., & Damasio, A. (1994). Impaired recognition of emotion in facial expressions following bilateral damage to the human amygdala. *Nature, 372,* 669–672.

Allison, T., Puce, A., & McCarthy, G. (2000). Social perception from visual cues: Role of the STS region. *Trends in Cognitive Sciences, 4,* 267–278.

Anderson, A. K., & Phelps, E. A. (2002). Is the human amygdala critical for the subjective experience of emotion? Evidence of intact dispositional affect in patients with amygdala lesions. *Journal of Cognitive Neuroscience, 14,* 709–720.

Archer, J., Hay, D. C., & Young, A. W. (1994). Movement, face processing and schizophrenia: Evidence of a differential deficit in expression analysis. *British Journal of Clinical Psychology, 33,* 517–528.

Atkinson, A. P. (in preparation). Face processing and empathy. In T .F. D. Farrow & P. W. R. Woodruff (Eds.), *Empathy in mental illness and health.* Cambridge, UK: Cambridge University Press.

Atkinson, A. P., Dittrich, W. H., Gemmell, A. J., & Young, A. W. (2004). Emotion perception from dynamic and static body expressions in point-light and full-light displays. *Perception, 33,* 717–746.

Baron-Cohen, S., Ring, H. A., Bullmore, E. T., Wheelwright, S., Ashwin, C., & Williams, S. C. R. (2000). The amygdala theory of autism. *Neuroscience and Biobehavioral Reviews, 24,* 355–364.

Baron-Cohen, S., Ring, H. A., Wheelwright, S., Bullmore, E. T., Brammer, M. J., Simmons, A., & Williams, S. C. R. (1999). Social intelligence in the normal and autistic brain: An fMRI study. *European Journal of Neuroscience, 11,* 1891–1898.

Baron-Cohen, S., Wheelwright, S., Hill, J., Raste, Y., & Plumb, I. (2001). The "reading the mind in the eyes" test revised version: A study with normal adults, and adults with Asperger syndrome or high-functioning autism. *Journal of Child Psychology and Psychiatry, 42,* 241–251.

Baron-Cohen, S., Wheelwright, S., & Joliffe, T. (1997). Is there a "language of the eyes"? Evidence from normal adults and adults with autism or Asperger syndrome. *Visual Cognition, 4,* 311–332.

Barsalou, L. W., Simmons, W. K., Barbey, A. K., & Wilson, C. D. (2003). Grounding conceptual knowledge in modality-specific systems. *Trends in Cognitive Sciences, 7,* 84–91.

Bassili, J. N. (1978). Facial motion in the perception of faces and of emotional expression. *Journal of Experimental Psychology: Human Perception and Performance, 4,* 373–379.

Berry, D. S., Misovich, S. J., Kean, K. J., & Baron, R. M. (1992). Effects of disruptions of structure and motion on perceptions of social causality. *Personality and Social Psychology Bulletin, 18,* 237–244.

Breiter, H. C., Etcoff, N. L., Whalen, P. J., Kennedy, W. A., Rauch, S. L., Buckner, R. L., Strauss, M. M., Hyman, S. E., & Rosen, B. R. (1996). Response and habituation of the human amygdala during visual processing of facial expression. *Neuron, 17,* 875–887.

Buccino, G., Binkofski, F., Fink, G. R., Fadiga, L., Fogassi, L., Gallese, V. V., Seitz, R. J., Zilles, K., Rizzolatti, G., & Freund, H.-J. (2001). Action observation activates premotor and parietal areas in a somatotopic manner: An fMRI study. *European Journal of Neuroscience, 13,* 400–404.

Cacioppo, J. T., Berntson, G. G., & Klein, D. J. (1992). What is an emotion? The role of somatovisceral afference, with special emphasis on somatovisceral "illusions." In M. S. Clark (Ed.), *Emotion and social behavior* (Vol. 14, pp. 63–98). Newbury Park, CA: Sage.

Cacioppo, J. T., Berntson, G. G., Larsen, J. T., Poehlmann, K. M., & Ito, T. A. (2000). The psychophysiology of emotion. In R. Lewis & J. M. Haviland-Jones (Eds.), *Handbook of emotions* (2nd ed., pp. 173–191). New York: Guilford Press.

Calder, A. J., Keane, J., Cole, J., Campbell, R., & Young, A. W. (2000). Facial expression recognition by people with Möbius syndrome. *Cognitive Neuropsychology, 17,* 73–87.

Calder, A. J., Keane, J., Lawrence, A. D., & Manes, F. (2004). Impaired recognition of anger following damage to the ventral striatum. *Brain, 127,* 1958–1969.

Calder, A. J., Keane, J., Manes, F., Antoun, N., & Young, A. W. (2000). Impaired recognition and experience of disgust following brain injury. *Nature Neuroscience, 3,* 1077–1078.

Calder, A. J., Lawrence, A. D., & Young, A. W. (2001). Neuropsychology of fear and loathing. *Nature Reviews Neuroscience, 2,* 352–363.

Calder, A. J., Young, A. W., Rowland, D., Perrett, D. I., Hodges, J. R., & Etcoff, N. L. (1996). Facial emotion recognition after bilateral amygdala damage: Differentially severe impairment of fear. *Cognitive Neuropsychology, 13,* 699–745.

Canli, T., Sivers, H., Whitfield, S. L., Gotlib, I. H., & Gabrieli, J. D. E. (2002). Amygdala response to happy faces as a function of extraversion. *Science, 296,* 2191–2191.

Carmichael, S. T., & Price, J. L. (1995). Limbic connections of the orbital and medial prefrontal cortex in macaque monkeys. *Journal of Comparative Neurology, 363,* 615–641.

Carr, L., Iacoboni, M., Dubeau, M. C., Mazziotta, J. C., & Lenzi, G. L. (2003). Neural mechanisms of empathy in humans: A relay from neural systems for imitation to limbic areas. *Proceedings of the National Academy of Sciences, 100,* 5497–5502.

Cosmides, L., & Tooby, J. (2000). Evolutionary psychology and the emotions. In M. Lewis & J. M. Haviland-Jones (Eds.), *Handbook of emotions* (2nd ed., pp. 91–115). New York: Guilford Press.

Cowey, A., & Stoerig, P. (1991). The neurobiology of blindsight. *Trends in Neurosciences, 14,* 140–145.

Craig, A. D. (2003). Interoception: The sense of the physiological condition of the body. *Current Opinion in Neurobiology, 13,* 500–505.

Crick, F. (1996). Visual perception: Rivalry and consciousness. *Nature, 379,* 485–486.

Cutting, J. E., & Kozlowski, L. T. (1977). Recognizing friends by their walk: Gait perception without familiarity cues. *Bulletin of the Psychonomic Society, 9,* 353–356.

Damasio, A. R. (1994). *Descartes' error: Emotion, reason, and the human brain.* New York: Grosset/Putnam.

Damasio, A. R. (1999). *The feeling of what happens: Body and emotion in the making of consciousness.* New York: Harcourt Brace.

Damasio, A. R., Grabowski, T. J., Bechara, A., Damasio, H., Ponto, L. L., Parvizi, J., et al. (2000). Subcortical and cortical brain activity during the feeling of self-generated emotions. *Nature Neuroscience, 3,* 1049–1056.

Darwin, C. (1998). *The expression of the emotions in man and animals* (3rd ed.; P. Ekman, Ed.). London: Harper Collins. (Original work published 1872)

Decety, J., & Chaminade, T. (2003). When the self represents the other: A new cognitive neuroscience view on psychological identification. *Consciousness and Cognition, 12,* 577–596.

de Gelder, B., Pourtois, G., & Weiskrantz, L. (2002). Fear recognition in the voice is modulated by unconsciously recognized facial expressions but not by unconsciously recognized affective pictures. *Proceedings of the National Academy of Sciences, 99,* 4121–4126.

de Gelder, B., Vroomen, J., Pourtois, G., & Weiskrantz, L. (1999). Non-conscious recognition of affect in the absence of striate cortex. *NeuroReport, 10,* 3759–3763.

Dimberg, U. (1982). Facial reactions to facial expressions. *Psychophysiology, 19,* 643–647.

Dimberg, U., Thunberg, M., & Elmehed, K. (2000). Unconscious facial reactions to emotional facial expressions. *Psychological Science, 11,* 86–89.

Dittrich, W. H., Troscianko, T., Lea, S. E. G., & Morgan, D. (1996). Perception of emotion from dynamic point-light displays represented in dance. *Perception, 25,* 727–738.

Dretske, F. I. (1969). *Seeing and knowing.* London: Routledge & Kegan Paul.

Ekman, P. (1992). An argument for basic emotions. *Cognition and Emotion, 6,* 169–200.

Ekman, P., & Davidson, R. J. (1993). Voluntary smiling changes regional brain activity. *Psychological Science, 4,* 342–345.

Esteves, F., Parra, C., Dimberg, U., & Öhman, A. (1994). Nonconscious associative learning: Pavlovian conditioning of skin conductance responses to masked fear-relevant facial stimuli. *Psychophysiology, 31,* 375–385.

Fox, R., & McDaniel, C. (1982). The perception of biological motion by human infants. *Science, 218,* 486–487.

Goldman, A. I., & Sripada, C. S. (2005). Simulationist models of face-based emotion recognition. *Cognition, 94,* 193–213.

Grossman, E. D., Donnelly, M., Price, R., Pickens, D., Morgan, V., Neighbor, G., & Blake, R. (2000). Brain areas involved in perception of biological motion. *Journal of Cognitive Neuroscience, 12,* 711–720.

Grossman, E. D., & Blake, R. (2002). Brain areas active during visual perception of biological motion. *Neuron, 35,* 1167–1175.

Gunns, R. E., Johnston, L., & Hudson, S. M. (2002). Victim selection and kinematics: A point-light investigation of vulnerability to attack. *Journal of Nonverbal Behavior, 26,* 129–158.

Hadjikhani, N., & de Gelder, B. (2003). Seeing fearful body expressions activates the fusiform cortex and amygdala. *Current Biology, 13,* 2201–2205.

Halgren, E., Walter, R. D., Cherlow, D. G., & Crandall, P. H. (1978). Mental phenomena evoked by electrical stimulation of the human hippocampal formation and amygdala. *Brain, 101,* 83–117.

Hari, R., Forss, N., Avikainen, S., Kirveskari, E., Salenius, S., & Rizzolatti, G. (1998). Activation of human primary motor cortex during action observation: A neuromagnetic study. *Proceedings of the National Academy of Sciences, 95,* 15061–15065.

Heberlein, A. S., Adolphs, R., Tranel, D., & Damasio, H. (2004). Cortical regions for judgments of emotions and personality traits from point-light walkers. *Journal of Cognitive Neuroscience, 16,* 1143–1158.

Heider, F., & Simmel, M. (1944). An experimental study of apparent behavior. *American Journal of Psychology, 57,* 243–259.

Hess, U., & Blairy, S. (2001). Facial mimicry and emotional contagion to dynamic emotional facial expressions and their influence on decoding accuracy. *International Journal of Psychophysiology, 40,* 129–141.

Hill, H., & Pollick, F. E. (2000). Exaggerating temporal differences enhance recognition of individuals from point light displays. *Psychological Science, 11,* 223–228.

Humphreys, G. W., Donnelly, N., & Riddoch, M. J. (1993). Expression is computed separately from facial identity, and it is computed separately for moving and static faces: Neuropsychological evidence. *Neuropsychologia, 31,* 173–181.

Iacoboni, M., Woods, R. P., Brass, M., Bekkering, H., Mazziotta, J. C., & Rizzolatti, G. (1999). Cortical mechanisms of human imitation. *Science, 286,* 2526–2528.

Iidaka, T., Omori, M., Murata, T., Kosaka, H., Yonekura, Y., Okada, T., & Sadato, N. (2001). Neural interaction of the amygdala with the prefrontal and temporal cortices in the processing of facial expressions as revealed by fMRI. *Journal of Cognitive Neuroscience, 13,* 1035–1047.

Johansson, G. (1973). Visual perception of biological motion and a model for its analysis. *Perception and Psychophysics, 14,* 201–211.

Kamachi, M., Bruce, V., Mukaida, S., Gyoba, J., Yoshikawa, S., & Akamatsu, S. (2001). Dynamic properties influence the perception of facial expressions. *Perception, 30,* 875–887.

Ketter, T. A., Andreason, P. J., George, M. S., Lee, C., Gill, D. S., Parekh, P. I., Willis, M. W., Herscovitch, P., & Post, R. M. (1996). Anterior paralimbic mediation of procaine-induced emotional and psychosensory experiences. *Archives of General Psychiatry, 53,* 59–69.

Killgore, W. D., & Yurgelun-Todd, D. A. (2004). Activation of the amygdala and anterior cingulate during nonconscious processing of sad versus happy faces. *NeuroImage, 21,* 1215–1223.

Kilts, C. D., Egan, G., Gideon, D. A., Ely, T. D., & Hoffman, J. M. (2003). Dissociable neural pathways are involved in the recognition of emotion in static and dynamic facial expressions. *NeuroImage, 18,* 156–168.

Klin, A. (2000). Attributing social meaning to ambiguous visual stimuli in higher-functioning autism and Asperger syndrome: The social attribution task. *Journal of Child Psychology and Psychiatry, 41,* 831–846.

Kozlowski, L. T., & Cutting, J. E. (1977). Recognizing the sex of a walker from a dynamic point-light display. *Perception and Psychophysics, 21,* 575–580.

Krolak-Salmon, P., Henaff, M. A., Isnard, J., Tallon-Baudry, C., Guenot, M., Vighetto, A., Bertrand, O., & Mauguiere, F. (2003). An attention modulated response to disgust in human ventral anterior insula. *Annals of Neurology, 53,* 446–453.

LaBar, K. S., Crupain, M. J., Voyvodic, J. T., & McCarthy, G. (2003). Dynamic perception of facial affect and identity in the human brain. *Cerebral Cortex, 13,* 1023–1033.

Lane, R. D., Reiman, E. M., Ahern, G. L., Schwartz, G. E., & Davidson, R. J. (1997). Neuroanatomical correlates of happiness, sadness, and disgust. *American Journal of Psychiatry, 154,* 926–933.

Lane, R. D., Reiman, E. M., Bradley, M. M., Lang, P. J., Ahern, G. L., Davidson, R. J., & Schwartz, G. E. (1997). Neuroanatomical correlates of pleasant and unpleasant emotion. *Neuropsychologia, 35,* 1437–1444.

Lange, K., Williams, L. M., Young, A. W., Bullmore, E. T., Brammer, M. J., Williams, S. C., Gray, J. A., & Phillips, M. L. (2003). Task instructions modulate neural responses to fearful facial expressions. *Biological Psychiatry, 53,* 226–232.

Lawrence, A. D., Calder, A. J., McGowan, S. W., & Grasby, P. M. (2002). Selective disruption of the recognition of facial expressions of anger. *NeuroReport, 13,* 881–884.

LeDoux, J. (1998). *The emotional brain: The mysterious underpinnings of emotional life.* New York: Simon & Schuster.

Leslie, K. R., Johnson-Frey, S. H., & Grafton, S. T. (2004). Functional imaging of face and hand imitation: Towards a motor theory of empathy. *NeuroImage, 21,* 601–607.

Levenson, R. W., Ekman, P., & Friesen, W. V. (1990). Voluntary facial action generates emotion-specific autonomic nervous system activity. *Psychophysiology, 27,* 363–384.

Libet, B. (1981). The experimental evidence for subjective referral of a sensory experience backwards in time: Reply to P. S. Churchland. *Philosophy of Science, 48,* 182–197.

Morris, J. S., de Gelder, B., Weiskrantz, L., & Dolan, R. J. (2001). Differential extrageniculostriate and amygdala responses to presentation of emotional faces in a cortically blind field. *Brain, 124,* 1241–1252.

Morris, J. S., Öhman, A., & Dolan, R. J. (1998). Conscious and unconscious emotional learning in the human amygdala. *Nature, 393,* 467–470.

Morris, J. S., Öhman, A., & Dolan, R. J. (1999). A subcortical pathway to the right amygdala mediating "unseen" fear. *Proceedings of the National Academy of Sciences, 96,* 1680–1685.

Murphy, F. C., Nimmo-Smith, I., & Lawrence, A. D. (2003). Functional neuroanatomy of emotions: A meta-analysis. *Cognitive, Affective, and Behavioral Neuroscience, 3,* 207–233.

Narumoto, J., Okada, T., Sadato, N., Fukui, K., & Yonekura, Y. (2001). Attention to emotion modulates fMRI activity in human right superior temporal sulcus. *Cognitive Brain Research, 12,* 225–231.

Niedenthal, P. M., Barsalou, L. W., Winkielman, P., Krauth-Gruber, S., & Ric, F. (in press). Embodiment in attitudes, social perception, and emotion. *Personality and Social Psychology Review.*

Owren, M. J., & Bachorowski, J.-A. (2001). The evolution of emotional expression: A "selfish-gene" account of smiling and laughter in early hominids and humans. In T. J. Mayne & G. A. Bonanno (Eds.), *Emotions: Current issues and future directions* (pp. 152–191). New York: Guilford Press.

Panksepp, J. (1998). *Affective neuroscience.* New York: Oxford University Press.

Pascual-Leone, A., & Walsh, V. (2001). Fast backprojections from the motion to the primary visual area necessary for visual awareness. *Science, 292,* 510–512.

Pasley, B. N., Mayes, L. C., & Schultz, R. T. (2004). Subcortical discrimination of unperceived objects during binocular rivalry. *Neuron, 42,* 163–172.

Pessoa, L., Kastner, S., & Ungerleider, L. G. (2002). Attentional control of the processing of neutral and emotional stimuli. *Cognitive Brain Research, 15,* 31–45.

Phan, K. L., Wager, T., Taylor, S. F., & Liberzon, I. (2002). Functional neuroanatomy of emotion: a meta-analysis of emotion activation studies in PET and fMRI. *NeuroImage, 16,* 331–348.

Phillips, M. L., Williams, L. M., Heining, M., Herba, C. M., Russell, T., Andrew, C., et al. (2004). Differential neural responses to overt and covert presentations of facial expressions of fear and disgust. *NeuroImage, 21,* 1484–1496.

Phillips, M. L., Young, A. W., Senior, C., Brammer, M., Andrew, C., Calder, A. J., Bullmore, E. T., Perrett, D. I., Rowland, D., Williams, S. C., Gray, J. A., & David, A. S. (1997). A specific neural substrate for perceiving facial expressions of disgust. *Nature, 389,* 495–498.

Plutchik, R. (1980). *Emotion: A psychoevolutionary synthesis.* New York: Harper Row.

Pollick, F. E., Paterson, H. M., Bruderlin, A., & Sanford, A. J. (2001). Perceiving affect from arm movement. *Cognition, 82,* B51–61.

Pollick, F. E., Hill, H., Calder, A., & Paterson, H. (2003). Recognising facial expression from spatially and temporally modified movements. *Perception, 32,* 813–826.

Puce, A., & Perrett, D. (2003). Electrophysiology and brain imaging of biological motion. *Philosophical Transactions of the Royal Society of London, B, 358,* 435–445.

Rapcsak, S. Z., Galper, S. R., Comer, J. F., Reminger, S. L., Nielsen, L., Kaszniak, A. W., et al. (2000). Fear recognition deficits after focal brain damage. *Neurology, 54,* 575–581.

Reingold, E. M., & Merikle, P. M. (1988). Using direct and indirect measures to study perception without awareness. *Perception and Psychophysics, 44,* 563–575.

Rizzolatti, G., Fadiga, L., Gallese, V., & Fogassi, L. (1996). Premotor cortex and the recognition of motor actions. *Cognitive Brain Research, 3,* 131–141.

Rolls, E. T. (1999). *The brain and emotion.* Oxford: Oxford University Press.

Rosenberg, E. L., & Ekman, P. (1994). Coherence between expressive and experiential systems in emotion. *Cognition and Emotion, 8,* 201–230.

Rossion, B., de Gelder, B., Pourtois, G., Guerit, J. M., & Weiskrantz, L. (2000). Early extrastriate activity without primary visual cortex in humans. *Neuroscience Letters, 279,* 25–28.

Russell, J. A. (2003). Core affect and the psychological construction of emotion. *Psychological Review, 110,* 145–172.

Sato, W., Kochiyama, T., Yoshikawa, S., Naito, E., & Matsumura, M. (2004). Enhanced neural activity in response to dynamic facial expressions of emotion: An fMRI study. *Cognitive Brain Research, 20,* 81–91.

Schneider, F., Gur, R. C., Gur, R. E., & Muenz, L. R. (1994). Standardized mood induction with happy and sad facial expressions. *Psychiatry Research, 51,* 19–31.

Schultz, R. T., Grelotti, D. J., Klin, A., Kleinman, J., Van der Gaag, C., Marois, R., et al. (2003). The role of the fusiform face area in social cognition: Implications for the pathobiology of autism. *Philosophical Transactions of the Royal Society of London, B, 358,* 415–427.

Servos, P., Osu, R., Santi, A., & Kawato, M. (2002). The neural substrates of biological motion perception: An fMRI study. *Cerebral Cortex, 12,* 772–782.

Sprengelmeyer, R., Rausch, M., Eysel, U. T., & Przuntek, H. (1998). Neural structures associated with recognition of facial expressions of basic emotions. *Proceedings of the Royal Society of London, B, 265,* 1927–1931.

Sprengelmeyer, R., Young, A. W., Schroeder, U., Grossenbacher, P. G., Federlein, J., Buttner, T., et al. (1999). Knowing no fear. *Proceedings of the Royal Society of London, B: Biological Sciences, 266,* 2451–2456.

Sprengelmeyer, R., Young, A. W., Sprengelmeyer, A., Calder, A. J., Rowland, D., Perrett, D. I., et al. (1997). Recognition of facial expressions: Selective impairment of specific emotions in Huntington's disease. *Cognitive Neuropsychology, 14,* 839–879.

Strafella, A. P., & Paus, T. (2000). Modulation of cortical excitability during action observation: A transcranial magnetic stimulation study. *Experimental Brain Research, 11,* 2289–2292.

Thornton, I. M., & Kourtzi, Z. (2002). A matching advantage for dynamic human faces. *Perception, 31,* 113–132.

Vaina, L. M., Solomon, J., Chowdhury, S., Sinha, P., & Belliveau, J. W. (2001). Functional neuroanatomy of biological motion perception in humans. *Proceedings of the National Academy of Sciences, 98,* 11656–11661.

Vuilleumier, P., Armony, J. L., Driver, J., & Dolan, R. J. (2003). Distinct spatial frequency sensitivities for processing faces and emotional expressions. *Nature Neuroscience, 6,* 624–631.

Vuilleumier, P., Richardson, M. P., Armony, J. L., Driver, J., & Dolan, R. J. (2004). Distant influences of amygdala lesion on visual cortical activation during emotional face processing. *Nature Neuroscience, 7,* 1271–1278.

Wallbott, H. G. (1998). Bodily expression of emotion. *European Journal of Social Psychology, 28,* 879–896.

Wehrle, T., Kaiser, S., Schmidt, S., & Scherer, K. R. (2000). Studying the dynamics of emotional expression using synthesized facial muscle movements. *Journal of Personality and Social Psychology, 78,* 105–119.

Weiskrantz, L. (1990). Outlooks for blindsight: Explicit methodologies for implicit processes. *Proceedings of the Royal Society of London, B, 239,* 247–278.

Whalen, P. J., Rauch, S. L., Etcoff, N. L., McInerney, S. C., Lee, M. B., & Jenike, M. A. (1998). Masked presentations of emotional facial expressions modulate amygdala activity without explicit knowledge. *Journal of Neuroscience, 18,* 411–418.

Wicker, B., Keysers, C., Plailly, J., Royet, J. P., Gallese, V., & Rizzolatti, G. (2003). Both of us disgusted in My insula: The common neural basis of seeing and feeling disgust. *Neuron, 40,* 655–664.

Wild, B., Erb, M., & Bartels, M. (2001). Are emotions contagious? Evoked emotions while viewing emotionally expressive faces: Quality, quantity, time course and gender differences. *Psychiatry Research, 102,* 109–124.

Williams, L. M., Phillips, M. L., Brammer, M. J., Skerrett, D., Lagopoulos, J., Rennie, C., et al. (2001). Arousal dissociates amygdala and hippocampal fear responses: Evidence from simultaneous fMRI and skin conductance recording. *NeuroImage, 14,* 1070–1079.

Williams, M. A., Morris, A. P., McGlone, F., Abbott, D. F., & Mattingley, J. B. (2004). Amygdala responses to fearful and happy facial expressions under conditions of binocular suppression. *Journal of Neuroscience, 24,* 2898–2904.

Winston, J. S., O'Doherty, J., & Dolan, R. J. (2003). Common and distinct neural responses during direct and incidental processing of multiple facial emotions. *NeuroImage, 20,* 84–97.

Young, A. W., Hellawell, D. J., Van De Wal, C., & Johnson, M. (1996). Facial expression processing after amygdalotomy. *Neuropsychologia, 34,* 31–39.

PART III

Unconscious
Emotional Behavior

CHAPTER 8

Conscious and Unconscious Emotion in Nonlinguistic Vocal Communication

MICHAEL J. OWREN

DREW RENDALL

JO-ANNE BACHOROWSKI

Human and nonhuman communication occurs in many forms, across diverse modalities, and likely representing a wide variety of mechanisms and functions. In spite of this diversity, researchers and laypeople alike tend to understand communication from a particular standpoint; namely, that signals have content, convey messages, and have meaning. This standpoint is the canonical approach in linguistic communication, where words are arbitrary constructions that convey a specific message by virtue of their symbolic relation to objects and events in the world. Although different in many respects, an emotion-related signal, or expression, is nevertheless often conceived of in the same way. It is, for example, often considered the outward manifestation of a specific internal emotional state. In this chapter we attempt to account for the phenomenon of nonlinguistic vocal behavior from a different perspective. Rather than conceiving of these signals as vehicles for conveying encoded messages, we argue that they function first and foremost by engaging low-level psychological processes in the listener, such as attention, arousal, emotion, and motivation. This approach is dis-

1. *What is the scope of your proposed model? When you use the term* emotion, *how do you use it? What do you mean by terms such as* fear, anxiety, *or* happiness?

The affect-induction model is meant to have broad scope, applying to nonlinguistic vocal communication in both humans and other mammals. The basic claim is that all such signaling is fundamentally rooted in the affective impact that the sounds have on listeners. This interpretation contrasts with those arguing that the primary function of signaling is to activate cognitive representations. The affect-induction model thus conceives of emotions as foundational processes of attention, arousal, valenced affect, and motivation. These very basic processes can include both conscious and unconscious components and are critical in guiding an individual's moment-to-moment decision making and behavior. This concept of emotion is meant to contrast with the classic view of cognition as elaborated, abstract, and amodal processing. However, we deem affective processes to be fundamental to the psychological and physiological scaffolding that precedes, underlies, and supports cognitive representations (see Niedenthal, Barsalou, Ric & Krauth-Gruber, Chapter 2). A term such as *fear* can be conceived as a label of a region in a multidimensional state–space of psychological and physiological processes, whose common consequence is an increase in the probability of avoidant behavior (see Barrett, Chapter 11). Contributing dimensions include increased attention, heightened arousal, a negatively valenced subjective experience, and a concomitant goal of evading the triggering stimulus.

2. *Define your terms:* conscious, unconscious, awareness. *Or say why you do not use these terms.*

Definitions of conscious and unconscious used in this chapter follow the spirit of Öhman's (1999) discussion of these concepts. The term *unconscious* is used to refer to processes that underlie a behavior or a feeling state but that are not accessible to introspection or perceptible as causes of that behavior or state. Conversely, the process is considered *conscious* if it is accessible to examination through introspection and is perceptible. The conscious processing of external stimuli implies that these events are attended to, noticed, and trigger awareness. In contrast, unconscious processing includes learning about stimuli and events that may be noticed as they occur, but either do not form explicit memories or are not retained as such. The contrast between conscious and unconscious is used synonymously with the distinction between implicit and explicit, and between automatic and controlled. We consider the difference to be important both for the affective processes driving nonlinguistic vocal production and for those shaping perception of these kinds of vocalizations.

3. *Does your model deal with what is conscious, what is unconscious, or their relationship? If you do not address this area specifically, can you speculate on the relationship between what is conscious and unconscious? Or if you do not*

(continued)

like the conscious–unconscious distinction, or if you do not think this is a good question to ask, can you say why?

The affect-induction framework relies on a basic distinction that is aligned with, if not identical to, conscious versus unconscious, explicit versus implicit, and controlled versus automatic processing. This account particularly stresses signaler exploitation of unconscious perceiver biases, over which the perceiver has little direct control. Specifically, sound stimuli are proposed to routinely induce affective responses rooted in foundational nervous-system properties, over which listeners have little or no conscious or explicit control. Try as one might, for example, it is difficult to suppress psychological and autonomic responses when hearing fingernails on a chalkboard, a wailing baby, a noxious car alarm, or a cat screaming when its tail is stepped on. Some of the neural circuits involved may lie both literally and figuratively close to those that maintain unconscious vegetative functions such as breathing, heartbeat, and alertness. The framework also stresses the importance of learned responses in listeners, in whom crucial conditioning processes are unconscious, implicit, and automatic.

However, both unconditioned and conditioned effects of sounds also bring the listener's conscious, explicit, and controlled processes into play. These are processes through which listeners may attempt to minimize the sound's impact or execute planful behavior as a result of that impact. Similar points also can be made about signalers who unconsciously use vocalizations to exert influence over listeners. To the extent that vocal production can become subject to conscious, explicit, or controlled processes, individuals who learn that producing calls can affect the behavior of others may come to deploy their sounds more deliberately or reflectively. On both the perception and production sides, then, the conscious–unconscious distinction likely reflects a continuum of states that can gradate from one to another, both developmentally and evolutionarily.

cussed in the context of vocalizations produced by both nonhuman primates and humans, where the interplay of conscious and unconscious emotion processes exerts a critical role.

AN AFFECT-INDUCTION APPROACH
TO NONLINGUISTIC VOCAL SIGNALING

Whether produced by humans or nonhumans, and occurring in the visual, auditory, or other modalities, communication signals are commonly understood to stand for, or be about, something. This approach has been important in interpreting human facial affect, where particular expressions have been argued to be linked to particular signaler emotions (e.g., Keltner & Ekman, 2000; Keltner, Ekman, Gonzaga, & Beer, 2003) or social intentions (Fridlund, 1997). A proposed function of a facial expression is that, through such expression, signalers are conveying information about their emotional or intentional states to perceivers, thereby allowing more effective interaction for both parties (see Lundqvist & Öhman, Chapter 5). A similar interpretation is common in animal research (reviewed by Hauser, 1996), where such expressions are referred to as motivational signaling. The underlying explanatory metaphor in both cases is that the physical signal is a medium by which signalers can transmit encoded information to perceivers.

A recognized problem for this view is that both human "emotional expressions" and nonhuman "motivational signals" are often much less tied to specific underlying states or external contexts than one would expect. That problem led Frijda and Tcherkassof (1997) to argue that human facial expressions show only general affinities, rather than specific or exclusive relationships, with particular emotions. In fact, a given emotion may be associated with a variety of expressions at different times, whereas various expressions may be associated with the same underlying emotion (see also Russell & Fernández-Dols, 1997). Similarly, Owren and Rendall (2001) point out that although a few primate vocalizations are linked to quite specific triggering circumstances, many are not. Indeed, examples of acoustically similar vocalizations that occur across contexts, and of dissimilar calls that appear in the same context, are readily available (e.g., Owren, Rendall, & Bachorowski, 2003).

Focusing on vocal signals, in particular, we suggest that the properties of sound as a medium allow vocalizers to influence perceivers in immediate ways, and that the strategies involved can explain the observed lack of specificity. One proposed strategy is that vocalizers can contact low-level nervous-system processes in listeners through the direct, unconditioned impact of the acoustic signal itself. A second strategy is that vocalizers can create indirect, conditioned responses in listeners by pairing their own distinctive sounds with affectively significant outcomes experienced by those listeners. These are functions that likely emerged early in the evolution of mammalian vocal communication, given that neither require agreed-upon meanings, encoding and decoding processes in signaler and perceiver, or even coincident fitness interests for the two parties (Owren & Rendall, 2001).

Sound Induces Affect

A striking feature of sound is that it can powerfully influence a listener's affective state. As a simple example in humans, tapping a pencil in an otherwise quiet room can be remarkably distracting and annoying to others. Another common experience is that sounds can be so noxiously intrusive as to become viscerally disturbing, such as when a human infant's shrieks and cries aggravate everyone within earshot. Sound is also a highly effective medium to use to make warning signals, such as fire alarms, because it can be used to divert attention instantly from whatever task is at hand and to virtually compel a response, such as exiting the premises. In these cases, sound works as a medium of communication, first and foremost, because it directly engages the listener's nervous system and does not require learning or symbolic value in order to be effective. Sound is also a ready mediator of emotional learning, as demonstrated over decades of animal research in which tones and buzzers have been used as cues of upcoming events such as food or shock delivery. Humans also routinely acquire affective responses to particular sounds through simple associative learning, for instance, to stimuli such as school bells, police sirens, or even the theme music of a favorite television program.

Recent empirical work on sound-induced affect has confirmed that sound can both modify arousal levels and elicit valenced (positive vs. negative) emotional responses in human listeners (Bradley & Lang, 2000). In these studies, participants first provided explicit ratings of a variety of common sounds, with separate characterizations of the arousal and valenced emotions experienced upon hearing each stimulus. Their ratings were then found to be aligned with the psychophysiological reactions that occurred in response to the sounds. Using stimuli as disparate as machine noises, non-human vocalizations, nonlinguistic human vocalizations, and sounds associated with appetitive human behaviors, Bradley and Lang's work reported that listeners experienced both nonspecific nervous-system activation effects and specifically positively or negatively valenced reactions. Responses to the sound of beer being poured was one particularly compelling example of the accrual of salient associations to an affectively significant stimulus. Although unremarkable and unobtrusive as an acoustic event, this distinctive sound is routinely paired with the very pleasant behavior of ingesting beer. Participant responses revealed that the sound alone induced unequivocally positive emotion.

Using Nonlinguistic Vocalizations for Affect Induction

Initially inspired by demonstrations of highly diverse acoustics and usage in the calls of various primate species, Owren and Rendall (1997, 2001; Rendall & Owren, 2002) have suggested that affect induction may play a key role in the normative vocalizations of many mammalian species (see Owren & Bachorowski, 2003, where they apply the model to human laughter). Here the term "affect" was broadly construed to include perceiver processes that mediate the psychological dimensions commonly characterized as attention, arousal, emotion, and motivation. This affect-induction, or affect-conditioning, approach notes that these low-level psychological processes in perceivers can become an avenue of influence for signalers. By changing the affective states of listeners, vocalizers can thereby also influence their behavior. In this view, the nature of the auditory system itself creates opportunities for signalers, the most basic of which are to capitalize on direct and indirect impacts on perceiver affect.

Direct (Unconditioned) Effects of Vocalizations

The simplest way that one individual can influence another by vocalizing is to produce acoustic energy that elicits an affective response, in and of itself. The cross-species generality of that claim is illustrated by the acoustic startle phenomenon (Davis, 1984). This response is a reflexive interruption of ongoing behavior elicited by features such as abrupt onsets and high amplitudes, and is believed to occur in all hearing species (Eaton, 1984). Although vocalizations are unlikely to have evolved specifically to evoke startle, its occurrence demonstrates that sound can affect listeners at foundational levels. Abrupt onsets and phenomena such as rapid upward frequency sweeps have been linked to increased arousal in both humans and other mammals, in which slow-onset sounds with gradually falling frequencies are found to decrease arousal levels (reviewed by Owren & Rendall, 2001). In the affect-induction view, these links indicate that callers can potentially modulate listener affect by producing sounds with particular kinds of acoustic properties—regardless of other aspects of the vocal or social circumstances.

In fact, producing direct-impact vocalizations may be one of the few ways in which socially impotent vocalizers can influence the behavior of more powerful individuals. A classic example is the plethora of shrieks, screams, wails, and whines that human and nonhuman youngsters produce when attempting to shape caregiver behavior. In the human case, infants can use crying to draw attention, induce response motivation, and even "train" caregivers in how to "turn off" these sounds. Infant crying is typically perceived as a markedly negative event, routinely described as grating, aversive, and distressing by adult listeners (Zeskind & Lester, 1978). It also has marked impact on listener arousal (Bradley & Lang, 2000). This strategy of producing noxious sounds is indisputably crude, one that can only work because caregivers are usually deeply invested in the infant's well-being. When that bias is absent—for example, with biologically unrelated stepparents or adoptive caregivers—crying, in particular, places the infant at risk of physical abuse (e.g., Frodi, 1985; Murry, 1985). Although it is commonly contended that caregivers can distinguish among putative variants of crying that are specific to experiences of pain, hunger, and a wet diaper (Berry, 1975), there is little evidence to support this contention of language-like function (Gustafson, Wood, & Green, 2000). Instead, these potent sounds appear to be effective primarily due to their direct impact on listener arousal and affect, with acoustic variability in crying being most strongly correlated with perceptions of urgency and infant distress (Barr, Hopkins, & Green, 2000; Dessureau, Kurowski, & Thompson, 1998; Gustafson & Green, 1989; Gustafson et al., 2000; Protopapas & Eimas, 1997).

Nonlinguistic aspects of spoken language also likely exert effects via their direct impact. For example, adult humans routinely rely on the direct effects of vocalizations in infant-directed speech, thereby capitalizing on infant sensitivity to auditory stimulation (Fernald, 1991; Papoucek, Bornstein, Nuzzo, Papoucek, & Symmes, 1990). Sounds with pronounced upward frequency sweeps engage and arouse an infant, whereas sounds with marked downward sweeping frequencies are quieting (e.g., Fernald, 1992). Equivalent impacts on infant state have been found using synthetic stimuli (Kaplan & Owren, 1994), indicating that infant responsiveness derives from the direct effects of the acoustics themselves. In adult-directed speech, it is likely no coincidence that features such as pitch, amplitude, and rate are the ones that consistently emerge as emotion-related cues to talker affect (reviewed by Banse & Scherer, 1996). The affect-induction perspective is that when listeners are able to draw inferences about talker affect from emotion-related acoustics, they do so based on the impact of acoustics on their own affect-response systems (Bachorowski & Owren, 2002; Russell, Bachorowski, & Fernández-Dols, 2003; also see Hietanen, Surakka, & Linnankoski, 1998).

Indirect (Conditioned) Effects of Vocalizations

A second simple strategy is for signalers to pair their individually distinctive vocalizations with the occurrence of affect-inducing actions or events, thereafter being able to use those sounds to elicit corresponding learned responses in perceivers. In other words, if vocalizers can associate their calls with the salient, affective responses occurring in others, conditioning effects can give them leverage over those individuals' emotional states. Dominant primates thus routinely vocalize before attacking subordinates, which we propose makes them able thereafter to use their threat calls to elicit learned fear. Affiliative calls are also common, for example, when a dominant animal approaches a subordinate for grooming. If the calls have been paired with friendly grooming episodes in the past, hearing these sounds will elicit decreased arousal and fear in the wary subordinate, thereby making it more likely to tolerate the dominant animal's approach without moving away.

These examples involve a vocalizer that inherently has control over the likely outcome of an interaction. That control allows it to take advantage of basic conditioning processes in another to influence that individual's affective state and expectations, and thereby make this listener more likely to behave as the caller desires. This strategy can thus best be used by socially potent vocalizers, such as mothers of dependent offspring or higher- rather than lower-ranking group members. However, it is also available to any creature that can reliably associate its particular calls with a salient affect occurring in a listener.

Human vocalizers regularly produce individually distinctive sounds paired with behaviors that affect others in important ways. For example, a parent's comforting tone can effectively soothe a distressed child, in part, because that tone has been paired with past nurturing behaviors and the gradual calming effects the child experienced at those times. The distinctive features of the caregiver's voice play an important role; the calming response will not occur in relation to any vocalizer who might adopt a similar tone. Repeated pairings of individually distinctive laugh sounds with affiliative behavior on the part of the laugher and positive affect on the part of the listener should also support the development of learned emotional responses to those laugh acoustics (Owren & Bachorowski, 2003). Corroborative evidence for such learning includes finding that pairs of friends who interact while performing tasks that elicit frequent laughter are more likely to laugh in close temporal proximity than are stranger pairs (Smoski & Bachorowski, 2003). This result suggests that the participants who were friends rather than strangers experienced laughter-induced affect learned during past interactions in which their partners' laughter had been paired with positive emotions in themselves.

The Lack of Specificity Problem

The affect-induction approach has a number of implications for non-linguistic vocal signaling (Owren & Rendall, 1997, 2001), one of which is that signals are not expected to routinely show specific and exclusive relationships with particular vocalizer states. For example, many sounds are proposed to be effective through the direct impact they have on listener affect rather than because they provide veridical information about signaler state. Any of a variety of acoustic features might have the desired effect in a particular situation, or using a diversity of sounds may be the most effective. Vocal variability is particularly likely when a listener fails to behave as the vocalizer desires. Socially impotent individuals who are not getting what they want are thus predicted to produce ongoing streams of variable vocalizations that both take advantage of the impact of diverse forms of acoustic energy and that help avoid or overcome listener habituation. This variability is undeniably evident in vocalizations of socially impotent individuals, both human and primate (reviewed by Owren et al., 2003).

Vocalizations by socially potent individuals, on the other hand, are predicted to show marked individual distinctiveness rather than affective or context specificity. Here the mechanism of influence is the perceiver's conditioned response to the vocalization, occurring both as a generalized reaction to hearing sounds from many different vocalizers, and through specific associations with the distinctive properties of these sounds when produced by particular vocalizers. These expectations result from basic learning principles. For example, a given monkey hears threat calls produced by many different individuals through the course of the day, some of which have been previously followed by attack (higher-ranking animals), and some of which have not (lower-ranking animals). Overall, there may be a modest affective response to threat calls, in general. However, affective responses to calls from higher-ranking animals will be strong and specific, if the threats of these animals are individually distinctive. Stated as a prediction, the claim is that nonlinguistic vocalizations used by socially potent individuals should occur in forms that readily include cues to the identity of the signaler. We suggest that this is the case for many of the most common calls in the vocal repertoires of primates (Owren et al., 2003).

It also follows that if socially potent vocalizers are not having the desired effect in a given situation, they will increasingly fall back on the strategy of direct acoustic impact. In primates, for example, threat calls should become louder and occur at a higher rate when a subordinate is not backing down, as desired. In humans, linguistic components of speech are routinely supplemented by direct-impact acoustics such as increased loudness, pitch, and sharpness of attack when targets of an utterance are unresponsive. For instance, when unruly offspring fail to heed the linguistic commands of adults, conversational tones (e.g., "Stop that, right now") became high-impact ones (*"STOP THAT—RIGHT NOW!"*). This strategy appears to be so deeply ingrained that it occurs even in circumstances in which it cannot possibly be effective, such as when tourists who are unable to speak the local language resort to speaking their own language more loudly.

CONSCIOUS AND UNCONSCIOUS PROCESSES
IN EMOTION-RELATED VOCALIZATIONS

The remainder of the chapter examines the roles played by conscious and unconscious emotional processes in the affect-based interpretation of the nonlinguistic vocal behavior we have presented. There are points to make about both production and perception of vocalization, and we particularly draw on Öhman's (1999) distinctions between the conscious and unconscious (and see Smith & Neumann, Chapter 12). It will also be convenient and illustrative to compare and contrast the processes critical to nonlinguistic vocalization with those underlying human spoken language.

Nonlinguistic Vocal Production

Öhman (1999) suggests a conceptual separation between unconscious processes that can underlie a consciously experienced event and the conscious processes that make up the experience. That distinction is applicable to both the production and perception sides of the communicative equation, and it is particularly apt for the former. Whether vocalizers are human or nonhuman, there are important differences between nonlinguistic vocalization and human language production. The semantic and syntactic knowledge involved in language competence are, of course, unconscious or implicit. However, language behavior is nonetheless importantly different from nonlinguistic vocalizing in showing intentionality or theory of mind— meaning that talkers tacitly attribute mental states to perceivers and produce signals that are specifically designed to alter those states (Dennett, 1983).

On one hand, the low-level machinery involved in representing, selecting, and sequencing words is itself not directly accessible, nor are talkers likely to be consistently aware of the motivations that underlie saying particular things at particular times. On the other hand, the decision to speak or not to speak, to discuss a particular topic or some other, to select some words or word sequences over others, and to sometimes inflect a sentence in a particular way that alters its perceived significance are all explicitly controlled by the talker. Sentences can be spoken aloud or merely in one's head; talkers can thus be said to have a conscious intention to use speech specifically so as to activate representations in listeners that are fundamentally similar to those occurring in their own minds (Rendall & Owren, 2002).

Research on primates suggests something quite different. Here, vocalizing appears to be rooted almost exclusively in the signaler's own circumstances, with surprisingly little impact on the circumstances and mental states of perceivers (reviewed in Seyfarth & Cheney, 2003). For example, producing alarm calls would seem a prime instance in which the vulnerability of other primates is critical to either producing or not producing a call. Instead, call production is often orthogonal to listener needs, with alarm callers routinely continuing long after everyone in the group has already escaped to safety and begun calling themselves. Even primate mothers appear to call based solely on their own vulnerability, as dramatically illustrated by a failure to call to predators that are a threat to their infants but not to themselves. This phenomenon has been observed both under natural circumstances (Cheney & Seyfarth, 1990a; Rendall, personal observation) and in experiments with captive animals (Cheney & Seyfarth, 1990b). Evidence of intentionality is also absent in contact calling that occurs when primates (1) are out of sight of one another (Cheney, Seyfarth, & Palombit, 1996; Rendall, Cheney, & Seyfarth, 2000) or (2) produce food-discovery vocalizations (Clark & Wrangham, 1993; Chapman & Lefebvre, 1990). Overall, primates exhibit surprisingly circumscribed attributional or perspective-taking capacity (e.g., Povinelli & Bering, 2003; Tomasello & Call, 1997), whereas humans routinely show these abilities both as a prerequisite for effective language use and in other aspects of everyday life.

Neural Mechanisms in Production

Results such as these suggest important differences between the mechanisms involved in nonlinguistic primate vocalizations versus human language. In regard to the former, the available neurobiological evidence indicates a primary role of subcortical structures (e.g., Jürgens, 1998) that are unlikely to be under volitional control (e.g., Kappas & Scherer, 1995). In contrast, whereas spoken language relies on subsystems distributed throughout the brain (e.g., Lieberman, 2002), consciously accessible cortical circuitry is central. Human–nonhuman similarities are much greater for nonlinguistic vocalizations, as exemplified by spontaneous human laughter. Here the critical neural structures and motor programs are not only believed to be primarily subcortical, but also to be homologous with those of primates (Deacon, 1997; although see Fried, Wilson, MacDonald, & Behnke, 1998). The emergence of intentional communication through language is thus connected to the emergence of volitional control of the vocal apparatus as well as to a more sophisticated understanding of the psychological states of others—with conscious processing and the cerebral cortex likely being central contributors in each case.

Nonlinguistic Vocal Perception

Öhman's (1999) distinction between unconscious underpinnings and conscious experience also applies to vocal perception, in which, for instance, a sound may trigger inaccessible perceptual and appraisal responses that then give rise to conscious feeling states (see Scherer, Chapter 13). Öhman further notes that although external stimuli such as sounds may fully engage the perceiver as they happen, their occurrence may subsequently be retained only as an implicit, rather than explicit, memory. Both points are central to the affect-induction view, in which implicit and learned affective responses in listeners are primary contributors to the effectiveness of nonlinguistic communication for vocalizers. Tulving (2002) goes so far as to argue that nonhuman animals are entirely lacking in episodic memory, meaning that they cannot retain the particulars of individual events or form broader associations and generalized knowledge. This argument is particularly relevant in that autobiographical episodes from the past are likely to be the most consciously experienced of all memories. Whether or not Tulving's claim is literally correct for all species, nonhumans and humans are clearly alike in showing powerful and pervasive implicit learning processes, while being much less similar in the domain of episodic memory.

Neural Mechanisms in Perception

In perception, as in production, neurobiological evidence reveals a primary role of subcortical circuitry. As a result, our characterizations of conscious and unconscious locate the major effects highlighted in the affect-induction approach squarely on the unconscious side. Although vocal communication events may be salient and attended to by perceivers as they occur, from the vocalizer's point of view the locus of action lies in automatic, inaccessible processes that originate as early as the brainstem level (e.g., attentional and arousal effects mediated in the medulla and pons) and, importantly, involve subcortical forebrain nuclei that mediate affective learning (e.g., limbic system). The amygdala, in particular, has been found to be central in learned fear (e.g., LeDoux, 1996, 2000; see Bouton, Chapter 9) and is suspected of being critical in other forms of affective conditioning as well (e.g., Aggleton & Young, 2000).

There are, of course, many contributors to affective learning, which may nonetheless place the amygdala in a central role. This structure has reciprocal connections to a variety of other centers, including the thalamus, hypothalamus, hippocampus, and multiple cortical areas (e.g., Emery & Amaral, 2000). The amygdala is thus likely to affect memory formation mediated by the hippocampus, as well as to modulate cortical processing through its effects on general arousal in multiple forebrain regions and by altering processing in primary and secondary sensory cortical areas (also see Phelps, Chapter 3). Cortical inputs to the amygdala are, in turn, believed to reflect the later, more sophisticated stages of sensory-perceptual processing and the results of more complex evaluative and social–cognitive processing. The important point for us is that the amygdala, a low-level and likely consciously inaccessible structure, is both shaping and responding to processing occurring in a variety of higher-level neural structures, whose activities are much more likely to be wholly or partially subject to conscious awareness.

SPIRALING TOWARD CONSCIOUS, CONTROLLED PROCESSES

Summarizing previous points, both we and other authors have argued that unconsciously controlled emotional and motivational processes are critical in the production of nonlinguistic vocalizations; we have also noted that it can be difficult to find exclusive, one-to-one relationships between these signaler states and vocal acoustics. The spontaneous, egocentric nature of these signals is further underscored by the finding that subcortical rather than cortical circuitry is primary in producing the sounds. We have also placed subcortically mediated unconscious processing in a central role in perceivers, arguing that nonlinguistic vocalizations work from the signaler's point of view, first and foremost, because they can be used to influence listener behavior through these low-level systems. The overarching view is that the evolutionary origins of nonlinguistic vocal communication largely involve automatic systems in which unconscious processes in vocalizers trigger production, and implicit responses in perceivers play a primary role in mediating the influences that these sounds exert on their behavior.

However, an important component of the affect-induction approach is also that signaler and perceiver interests cannot be assumed to be coincident under all, or even most, circumstances. Rather, a fundamental tenet of contemporary evolutionary theory is that two organisms never have exactly the same reproductive interests (unless they are genetically identical). In the face of divergent fitness interests, signaling among biologically unrelated individuals cannot be assumed to evolve as inherently cooperative, information-sharing events (Owren & Rendall, 2001). Even when signaling is parent-to-offspring or sibling-to-sibling, a situationally dependent mosaic of overlapping and conflicting interests is involved. As a result, any success that vocalizers have in influencing perceivers also creates selection pressure on those individuals. Those pressures trigger changes whose outcomes depend on whether the effects either benefit or detract from perceiver fitness, and in turn create selection pressure that feeds back onto signaler behavior. Our conclusion is that this reciprocally driven spiral of selective pressures is likely a key mechanism by which cortically mediated and explicit cognitive operations come into play in the emergence of controlled and consciously modulated communicative behavior.

Signaler Success Creates Selection Pressure on Listeners

The affect-induction view argues that signaler vocal behavior is not predicated either on listener decoding processes or an ability to infer vocalizer intentions. Instead, the claim is that the evolutionary origins of vocal signaling ultimately lie in the impact that vocalizers could have on listener affect due to preexisting, unconscious mechanisms. These underlying processes would specifically involve attention, arousal, positive or negative emotional responses, and motivational or appraisal processes that mediate behavior such as approach or avoidance. This argument, in turn, rests on viewing audition as a preattentive, sentinel-like system designed to detect, localize, and identify functionally significant sounds related to imperatives such as evading predators and capturing prey by commandeering listener attention and marshaling the physiological resources needed for rapid action.

The upshot is that signal evolution does not require a foundation of mutual benefit for signaler and perceiver—signals can evolve regardless of the net fitness impact on perceivers. However, any leverage that signalers gain over perceivers also necessarily creates selection pressure on those individuals. Listeners may benefit from signal impact in some circumstances, such as when a mother responds to her infant's piercing shrieks or a subordinate shies away from a formidable, threat-calling opponent. But the situation can also be quite different, as illustrated by infants that shriek incessantly during weaning or a formerly unbeatable but now vulnerable foe continuing to elicit conditioned fear responses with its threat calls.

Signaler success in influencing others therefore inevitably selects for more effective perceiver appraisal of such events and their significance. For example, whereas infants may selfishly benefit from crying, screaming, and shrieking in order to elicit maternal resources in excess of actual need, mothers benefit by becoming better able to habituate more effectively to the jarring effects of these sounds, and to "see through" their unconditioned and conditioned power. In nonhumans, that argument can be cast in terms of selfish gene selection, whereas in humans it has also been considered a form of emotional intelligence (Bachorowski & Owren, 2002). In both cases, signaler behavior could prompt the emergence of automatic as well as controlled, effortful, and evaluative processes in perceivers (see Gray, Schaefer, Braver, & Most, Chapter 4; Clore, Storbeck, Robinson, & Centerbar, Chapter 16). These observations thus suggest that an escalating evolutionary process, initiated by vocalizers leveraging listeners via their unconscious processes, could create the selection pressure that ultimately gives rise to explicit, consciously controlled countermeasures.

Perceiver Success Creates Selection Pressure on Signalers

Although selection pressure exerted on listeners is thus separable from the mechanisms and functions of vocalizing, resulting changes in these perceivers can, in turn, feed back on the unconscious and conscious processes in signalers. The reciprocal nature of the selection pressures may be a major contributor to the confusing variety of relationships that seem to exist between spontaneous emotional signals and affective states. Although theorists have disagreed over the extent to which there are one-to-one relationships between the two, there is little doubt that signaler arousal, emotion, and motivation all play a central mechanistic role in nonlinguistic signaling (e.g., Kappas & Scherer, 1995; Keltner et al., 2003; Russell et al., 2003). One interpretation is that signaler state is crucial both as mechanism and function: An affective state mechanistically triggers a corresponding outward expression, the function of which is to convey that the state has occurred. However, the picture is different if mechanism and function are recognized as separable components. Logically, one should no more infer that the function of vocalizing is to signal affect than, for instance, to show that the vocalizer's laryngeal motor neurons are active.

An alternative is to view the connection between affect and signal as a causal but purely mechanical link that has no necessary implications for function. Again, we argue for assuming only that the function of signaling is to influence listener behavior in a manner that, on average, has some net benefit to the vocalizer. Instead of viewing affect as being manifested in signaling, we suggest viewing affective states as having "access" to the motor neurons and programs that are the proximal cause of vocal production. The evidence suggests that various affective states show differential probabilities of triggering a given vocalization program, with those probabilities likely being adjusted by natural selection. The relationship between a particular state and a given kind of motor output might thus be one-to-one, many-to-one, one-to-many, or many-to-many—depending on historical factors in the evolution of the behavior.

If the connection begins as a one-to-one relationship in a vocalizer, it could, but need not, remain that way. For example, if fitness interests in signalers and perceivers are closely aligned, then both parties benefit from the latter being able to draw increasingly accurate inferences concerning states and likely behaviors in the former. However, if the impact of the signal more routinely benefits vocalizers than it does listeners, then perceivers eventually will become able to modulate the effects being exerted on them. In this case, the resulting changes will create selection pressure on signalers to decrease specificity and predictably in accordance with the selfish interests in the parties involved. Signaling might also begin as a relatively undifferentiated event, with a single affective state being able to trigger more than one vocalization-producing motor program, or with many affective states having access to multiple programs. Here again, the degree of specificity would likely change over evolutionary time, reflecting complex interactions between vocalizer and listener interests, resulting effects on conscious and unconscious mechanisms in perceivers, and the degree to which these changes are beneficial or detrimental to signaler interests.

As a final point, this interaction through evolutionary time may also produce changes in signalers' conscious control of vocalization. There is only modest evidence of such outcomes among primates, whose vocal behavior appears to be unconsciously controlled, as discussed above. However, both primates and humans can suppress affectively related vocal behavior to some degree (e.g., Cheney & Seyfarth, 1990a; Deacon, 1997), whereas humans can also produce, to some degree, volitional simulations of otherwise spontaneous sounds such as laughter and crying. Owren and Bachorowski (2001) have argued that the emergence of an unconsciously based mechanistic connection between positive affect and the motor program underlying spontaneous, emotion-dependent, and subcortically mediated smiling in early hominids also made the evolution of a volitional, conscious, and cortically mediated version of this expression virtually inevitable. Although modern humans do not appear to have gained the same degree of volitional control over affect-related vocal expressions, there is little doubt that conscious processes play a role here as well.

FINAL THOUGHTS

Whether or not the perspective described here ultimately proves to be correct, we suggest that some of its underlying points at least should have some lasting value. The first underlying point is that there is good reason to avoid making the common but mistaken assumption that there is an inevitable symmetry between signalers and perceivers in communicative events. On the contrary, the fitness interests, neural mechanisms, psychological processes, and affect-related links involved may all be significantly different and should always be considered separately for the two parties. Second is that both parties show an undeniable and intimate connection between internal state and vocal signaling, and that connection becomes all the more interesting when one has abandoned implicit and explicit assumptions of coincident interests and mutual benefits in signaling. We believe that working to understand the complexities of how conscious and unconscious processes give rise to vocal signals will eventually be much more revealing about both topics than proceeding by force-fitting preconceived notions of function in emotion-related signaling. In a similar vein, our final point is that nonlinguistic vocal signals and human speech are obviously and importantly different, and it was specifically language that came later. In other words, it seems most sensible to work toward understanding affectively related vocalization in its own right, and to avoid implicitly or explicitly relying on language as a general model of communication. We believe that grappling with affect-related signaling is much more likely to produce insights into language than the converse approach, with even the most sophisticated linguistic representations being importantly grounded in the interplay of conscious and unconscious emotion.

REFERENCES

Aggleton, J. P., & Young, A. W. (2000). The enigma of the amygdala: On its contribution to human emotion. In R. D. Lane & L. Nadel (Eds.), *Cognitive neuroscience of emotion* (pp. 106–128). New York: Oxford University Press.

Bachorowski, J.-A., & Owren, M. J. (2002). The role of vocal acoustics in emotional intelligence. In L. F. Barrett & P. Salovey (Eds.), *The wisdom in feeling: Psychological processes in emotional intelligence* (pp. 11–36). New York: Guilford Press.

Banse, R., & Scherer, K. R. (1996). Acoustic profiles in vocal emotion expression. *Journal of Personality and Social Psychology, 70,* 614–636.

Barr, R. G., Hopkins, J. A., & Green, J. A. (2000). Crying as a sign, a symptom and a signal: Evolving concepts of crying behavior. In R. G. Barr, B. Hopkins, & J. A. Green (Eds.), *Crying as a sign, a symptom, and a signal* (pp. 1–7). New York: Cambridge University Press.

Berry, K. K. (1975). Developmental study of recognition of antecedents of infant vocalizations. *Perceptual and Motor Skills, 41,* 400–402.

Bradley, M. M., & Lang, P. J. (2000). Affective reactions to acoustic stimuli. *Psychophysiology, 37,* 204–215.

Chapman, C. A., & Lefebvre, L. (1990). Manipulating foraging group size: Spider monkey food calls at fruiting trees. *Animal Behaviour, 39,* 891–896.

Cheney, D. L., & Seyfarth, R. M. (1990a). *How monkeys see the world.* Chicago: University of Chicago Press.

Cheney, D. L., & Seyfarth, R. M. (1990b). Attending to behaviour versus attending to knowledge: Examining monkeys' attribution of mental states. *Animal Behaviour, 40,* 742–753.

Cheney, D. L., Seyfarth, R. M., & Palombit, R. (1996). The function and mechanisms underlying baboon "contact" barks. *Animal Behaviour, 52,* 507–518.

Clark, A. P., & Wrangham, R. W. (1993). Acoustic analysis of chimpanzee pant hoots: Do chimpanzees have an acoustically distinct food arrival pant hoot? *American Journal of Primatology, 31,* 99–109.

Davis, M. (1984). The mammalian startle reflex. In R. C. Eaton (Ed.), *Neural mechanisms of startle behavior* (pp. 287–351). New York: Plenum Press.

Deacon, T. W. (1997). *The symbolic species.* New York: Norton.

Dennett, D. C. (1983). Intentional systems in cognitive ethology: The "Panglossian paradigm" defended. *The Behavioral and Brain Sciences, 6,* 343–390.

Dessureau, B. K., Kurowski, C. O., & Thompson, N. S. (1998). A reassessment of the role of pitch and duration in adults' responses to infant crying. *Infant Behavior and Development, 21,* 367–371.

Eaton, R. C. (Ed.) (1984). *Neural mechanisms of startle behavior.* New York: Plenum Press.

Emery, N. J., & Amaral, D. G. (2000). The role of the amygdala in primate social cognition. In R. D. Lane & L. Nadel (Eds.), *Cognitive neuroscience of emotion* (pp. 156–191). New York: Oxford University Press.

Fernald, A. (1991). Prosody in speech to children: Prelinguistic and linguistic functions. In R. Vasta (Ed.), *Annals of child development* (Vol. 8, pp. 43–80). Philadelphia: Kingsley.

Fernald, A. (1992). Human maternal vocalizations to infants as biologically relevant signals: An evolutionary perspective. In J. H. Barkow, L. Cosmides, & J. Tooby (Eds.), *The adapted mind* (pp. 391–428). New York: Oxford University Press.

Fridlund, A. (1997). The new ethology of human facial expressions. In J. M. Russell & J. M. Fernández-Dols (Eds.), *The psychology of facial expression* (pp. 103–129). New York: Cambridge University Press.

Fried, I., Wilson, C. L., MacDonald, K. A., & Behnke, E. J. (1998). Electric current stimulates laughter. *Nature, 391,* 650.

Frijda, N. H., & Tcherkassof, A. (1997). Facial expressions as modes of action readiness. In J. M. Russell & J. M. Fernández-Dols (Eds.), *The psychology of facial expression* (pp. 78–102). New York: Cambridge University Press.

Frodi, A. (1985). When empathy fails: Aversive infant crying and child abuse. In B. M. Lester, & C. F. Zachariah Boukydis (Eds.), *Infant crying: Theoretical and research perspectives* (pp. 263–277). New York: Plenum Press.

Gustafson, G. E., & Green, J. A. (1989). On the importance of fundamental frequency and other acoustic features in cry perception and infant development. *Child Development, 60,* 772–780.

Gustafson, G. E., Wood, R. M., & Green, J. A. (2000). Can we hear the causes of infant crying? In R. G. Barr, B. Hopkins, & J. A. Green (Eds.), *Crying as a sign, a symptom, and a signal* (pp. 8–22). New York: Cambridge University Press.

Hauser, M. D. (1996). *The evolution of communication.* Cambridge, MA: Harvard University Press.

Hietanen, J. K., Surakka, V., & Linnankoski, I. (1998). Facial electromyographic responses to vocal affect expressions. *Psychophysiology, 35,* 530–536.

Jürgens, U. (1998). Neuronal control of mammalian vocalization with special reference to the squirrel monkey. *Naturwissenshaften, 85,* 376–388.

Kaplan, P. S., & Owren, M. J. (1994) Dishabituation of visual attention in 4–month-olds by infant-directed frequency sweeps. *Infant Behavior and Development, 17,* 347–358.

Kappas, A., & Scherer, K. R. (1995). Primate vocal expression of affective state. In D. Todt, P. Goedeking, & D. Symmes (Eds.), *Primate vocal communication* (pp. 123–132). Berlin: Springer-Verlag.

Keltner, D., & Ekman, P. (2000). Facial expression of emotion. In M. Lewis & J. M. Haviland-Jones (Eds.), *Handbook of emotions* (2nd ed., pp. 236–249). New York: Guilford Press.

Keltner, D., Ekman, P., Gonzaga, G. C., & Beer, J. (2003). Facial expression of emotion. In R. J. Davidson, K. R. Scherer, & H. H. Goldsmith (Eds.), *Handbook of affective sciences* (pp. 415–432). New York: Oxford University Press.

LeDoux, J. (1996). *The emotional brain.* New York: Simon & Schuster.

LeDoux, J. (2000). Cognitive–emotional interactions: Listen to the brain. In R. D. Lane & L. Nadel (Eds.), *Cognitive neuroscience of emotion* (pp. 129–155). New York: Oxford University Press.

Lieberman, P. (2002). The neural bases of language. *Yearbook of Physical Anthropology, 45,* 36–62.

Murry, A. D. (1985). Aversiveness is in the mind of the beholder: Perception of infant crying by adults. In B. M. Lester & C. F. Zachariah Boukydis (Eds.), *Infant crying: Theoretical and research perspectives* (pp. 217–239). New York: Plenum Press.

Öhman, A. (1999). Distinguishing unconscious from conscious emotional processes: Methodological considerations and theoretical implications. In T. Dalgleish & M. Power (Eds.), *Handbook of cognition and emotion* (pp. 321–352). New York: Wiley.

Owren, M. J., & Bachorowski, J.-A. (2001). The evolution of emotional expression: A "selfish-gene" account of smiling and laughter in early hominids and humans. In T. J. Mayne & G. A. Bonanno (Eds.), *Emotions: Current issues and future directions* (pp. 152–191). New York: Guilford Press.

Owren, M. J., & Bachorowski, J.-A. (2003). Reconsidering the evolution of nonlinguistic communication: The case of laughter. *Journal of Nonverbal Behavior, 27,* 108–200.

Owren, M. J., & Rendall, D. (1997). An affect-conditioning model of nonhuman primate signaling. In D. H. Owings, M. D. Beecher, & N. S. Thompson (Eds.), *Perspectives in ethology: Vol. 12. Communication* (pp. 299–346). New York: Plenum Press.

Owren, M. J., & Rendall, D. (2001). Sound on the rebound: Bringing form and function back to the forefront in understanding nonhuman primate vocal signaling. *Evolutionary Anthropology, 10,* 58–71.

Owren, M. J., Rendall, D., & Bachorowski, J.-A. (2003). Nonlinguistic vocal communication. In D. Maestripieri (Ed.), *Primate psychology* (pp. 353–395). Cambridge, MA: Harvard University Press.

Papoucek, M., Bornstein, M. H., Nuzzo, C., Papoucek, H., & Symmes, D. (1990). Infant responses to prototypical melodic contours in parental speech. *Infant Behavior and Development, 13,* 539–545.

Povinelli, D. J., & Bering, J. M. (2003). The mentality of apes revisited. *Current Directions in Psychological Science, 11,* 115–119.

Protopapas, A., & Eimas, P. D. (1997). Perceptual differences in infant cries revealed by modifications of acoustic features. *Journal of the Acoustical Society of America, 102,* 3723–3734.

Rendall, D., Cheney D. L., & Seyfarth R. M. (2000). Proximate factors mediating "contact" calls in adult female baboons and their infants. *Journal of Comparative Psychology, 114,* 36–46.

Rendall, D., & Owren, M. J. (2002). Animal vocal communication: Say what? In M. Bekoff, C. Allen, & G. Burghardt (Eds.), *The cognitive animal* (pp. 307–313). Cambridge, MA: MIT Press.

Russell, J. A., Bachorowski, J. A., & Fernández-Dols, J. M. (2003). Facial and vocal expressions of emotion. *Annual Review of Psychology, 54,* 329–349.

Russell, J. M., & Fernández-Dols, J. M. (1997). What does a facial expression mean? In J. M. Russell & J. M. Fernández-Dols (Eds.), *The psychology of facial expression* (pp. 3–30). New York: Cambridge University Press.

Seyfarth, R. M., & Cheney, D. L. (2003). Signalers and receivers in animal communication. *Annual Review of Psychology, 54,* 145–173.

Smoski, M.J., & Bachorowski, J.-A. (2003). Antiphonal laughter between friends and strangers. *Cognition and Emotion, 17,* 327–340.

Tomasello, M., & Call, J. (1997). *Primate cognition.* New York: Oxford University Press.

Tulving E. (2002). Chronesthesia: Conscious awareness of subjective time. In D. T. Stuss & R. T. Knight (Eds.), *Principles of frontal lobe function* (pp. 311–325). New York: Oxford University Press.

Zeskind, P. S., & Lester, B. (1978). Acoustic features and auditory perceptions of the cries of newborns with prenatal and perinatal complications. *Child Development, 49,* 580–589.

CHAPTER 9

Behavior Systems and the Contextual Control of Anxiety, Fear, and Panic

Mark E. Bouton

There is little question that classical conditioning can influence emotions and emotional behavior. Ever since Watson and Rayner's (1920) famous experiment demonstrating emotional conditioning in an infant boy, classical conditioning has been seen as a mechanism that allows emotions to be triggered by new stimuli. Today, conditioning is still viewed as central to the learning of emotional triggers (see Owren, Rendall, & Bachorowski, Chapter 8; Barrett, Chapter 11) and emotional disorders (e.g., Barlow, 2002; Bouton, Mineka, & Barlow, 2001; Lang, 1995; LeDoux, 1996; Nelson & Bouton, 2002; Öhman & Mineka, 2001). Conditioning has also become an important methodological tool allowing investigators to study the neuroscience of emotion (e.g., LeDoux, 1996; see also Phelps, Chapter 3; Lundqvist & Öhman, Chapter 5).

The present chapter addresses a specific topic within the general study of emotional conditioning—namely, how the *context* in which conditioning occurs controls the triggering of emotional behavior. In a typical fear conditioning experiment with rats, a signal such as a tone (a conditional stimulus, or CS) might elicit fear once it has been paired with an electric foot shock (an unconditional stimulus, or US) on several occasions. The context is typically defined as the experimental chamber the rat is placed in before it

1. *What is the scope of your proposed model? When you use the term* emotion, *how do you use it? What do you mean by terms such as* fear, anxiety, *or* happiness?

In this chapter emotion is defined in terms of its behavioral aspects; emotions are viewed as loosely coordinated sets of behavioral, physiological, and cognitive responses that function to cope with events in the environment (see Scherer, Chapter 13; for an alternate view, see Barrett, Chapter 11). Because much of the research described in this chapter focuses on behavior elicited in nonhuman animals, it may be taken as an illustration of the richness inherent in the organization of emotions in the absence of consciousness or conscious awareness.

2. *Define your terms*: conscious, unconscious, awareness. *Or say why you do not use these terms.*

This chapter focuses on emotional behavior in nonhuman animals, such that distinctions between consciousness, awareness, and so on, are not relevant for this chapter.

3. *Does your model deal with what is conscious, what is unconscious, or their relationship? If you do not address this area specifically, can you speculate on the relationship between what is conscious and unconscious? Or if you do not like the conscious–unconscious distinction, or if you do not think this is a good question to ask, can you say why?*

Humans produce behavioral and interoceptive states to emotional challenges that are homologous to those in animals, as discussed in this chapter. It is possible to speculate that in humans, these states can be consciously experienced and represented in awareness, either as affect or emotion.

receives these crucial conditioning events. Quite a lot is now known about the associative learning that goes into Pavlovian conditioning (see Pearce & Bouton, 2001, for one review). Here I provide a somewhat selective review of what we know about how the context in which the CS is presented further influences how the organism responds to it. The fact that emotion triggered by the CS is itself modulated by the context may have important implications for an understanding of emotion and emotional disorders.

In typical fear conditioning experiments in my own laboratory, a rat is put in an experimental chamber each day for a 90-minute session. In these sessions, four to eight 60-second tones might be presented; some of these might end in a brief, 0.5-second foot shock. The animal is usually in the box for 10–20 minutes before the first tone occurs. The context—the experimental chamber—is thus a long-duration stimulus that has an onset long before the crucial conditioning events occur. There is a sense in which the chamber embeds the conditioning events in time and space. I mention this to make it clear that the context in a typical conditioning experiment truly is a background stimulus. Its temporal duration makes it somewhat different from the 60-second tone that directly elicits fear. This difference could have implications for how it might influence anxiety, fear, and panic.

CONDITIONING AND BEHAVIOR SYSTEMS

Time is unquestionably important in conditioning. To develop the point I want to make, however, it is necessary to observe that classical conditioning is a richer and more complex phenomenon than many people appreciate. Once conditioning has occurred, the CS triggers more than a simple unitary reflex; it elicits a large and interesting system or constellation of responses. All psychology students know about Pavlov's original experiment, in which a bell CS was paired with a food US. They also know that thanks to conditioning, the bell acquired the ability to elicit a salivary response. Modern researchers recognize that conditioning is an important means by which humans and other animals adapt to biologically significant events (e.g., Hollis, 1982, 1997); the salivary response is clearly functional in the sense that it helps the animal digest the upcoming meal. But a CS for food can elicit much more than this solitary response. Signals for food can evoke an entire set of behaviors and physiological reactions that prepare the organism to digest food. For example, in addition to the well-known salivary response, Pavlov's bell probably also elicited the secretion of gastric acid, pancreatic enzymes, and insulin. All of these facilitate food absorption, so that animals that have signaled meals are better at digesting them than animals that have unsignaled meals (e.g., Woods & Strubbe, 1994). In freely moving animals, signals for food can also elicit approach behaviors, and thus they guide and direct foraging. Food signals also elicit eating, if food is available, even in the satiated rat (e.g., Weingarten, 1983). CSs for food evoke a whole "behavior system," a set of behaviors and responses that are functionally organized to capture and consume food (e.g., Timberlake, 1994, 2001).

The same is true in fear conditioning. CSs associated with foot shock can elicit a whole system of conditioned fear responses that is, once again, organized to help the animal deal with the US (e.g., Bolles & Fanselow, 1980; Fanselow, 1994). A CS may evoke several behavioral responses that have evolved to prevent attack by predators. The most familiar one is freezing; when a CS for shock is presented, the animal becomes motionless. Freezing in the presence of a predator decreases the likelihood of death by attack—it thus has a documented payoff (Hirsch & Bolles, 1980). In the presence of stimuli that support alternative behaviors, the rat might flee from the situation or, when shock is delivered from a small prod attached to the wall of the chamber, it might bury the stimulus with sawdust (e.g., Treit, Pesold, & Rotzinger, 1993). CSs for shock also elicit corresponding changes in respiration, heart rate, blood pressure, and an endorphin response that decreases sensitivity to pain (e.g., Fanselow, 1979). Fear conditioning gives rise to a whole system of behaviors that are designed, through evolution, to help the organism adapt. When we say that an organism is afraid, we usually mean that some aspect of this system has been mobilized.

Behavior systems are often organized such that different behaviors come into play depending on how close in space and time the organism is to the US. For example, Fanselow and Lester (1988) argued that the defensive (fear) system is organized such that different behaviors are called forth depending on the animal's psychological distance from a predator—"predatory imminence." When imminence is low, the animal goes about its daily business, finding food sources and mates. (These behaviors might actually be timed and coordinated to minimize detection by predators.) But when predatory imminence increases, as it does when the animal detects a predator nearby, a different set of behaviors becomes functional. At this point, the rat might freeze, and to support the freeze, the heart rate might slow down and respiration become shallower. At a still higher point on the imminence scale, when a predator actually strikes, still other behaviors may come into play. At this point, the animal might jump, return the attack, and/or flee, with all the supporting physiological responses, such as increased heart rate and deeper breathing. The point is that qualitatively different defensive behaviors are available to the animal and are evoked according to when they are most functional. Fanselow and Lester suggest that each type of defensive behavior is designed (i.e., selected through evolution) to prevent movement to the next higher point on the imminence scale.

Timberlake (e.g., 1994, 2001) has written extensively about the rat's feeding behavior system. Here again the system is organized according to the imminence of the motivational object, although in this case the goal is to increase (rather than decrease) contact. When food is distant, there are general search behaviors that function to find it. When the possibility of food is detected, there may be focal search behaviors that function to locate and apprehend it. And finally, there are consumption and handling behaviors. Interestingly, in Timberlake's system, CSs that predict food at long, medium, or short time intervals will theoretically evoke different behaviors that correspond to general search, focal search, and consumption. Timberlake's system thus explicitly recognizes an important, but often overlooked, fact about conditioning: that the form of the conditioned response depends on the duration of the CS (Holland, 1980; Silva & Timberlake, 1997; Timberlake, Wahl, & King, 1982).

The last point is made extremely clear in studies of sexual behavior in the male Japanese quail. Michael Domjan and his students have studied this behavior system in detail (e.g., Domjan, 1994, 1997). In a typical experiment, a male quail is presented with a visual CS that is paired with the opportunity to copulate with a female. The response that comes to be evoked by the CS as a consequence of the pairings depends crucially on the duration and nature of the CS. For example, if a localized visual CS (presentation of a foam object with terrycloth or feathers on it) is presented for 20 minutes and then copulation with a female occurs, the CS will come to evoke pacing back and forth over trials (Akins, 2000; Akins, Domjan, & Gutierrez, 1994). However, if the same CS is presented for just 30–60 seconds immediately prior to copulation on each trial, it comes to evoke simple approach (e.g., Akins, 2000; Akins et al., 1994). It is as if the long stimulus elicits a general search behavior, whereas the shorter one elicits focal search. Further, when the CS is a 30–60 second presentation of a taxidermically prepared model that includes the head and neck of a female, the CS comes to evoke consummatory behavior—i.e., copulation responses (e.g., Akins, 2000; Domjan, Huber-McDonald, & Holloway, 1992; Cusato & Domjan, 2000). And interestingly, the strength of copulatory responses is increased when the model is presented in a context that has been separately associated with copulation (Domjan, Greene, & North, 1989; see also Hilliard, Nguyen, & Domjan, 1997). The result is consistent with the idea that conditioned "preparatory" responses, presumably elicited by the context, can augment or potentiate "consummatory" responses elicited by other stimuli (Domjan, 1994, 1997; Konorski, 1967).

The same point has been made for defensive conditioning. Following Konorski (1967), Wagner and Brandon (1989) have emphasized that animals associate a CS with both the emotional and sensory aspects of the US, and that the associations with these different aspects of the US evoke different responses. The emotional response is especially likely to be elicited by a long-duration CS. Consistent with this idea, in rabbit eyeblink conditioning, a mild shock delivered near the eye will elicit both a blink response and fear (indexed, in part, by a change in heart rate). With short CSs (typically those terminating in a US less than 1 second after CS onset), the CS elicits a protective blink of the eye near the site where the US is delivered. With longer CSs (e.g., 6.75 seconds or more), the CS elicits a change of heart-rate response (instead of the blink) that suggests fear (VanDercar & Schneiderman, 1967). Unlike the blink response, conditioned fear does not depend on where the US is actually delivered (either eye or a hindleg will do). One effect of fear is to potentiate the blink. Bombace, Brandon, and Wagner (1991) found that when a 1-second CS that elicited the blink was presented within a 30-second CS that was separately associated with shock, it elicited the blink more strongly (see also Brandon & Wagner, 1991). The phenomenon is similar to fear potentiated startle, in which a fear CS potentiates the acoustic startle reflex (e.g., Davis, 1992; see also Brandon, Bombace, Falls, & Wagner, 1991; McNish, Betts, Brandon, & Wagner, 1997). Although the long CS elicited no blink, it presumably elicited fear. In the defensive system, as in others, the nature of the conditioned response depends on CS duration, and CSs that have a distal temporal relation with the US can potentiate responding to CSs with a more proximate relation.

Research on behavior systems thus suggests that the nature of the conditioned response depends on the duration and qualitative aspects of the signal, and that the strength of a response can be influenced by stimuli in the background.

CONTEXT, CS DURATION, AND THE NATURE OF THE AVERSIVE CR: ANXIETY, FEAR, AND PANIC

The general characteristics of how behavior systems are organized have implications for emotion. Like other parts of the behavior system, emotions function to deal with the US (cf. Scherer, Chapter 13). In this light, it seems apparent that the type of emotion elicited by a signal may depend on the temporal and qualitative nature of the signal that triggers it. Conceivably, such flexibility and variability may contribute to the difficulty in finding a stable physiological signature for the different emotions (e.g., Cacioppo, Berntson, Larsen, Poehlmann, & Ito, 2000; Zajonc & McIntosh, 1992).

Bouton et al. (2001) accepted a behavior systems view in a conditioning account of panic disorder, the anxiety disorder in which panic attacks occur, intensify, and become debilitating with experience. They assumed, as had others before them, that out-of-the-blue panic attacks can be potent USs that generate aversive conditioning. Panic disorder develops in vulnerable individuals at least in part because they learn to fear the next panic attack (e.g., Goldstein & Chambless, 1978; Wolpe & Rowan, 1988). But in considering the behavior systems literature, Bouton et al. suggested that the attacks may worsen for two reasons. First, proximate cues connected with the early onset of a panic attack (e.g., the feeling of a pounding heart, feeling dizzy) become associated with the rest of the attack. These proximate cues, which are closely correlated with, and even resemble aspects of, the panic attack, acquire the ability to evoke *panic* as a conditioned response. Recent work studying drug effects confirms that the onset of an event can serve as a CS for the rest of the event (e.g., Kim, Siegel, & Patenall, 1999; Sokolowska, Siegel, & Kim, 2002).

The second mechanism that increases the intensity of panic attacks is more like the one we have just seen in other behavior systems. Bouton et al. supposed that certain CSs that signal a panic attack more remotely in time (e.g., the shopping mall) might come to elicit a preparatory emotional conditioned response (CR), *anxiety*, a forward-looking fear reaction that "prepares" the organism for the next panic attack. Anxiety differs from the panic elicited by a shorter, proximate CS; the latter is designed to deal with a traumatic event that is highly imminent or even already in progress. But equally important, the conditioning of the long-duration anxiety CR would be expected to potentiate the next panic attack, in the same way that longer-duration cues potentiate copulatory, eyeblink, and startle responses.

A distinction between anxiety and panic is consistent with at least two types of evidence. First, quantitative analyses of patient symptoms have distinguished between states of extreme fear and autonomic arousal that seem consistent with panic and a different state of apprehension and worry with tension that appears more like anxiety (e.g., Brown, Chorpita, & Barlow, 1998). Second, research in behavioral neuroscience has begun to separate at least two aversive motivational systems. For example, Michael Davis and his colleagues have distinguished between anxiety and fear at both the behavioral and neural levels (e.g., Davis & Shi, 1999; Davis, Walker, & Lee, 1997). In the Davis conceptualization, although there is considerable overlap in the effects of these two states, fear is a relatively short-term state that is activated by Pavlovian CSs, whereas anxiety is a longer-term state that is activated by more diffuse and unlearned cues. Fear appears to be mediated by activity in the amygdala; for instance, lesions of the amygdala abolish fear conditioning, including fear conditioning as measured by the potentiated startle response (e.g., Hitchcock & Davis, 1986; Kim, Campeau, Falls, & Davis, 1993; see also Fanselow, 1994; Kapp, Whalen, Supple, & Pascoe, 1992; LeDoux, 1996). In contrast, amygdala lesions do *not* abolish the rat's preference for covered arms in a plus maze, a widely accepted measure of anxiety (Treit et al., 1993). Amygdala central nucleus lesions also do not abolish startle responding potentiated by extended exposure to a bright light or by the infusion of corticotropin releasing hormone (Davis et al., 1997), both of which create a longer-lasting anxiety, as suggested by the fact that they are reduced by anxiolytic drugs (Walker & Davis, 1997a; Swerdlow, Geyer, Vale, & Koob, 1986). Importantly, the latter two effects are abolished by similar lesions of another part of the extended amygdala, the bed nucleus of the stria terminalis (BNST; Davis et al., 1997; Walker & Davis, 1997b); these lesions have no effect on fear conditioning, however (Davis et al., 1997; Hitchcock & Davis, 1991; LeDoux, Iwata, Cicchetti, & Reis, 1988; Walker & Davis, 1997b). The pattern thus begins to suggest a double dissociation between behavioral tasks affected by lesions of the amygdala (fear) and the BNST (anxiety).

Although anxiety might not always depend on learning (e.g., a bright light might presumably evoke anxiety in a rat as an unconditioned response), recent research in my laboratory suggests that it can be learned and elicited by long-duration CSs. In recent experiments, Jaylyn Waddell, Richard Morris, and I have compared the effects of BNST lesions on aversive conditioning with short and long signals for shock (Waddell, Morris, & Bouton, submitted for publication). In one experiment, over a series of sessions, rats received presentations of a clicking noise that ended in a moderately intense, 1-mA, 0.5-second foot shock. For one set of animals, the duration of the noise was 60 seconds, the standard duration used in fear conditioning experiments in my laboratory. For another set of rats, the duration of each noise was 600 seconds. For these animals, the CS signaled the US at a long enough distance that we did not expect it to generate a strong fear CR; it might evoke conditioned anxiety. Several weeks before conditioning, some of the animals in each condition received excitotoxic lesions of the BNST. Control groups received sham lesions in which they underwent similar surgeries, but no excitotoxins were delivered to the brain. The experiment thus asked whether the BNST affects aversive conditioning, and more importantly, whether it selectively affects a CS that has a long temporal relationship with the US.

We used the conditioned suppression method in which aversive conditioning was measured in terms of the extent to which the CS suppressed an operant lever-pressing response reinforced by food (Estes & Skinner, 1941). With the 1-minute CS, the lesion did not have a significant impact on fear conditioning, as is consistent with previous research (Hitchcock & Davis, 1991; LeDoux et al., 1988; Walker & Davis, 1997b). But the picture was different with the 10-minute CS. In this case, the BNST lesion significantly reduced conditioning. The lesions had no effect on baseline lever-pressing rates. The results were thus consistent with the idea that long-duration signals, but not shorter-duration signals, arouse an anxiety state that might be mediated by the BNST. Although the 10-minute CS evoked less suppression than the 1-minute CS did, the results of an additional experiment suggested that the BNST lesion still had an impact on 10-minute CSs that evoked more suppression. If the BNST plays a role in aversive CR to long-duration stimuli, it may well be that the duration of the CS, rather than merely a weak level of conditioned suppression, is what matters.

Of course, long-duration contextual cues are also a candidate for anxiety conditioning. It would be especially interesting to identify a situation in which a contextual anxiety cue potentiates a conditioned fear response in a manner analogous to that suggested for panic disorder (Bouton et al., 2001). One situation in which a context's direct association with a US augments fear of a CS is *reinstatement* (e.g., Bouton & Bolles, 1979b; Rescorla & Heth, 1975). In reinstatement, the subject first receives fear conditioning (e.g., tone–shock pairings) and then extinction (tone alone presentations) in several daily sessions. Although the original tone–shock pairings allow the tone to trigger fear, extinction undoes that effect; it eliminates the learned fear. However, in reinstatement, the shock is presented several times alone—independently of any behavior, and independently of the tone CS. With our typical methods, these shock presentations are sparse and widely spaced in time (i.e., 4–8 shocks are presented in a 90-minute session). But when the tone is presented alone, typically the next day, it elicits fear again. After extinction, exposure to the US again reinstates fear of the CS.

Many experiments in my laboratory have shown that reinstatement is an effect of context conditioning. When the reinstating shocks are presented, the animal associates them with the current context. This creates a dangerous context, and the presence of that danger when the tone is next presented somehow triggers fear of the extinguished CS. The main evidence supporting this idea is that when the shocks are presented in a different, irrelevant context, they produce no reinstatement (e.g., Bouton, 1984; Bouton & Bolles, 1979b; Bouton & King, 1983; Frohard, Guarraci, & Bouton, 2000; Wilson, Brooks, & Bouton, 1995). Thus, for reinstatement to occur, the CS must be tested in the context that has been made dangerous by recent exposure to the US.

Despite clear evidence that the context was important, in our early reinstatement experiments few rats showed overt signs of fear when they were returned to the context on the test day. Baseline lever-pressing rate was not significantly suppressed (see also Rescorla & Heth, 1975), and the animals showed little freezing, the classic sign of fear in the frightened rat. To provide an independent measure of contextual conditioning, we therefore attached side compartments to the Skinner boxes. For the first 6 minutes of the session, we allowed the rats to choose between sitting in the side box or earning food pellets while lever pressing (on a variable interval reinforcement schedule) in the Skinner box. Access to the side box was prevented once the test was over. Compared with rats shocked in another box, the rats that had been shocked in the current Skinner box preferred to sit in the side compartment, and the degree of this preference was strongly correlated with the strength of reinstatement that was observed when the CS was presented a minimum of 15 minutes later (Bouton, 1984; Bouton & King, 1983). However, as usual, there was little overt freezing or suppression of the lever-pressing baseline.

I now see this pattern as a possible consequence of the fact that the long-duration context evoked anxiety rather than fear. Freezing is primarily a response of the rat when it perceives a relatively high level of shock imminence. As a test of this, we have further examined the effect of BNST lesions on the reinstatement effect (Waddell et al., submitted for publication; see also Frohardt, 2001). Excitotoxic lesions were created a few weeks before the behavioral part of the experiment. The lesion had no impact on either fear conditioning or extinction with the 60-second CS. However, it significantly attenuated the reinstatement effect: After fear conditioning and then extinction, eight shocks in a 90-minute session reinstated fear to the CS in control subjects. But animals with BNST lesions showed no reinstatement effect. The results are consistent with our idea that the context might evoke a conditioned anxiety state that can potentiate (reinstate) fear of an extinguished CS. The CS and the context thus appear to elicit different emotional states that (1) depend differentially on the BNST, a brain area linked to other indices of anxiety, and (2) interact in a way predicted by a behavior systems view (Bouton et al., 2001).

We had previously shown that lesions of the hippocampus (Frohardt et al., 2000) or disruption of one of its major outputs, the fimbria fornix (Wilson et al., 1995), could also abolish the reinstatement effect. Those results were consistent with a fair amount of research indicating that the hippocampus is involved in contextual learning (e.g., Kim & Fanselow, 1992). But our experiments also indicated that an intact hippocampus or fornix is not necessary for at least one other important context learning effect (the renewal effect, described below; Frohardt et al., 2000; Wilson et al., 1995). Details of the neural circuitry are beyond the scope of this chapter, but the point of our work with the BNST is that it is consistent with a role for contextually controlled conditioned anxiety. Like other possible behavioral indicators of anxiety, conditioning of the context (by our typical, fairly sparse reinstatement shock presentation schedule) or a long-duration noise CS, may depend on the BNST.

One question is whether there is a one-to-one correspondence between anxiety and fear dissociated here and in the Davis laboratory, on the one hand, and anxiety and panic emphasized by Bouton et al. (2001), on the other. The answer may be "no." It seems possible that the panic response elicited by an extremely proximate early-onset cue might be rather different from the anticipatory fear evoked by a CS whose onset precedes the US by 60 seconds. Fanselow (e.g., 1994) has emphasized the distinction between the freezing elicited by such a CS and the activity burst that is directly elicited by shock. The activity burst responds to an aversive US that is already in progress, which might also be true of panic responses. Future research may therefore support a separation between three aversive emotional states: anxiety (supported by a very long CS), fear (supported by a less distal CS), and panic (perhaps supported by an extremely proximate and biologically prepared CS). Interestingly, the three states loosely correspond to the general search, focal search, and consummatory modes that have been proposed in appetitive systems.

INHIBITION AND THE CONTEXTUAL CONTROL
OF CONDITIONED RESPONDING

Thus far I have focused on the emotional effects of contexts and CSs that are directly associated with a US. However, contexts can also control emotional behaviors through another mechanism that is less direct. To illustrate, consider the *renewal* effect, another important effect in which the context controls the response to the CS. In the simplest demonstration of renewal (e.g., Bouton & Bolles, 1979a; Bouton & King, 1983), rats receive fear conditioning with a tone in one context (Context A) and then extinction (tone-alone trials) in either the same context or a different context (Context B). Once extinction is complete, so that the animals are no longer afraid of the CS, they are returned to the original context, Context A, where they receive further tests of the CS. At this point, the animals extinguished in the other context (Context B) show a strong return (renewal) of fear. The renewal effect, like reinstatement, indicates that extinction does not destroy the original learning, but instead leaves the CS sensitive to the context.

One of the interesting things about renewal is that it does not require that Context A or B have demonstrable direct associations with the US. Many conditioning models would allow Context A to acquire direct associations with the US during conditioning, and Context B to acquire inhibitory associations with the US during extinction (e.g., Rescorla & Wagner, 1972). Such associations would then add or subtract from the associative strength of the CS to generate performance. Although direct context–US associations are no doubt learnable, none of our tests provided evidence that they are necessary (or sufficient) to influence response to the CS in our standard procedures (see Bouton, 1991, for a review). In this sense, the renewal effect is different from reinstatement, which is mediated by a direct association between the context and the US. In renewal, the contexts appear to work as cues that retrieve the current "meaning" of the CS, or its current relation to the US, in the way *occasion setters* do (e.g., Holland, 1992; Schmajuk & Holland, 1998; see Pearce & Bouton, 2001). Casually speaking, Context A retrieves or activates the CS–US association, and Context B retrieves or activates a CS–no-US association. In this sense, they "disambiguate" the CS's current meaning. A more detailed discussion of the mechanism is provided by Bouton and Nelson (1998).

There are several versions of the renewal effect. In the "ABA" effect just described, the animal is returned to the original conditioning context (Context A) after extinction in a different context (Context B). But we and others have also shown an ABC renewal effect, wherein tests in a neutral third context (C) also cause a renewal of the original conditioned response (Bouton & Bolles, 1979a; Bouton & Brooks, 1993). We have also observed an AAB renewal effect, wherein conditioning and extinction occur in the same context (A), and testing occurs in a second context (B) (Bouton & Ricker, 1994). The fact that ABC and AAB renewal can occur indicates that conditioning (fear of the CS) generalizes more readily to a new context than extinction (inhibition of the CS) does.

In fact, one especially important discovery in our work on the renewal effect is exactly that: Extinction is more specific to its context than conditioning is. This is also evident in the ABA renewal design. After conditioning in Context A, we find that the CS elicits just as much fear in the group that then receives extinction in Context B as the group that receives extinction in Context A. That is, switching the context after conditioning has surprisingly little impact on fear of the CS, even in the presence of independent evidence that the animals recognize the difference between the contexts (e.g., Bouton & Brooks, 1993). We have seen this pattern in many experiments, regardless of the motivational system. For example, even if we study appetitive (tone–food) conditioning instead of fear (tone–shock) conditioning, the switch after conditioning has no effect, but the switch after extinction does (e.g., Bouton & Peck, 1989). The context is more important after extinction than it is after original conditioning.

Interestingly, our research on reinstatement provides converging support for this conclusion. Although the contextual conditioning created by shocks delivered after extinction has a clear effect on *extinguished* fear of the CS, the same contextual conditioning created by the same shock exposure *after conditioning alone* has surprisingly little effect on fear of the CS. For example, we have compared groups that received a small number of fear conditioning trials with other groups that received conditioning and then partial extinction to a point where the CS elicited the same amount of fear (Bouton, 1984). Animals in both sets of groups then received shocking in the same or different contexts, and it created the pattern of contextual fear (context preference) that I described earlier. Although there was clear context-dependent reinstatement in the extinguished rats, there was no evidence that the same contextual conditioning had an effect on fear of the

CS that had not been extinguished. It was as if contextual conditioning was not relevant until after extinction. Subsequent experiments showed that the extent to which CS fear was increased by contextual conditioning depended on the extent to which fear of the CS was "depressed" by extinction during the test (Bouton & King, 1986). Anxiety conditioned to the context does not potentiate fear automatically or unconditionally; it seems to remove the inhibition created by extinction.

The fact that extinction is more context dependent than conditioning led us to ask whether inhibitory learning is generally context specific. Byron Nelson and I studied this question in experiments with the "feature-negative" procedure (Bouton & Nelson, 1994; Nelson & Bouton, 1997). In this procedure, one CS (X) is paired with a US on trials when it is presented alone, but without the US on trials when it is presented with another CS (Y), that is, X+, YX–. After repeating and intermixing the two types of trials, Y develops purely inhibitory properties—it predicts the absence of a US that is otherwise presented with X. But Nelson and I discovered that inhibition to Y is *not* disrupted by context change: Like simple excitation, inhibition to Y generalized nicely across contexts. Instead, the ease with which responding to X could be inhibited was reduced when the context was switched. Nelson (2002) then confirmed what we had long suspected: that it is the second thing learned about the CS that is specific to its context. Both inhibition and excitation generalized across contexts, unless they were the second thing learned about the CS. The system thus seems to code the second thing learned about the CS as a conditional exception to a rule. In effect, the context is especially important in controlling retroactive inhibition. The fact that the inhibitability of responding to X was lost is also consistent with this rule. Generally speaking, an association you have learned to inhibit in one context is more difficult to inhibit in another.

RELAPSE AND THE MAINTENANCE OF EMOTION

Renewal and reinstatement have clear implications for relapse after therapy (e.g., Bouton, 2000, 2002; see also Quigley & Barrett, 1999), which is theoretically based on extinction. One should be aware that an emotion generated by an extinguished trigger cue can always return, depending on the background. But the idea is more general than this. Up to this point, I have stuck with a fairly conventional definition of context, namely, the physical background cues provided by the room or apparatus in which the CS and US are presented. In reality, though, "context" is probably much more than that. For instance, I have argued that learning and remembering are also sensitive to the gradually changing context provided by the passage of time (e.g., Bouton, 1993). This is not a controversial idea within the area of human memory, where it is not uncommon to think of forgetting over time as due to a growing mismatch between the contexts present during learning and testing. In this light, the context dependency of extinction explains *spontaneous recovery*, one of the earliest phenomena connected with extinction that suggests that extinction is not unlearning (Pavlov, 1927). Our idea is that spontaneous recovery is merely the failure to retrieve extinction outside the temporal extinction context. That is, just as we find a renewal effect if conditioning, extinction, and testing are conducted in physical contexts A, B, and C, so we may find spontaneous recovery when conditioning, extinction, and testing are conducted at times 1, 2, and 3. Spontaneous recovery is the renewal effect that occurs when the animal fails to retrieve extinction in a new temporal context.

One prediction of this view is that, if spontaneous recovery and renewal both result from failures to retrieve extinction, then both should be abolished by presenting a retrieval cue that reminds the animal of extinction just before the test. Cody Brooks and I found this to be the case (Brooks & Bouton, 1993, 1994). We found that a cue that was presented during the intertrial intervals of extinction could attenuate the effects if it was presented just before the test (see also Brooks, 2000; Brooks & Bowker, 2001). That sort of result supports the idea that spontaneous recovery and renewal are caused by the same mechanism—that is, a failure to retrieve extinction. It also suggests that either form of relapse can be reduced or perhaps prevented by reminders of the extinction/therapy experience. Interestingly, Collins and Brandon (2002) also found that a retrieval cue reduced renewal in human social drinkers when they tested alcohol cues in a context that was different from the one in which extinction exposures had taken place.

Another kind of context that is important is the interoceptive context produced by ingestion of a drug. There is an extensive literature on state-dependent retention effects, in which memory for material learned while under the influence of a drug is best remembered in that drug state. We have shown state-dependent fear extinction effects. For example, when fear conditioning occurs while the animal is in the sober state but fear extinction is conducted while the animal is under a benzodiazepine tranquilizer chlordiazepoxide (Librium) or diazepam (Valium), there is a strong, dose-dependent renewal effect that occurs when the animal is tested again in the sober state (Bouton, Kenney, & Rosengard, 1990). In effect, the drug works as Context B in the ABA renewal design. Cunningham (1979) has shown a similar effect of alcohol, and we have recently replicated and extended the findings with midazolam, another benzodiazepine that is often used in human anesthesia protocols (Pain, Oberling, & Bouton, 2001). A recent study with human subjects suggests that caffeine can also function in a similar way when spider fear is extinguished while patients are under the influence of caffeine (Mystkowski, Mineka, Vernon, & Zinbarg, 2003). It thus seems clear that renewal effects can be obtained with interoceptive drug contexts.

Such results have an obvious clinical implication: Using a drug to facilitate anxiety therapy can potentially backfire, creating relapse when the client encounters the CS again in the absence of the drug. Perhaps consistent with this possibility, there is evidence that the combination of drug and cognitive behavior therapy is less effective at long-term follow-up than is cognitive behavior therapy alone (Barlow, Gorman, Shear, & Woods, 2000). There is a subtler implication as well. State-dependent extinction would serve to insulate a person from the beneficial effects of natural extinction. That is, a person might take an anxiolytic drug to reduce anxiety; drug taking would be reinforced by anxiety reduction. But state-dependent extinction might preserve the original anxiety, which might ordinarily undergo some extinction through natural exposure to the anxiety stimulus. Thus the drug might paradoxically maintain the anxiety that motivates drug use. Renewal effects might contribute to the long-term maintenance of the disorder in addition to generating relapse.

Recent studies in my laboratory have isolated a new kind of renewal effect that might also contribute to the maintenance of emotion and emotional disorders. Bouton, Frohardt, Sunsay, and Waddell (submitted for publication) gave rats repeated CS–shock pairings in one context over several sessions. (There were additional daily sessions in which a different CS received the same treatment in a different context.) What we often (but not always) observed is a phenomenon that sometimes reveals itself in fear conditioning experiments: The acquisition of fear reached a maximum at a point in training and then began to decline, as if the fear response began to extinguish a little, despite continued pairings of the CS and the shock. Although such "nonmonotonic" learning curves have been observed in several laboratories, we have an incomplete understanding of them at the present time. Our own experiments indicate that they do not depend on the gradual development of "inhibition of delay," in which the animal learns to time the shock and confine its fear to late parts of the CS and extinguish fear to early parts. In addition, the decline is not due to recruitment of an endorphin response that makes the shocks less painful; administration of the opiate antagonist naloxone does not appear to abolish the effect (Vigorito & Ayres, 1987). Instead, the effect is usually attributed to the acquisition of an ill-defined adaptation process that allows the rat to cope with the US and/or fear.

One of the interesting things about the adaptation process is that, like extinction, it appears to be specific to the context in which it develops. At the end of experiments in which we have observed nonmonotonic fear learning curves, a context switch caused a significant *increase* in fear of the CS. Over a series of experiments, we discovered that the strength of this increased fear was correlated with the degree to which fear had declined from its maximum point to the start of testing (Bouton, Frohardt, Sunsay, & Waddell, submitted for publication). That is, when adaptation was evident, there was an increase in fear when the context switched. When less adaptation was evident, there was less increase in fear. Thus what appears to be lost with a switch in context is the animal's adaptation response. And further, the adaptation is to the CS or to the fear that it elicits; notice that the tests were of the CS, not the US, in the different context. As in extinction, the animal's fear of the CS is renewed if the context is switched after adaptation has occurred. The second thing learned about a CS is again attenuated by a context switch.

These findings might have implications for how organisms express and regulate emotion. It is interesting to think about a panic patient who experiences repeated pairings of a pounding heart and panic attacks while at home. With repeated attacks, she learns to panic when her heart begins to race, but she might eventually also learn to cope and adapt to the fear, to some extent. On the other hand, if she were now to encounter the CS (the pounding heart) in another context such as the shopping mall, the coping process would be lost, and a very strong panic response might result. Stronger fear outside the conditioning context might motivate the person to stay at home—and thus provide a mechanism for agoraphobia. The fact that coping and extinction processes are relatively context-specific could easily contribute to the maintenance and persistence of emotional disorders.

SUMMARY

This chapter has sketched a fairly complex role for context in the control of emotion and behavior. In the first part I considered consequences of an organism associating a context with the US, arguing that classical conditioning, and the conditioning of emotional processes, engages whole-behavior systems. Based on what we know about the organization of such systems, cues that have different temporal relationships with the US will evoke different kinds of responses, because the type of response that pays when the US occurs immediately may not have the same value when the

US is due to occur more remotely in time. The argument suggests that long-duration contextual cues—with a relatively distal temporal relationship with a frightening US—might elicit emotional responses that are different from those evoked by more proximate cues. A context might elicit anxiety, a forward-looking response designed to deal with the threat sometime in the future, whereas proximate cues might elicit panic, a kind of response designed to deal with the traumatic US now (Bouton et al., 2001). The existence of at least two aversive motivational states is consistent with a behavior systems perspective, with the analysis of symptomatology in anxious patients (Brown et al., 1998), and with neurobiological evidence suggesting at least two dissociable aversive motivational states (e.g., Davis et al., 1997; Fanselow, 1994). I have also described preliminary evidence from my laboratory suggesting that long-duration cues, including contextual cues, can elicit an aversive motivational state that depends on the BNST, an area in the extended amygdala thought to mediate anxiety. Anxiety conditioned to a context may exacerbate the emotion elicited by a fear CS—especially one that has been through extinction.

Other research has uncovered a role for context that does not depend on a direct context–US association. Work in my laboratory suggests that extinction itself is coded as specific to its context, as if the system were designed to use contextual information primarily when the CS acquires a second meaning. This means that emotional responding evoked by an extinguished CS is *on* unless the context switches it *off*. This role of context may be played by many different kinds of background stimuli, which seem to be important in forms of retroactive interference other than extinction, including counterconditioning (see Bouton, 1994) and the adaptation and coping effect that appears to emerge with continued fear conditioning. Like other aspects of the behavior system, the context's role can be seen as adaptive; the learning and memory system seems designed to preserve first-learned information, which on a statistical basis might provide the better sample of the true state of the world than second-learned information (Bouton, 1994). All of these processes may be expected to contribute to the evocation of anxiety, fear, and panic.

ACKNOWLEDGMENTS

Manuscript preparation and the yet-unpublished research reported here were supported by Grant No. RO1 MH64847 from the U.S. National Institute of Mental Health. I thank Erik Moody, Ceyhun Sunsay, William Timberlake, Jaylyn Waddell, and Amanda Woods, along with Lisa Feldman Barrett and Piotr Winkielman, for their comments.

REFERENCES

Akins, C. K. (2000). Effects of species-specific cues and the CS–US interval on the topography of the sexually conditioned response. *Learning and Motivation, 31,* 211–235.

Akins, C. K., Domjan, M., & Gutierrez, G. (1994). Topography of sexually conditioned behavior in male Japanese quail (*Coturnix japonica*) depends on the CS–US interval. *Journal of Experimental Psychology: Animal Behavior Processes, 20,* 199–209.

Barlow, D. H. (2002). *Anxiety and its disorders: The nature and treatment of anxiety and panic* (2nd ed). New York: Guilford Press.

Barlow, D. H., Gorman, J. M., Shear, M. K., & Woods, S. W. (2000). Cognitive-behavioral therapy, imipramine, or their combination for panic disorder: A randomized controlled study. *Journal of the American Medical Association, 283,* 2529–2536.

Bolles, R. C., & Fanselow, M. S. (1980). A perceptual–defensive–recuperative model of fear and pain. *Behavioral and Brain Sciences, 3,* 291–323.

Bombace, J. C., Brandon, S. E., & Wagner, A. R. (1991). Modulation of a conditioned eyeblink response by a putative emotive stimulus conditioned with hindleg shock. *Journal of Experimental Psychology: Animal Behavior Processes, 17,* 323–333.

Bouton, M. E. (1984). Differential control by context in the inflation and reinstatement paradigms. *Journal of Experimental Psychology: Animal Behavior Processes, 10,* 56–74.

Bouton, M. E. (1991). Context and retrieval in extinction and in other examples of interference in simple associative learning. In L. Dachowski & C. F. Flaherty (Eds.), *Current topics in animal learning: Brain, emotion, and cognition* (pp. 25–53). Hillsdale, NJ: Erlbaum.

Bouton, M. E. (1993). Context, time, and memory retrieval in the interference paradigms of Pavlovian learning. *Psychological Bulletin, 114,* 80–99.

Bouton, M. E. (1994). Conditioning, remembering, and forgetting. *Journal of Experimental Psychology: Animal Behavior Processes, 20,* 219–231.

Bouton, M. E. (2000). A learning theory perspective on lapse, relapse, and the maintenance of behavior change. *Health Psychology, 19*(Suppl.), 57–63.

Bouton, M. E. (2002). Context, ambiguity, and unlearning: Sources of relapse after behavioral extinction. *Biological Psychiatry, 52,* 976–986.

Bouton, M. E., & Bolles, R. C. (1979a). Contextual control of the extinction of conditioned fear. *Learning and Motivation, 10,* 445466.

Bouton, M. E., & Bolles, R. C. (1979b). Role of conditioned contextual stimuli in reinstatement of extinguished fear. *Journal of Experimental Psychology: Animal Behavior Processes, 5,* 368–378.

Bouton, M. E., & Brooks, D. C. (1993). Time and context effects on performance in a Pavlovian discrimination reversal. *Journal of Experimental Psychology: Animal Behavior Processes, 19,* 165–179.

Bouton, M. E., Frohardt, R. J., Sunsay, C., & Waddell, J. (submitted for publication). *Contextual control of inhibition with reinforcement: Adaptation and timing mechanisms.*

Bouton, M. E., Kenney, F. A., & Rosengard, C. (1990). Statedependent fear extinction with two benzodiazepine tranquilizers. *Behavioral Neuroscience, 104,* 44–55.

Bouton, M. E., & King, D. A. (1983). Contextual control of the extinction of conditioned fear: Tests for the associative value of the context. *Journal of Experimental Psychology: Animal Behavior Processes, 9,* 248–265.

Bouton, M. E., & King, D. A. (1986). Effect of context on performance to conditioned stimuli with mixed histories of reinforcement and nonreinforcement. *Journal of Experimental Psychology: Animal Behavior Processes, 12,* 4–15.

Bouton, M. E., Mineka, S., & Barlow, D. H. (2001). A modern learning theory perspective on the etiology of panic disorder. *Psychological Review, 108,* 4–32.

Bouton, M. E., & Nelson, J. B. (1994). Context-specificity of target versus feature inhibition in a feature-negative discrimination. *Journal of Experimental Psychology: Animal Behavior Processes, 20,* 51–65.

Bouton, M. E., & Nelson, J. B. (1998). Mechanisms of feature-positive and feature-negative discrimination learning in an appetitive conditioning paradigm. In N. A. Schmajuk & P. C. Holland (Eds.), *Occasion setting: Associative learning and cognition in animals* (pp. 69–112). Washington, DC: American Psychological Association.

Bouton, M. E., & Peck, C. A. (1989). Context effects on conditioning, extinction, and reinstatement in an appetitive conditioning preparation. *Animal Learning and Behavior, 17,* 188–198.

Bouton, M. E., & Ricker, S. T. (1994). Renewal of extinguished responding in a second context. *Animal Learning and Behavior, 22,* 317–324.

Brandon, S. E., Bombace, J. C., Falls, W. A., & Wagner, A. R. (1991). Modulation of unconditioned defensive reflexes by a putative emotive Pavlovian conditioned stimulus. *Journal of Experimental Psychology: Animal Behavior Processes, 17,* 312–322.

Brandon, S. E., & Wagner, A. R. (1991). Modulation of a discrete Pavlovian conditioned reflex by a putative emotive Pavlovian conditioned stimulus. *Journal of Experimental Psychology: Animal Behavior Processes, 17,* 299–311.

Brooks, D. C. (2000). Recent and remote extinction cues reduce spontaneous recovery. *Quarterly Journal of Experimental Psychology, 53B,* 25–58.

Brooks, D. C., & Bouton, M. E. (1993). A retrieval cue for extinction attenuates spontaneous recovery. *Journal of Experimental Psychology: Animal Behavior Processes, 19,* 77–89.

Brooks, D. C., & Bouton, M. E. (1994). A retrieval cue for extinction attenuates response recovery (renewal) caused by a return to the conditioning context. *Journal of Experimental Psychology: Animal Behavior Processes, 20,* 366–379.

Brooks, D. C., & Bowker, J. L. (2001). Further evidence that conditioned inhibition is not the mechanism of an extinction cue's effect: A reinforced cue prevents spontaneous recovery. *Animal Learning and Behavior, 29,* 381–388.

Brown, T. A., Chorpita, B. F., & Barlow, D. H. (1998). Structural relationships among dimensions of the DSM-IV anxiety and mood disorders and dimensions of negative affect, positive affect, and autonomic arousal. *Journal of Abnormal Psychology, 107,* 179–192.

Cacioppo, J. T., Berntson, G. G., Larsen, J. T., Poehlmann, K. M., & Ito, T. A. (2000).

The psychophysiology of emotion. In R. Lewis & J. M. Haviland-Jones (Eds.), *Handbook of emotion* (2nd ed., pp. 173–191). New York: Guilford Press.

Collins, B. N., & Brandon, T. H. (2002). Effects of extinction context and retrieval cues on alcohol cue reactivity among nonalcoholic drinkers. *Journal of Consulting and Clinical Psychology, 70,* 390–397.

Cunningham, C. L. (1979). Alcohol as a cue for extinction: State dependency produced by conditioned inhibition. *Animal Learning and Behavior, 7,* 45–52.

Cusato, B., & Domjan, M. (2000). Facilitation of appetitive conditioning with naturalistic conditioned stimuli: CS and US factors. *Animal Learning and Behavior, 26,* 247–256.

Davis, M. (1992). The role of the amygdala in conditioned fear. In J. P. Aggleton (Ed.), *The amygdala: Neurobiological aspects of emotion, memory, and mental dysfunction* (pp. 255–305). New York: Wiley-Liss.

Davis, M., & Shi, C. (1999). The extended amygdala: Are the central nucleus of the amygdala and the bed nucleus of the stria terminalis differentially involved in fear versus anxiety? *Annals of the New York Academy of Sciences, 877,* 281–291.

Davis, M., Walker, D. L., & Yee, Y. (1997). Roles of the amygdala and bed nucleus of the stria terminalis in fear and anxiety measured with the acoustic startle reflex: Possible relevance to PTSD. *Annals of the New York Academy of Sciences, 821,* 305–331.

Domjan, M. (1994). Formulation of a behavior system for sexual conditioning. *Psychonomic Bulletin and Review, 1,* 421–428.

Domjan, M. (1997). Behavior systems and the demise of equipotentiality: Historical antecedents and evidence from sexual conditioning. In M. E. Bouton & M. S. Fanselow (Eds.), *Learning, motivation, and cognition: The functional behaviorism of Robert C. Bolles* (pp. 31–51). Washington, DC: American Psychological Association.

Domjan, M., Greene, P., & North, N. C. (1989). Contextual conditioning and the control of copulatory behavior by species-specific sign stimuli in male Japanese quail. *Journal of Experimental Psychology: Animal Behavior Processes, 15,* 147–153.

Domjan, M., Huber-McDonald, M., & Holloway, K. S. (1992). Conditioning copulatory behavior to an artificial object: Efficacy of stimulus fading. *Animal Learning and Behavior, 20,* 350–362.

Estes, W. K., & Skinner, B. F. (1941). Some quantitative properties of anxiety. *Journal of Experimental Psychology, 29,* 390–400.

Fanselow, M. S. (1979). Naloxone attenuates rat's preference for signaled shock. *Physiological Psychology, 7,* 70–74.

Fanselow, M. S. (1994). Neural organization of the defensive behavior system responsible for fear. *Psychonomic Bulletin and Review, 1,* 429–438.

Fanselow, M. S., & Lester, L. S. (1988). A functional behavioristic approach to aversively motivated behavior: Predatory imminence as a determinant of the topography of defensive behavior. In R. C. Bolles & M. D. Beecher (Eds.), *Evolution and learning* (pp. 185–212). Hillsdale, NJ: Erlbaum.

Frohardt, R. J. (2001). *The role of the hippocampal formation, bed nucleus of the stria terminalis, and nucleus accumbens in contextual fear conditioning and reinstatement.* Unpublished doctoral dissertation, University of Vermont, Burlington.

Frohardt, R. J., Guarraci, F. A., & Bouton, M. E. (2000). The effects of neurotoxic hippocampal lesions on two effects of context after fear extinction. *Behavioral Neuroscience, 114,* 227–240.

Goldstein, A. J., & Chambless, D. L. (1978). A reanalysis of agoraphobia. *Behavior Therapy, 9,* 47–59.

Hilliard, S., Nguyen, M., & Domjan, M. (1997). One-trial appetitive conditioning in the sexual behavior system. *Psychonomic Bulletin and Review, 4,* 237–241.

Hirsch, S. M., & Bolles, R. C. (1980). On the ability of prey to recognize predators. *Zeitschrift Fuer Tierpsychologie, 54,* 71–84.

Hitchcock, J. M., & Davis, M. (1986). Lesions of the amygdala, but not of the cerebellum or red nucleus, block conditioned fear as measured with the potentiated startle paradigm. *Behavioral Neuroscience, 100,* 11–22.

Hitchcock, J. M., & Davis, M. (1991). The efferent pathway of the amygdala involved in conditioned fear as measured with the fear-potentiated startle paradigm. *Behavioral Neuroscience, 105,* 826–842.

Holland, P. C. (1980). CS–US interval as a determinant of the form of Pavlovian appetitive conditioned responses. *Journal of Experimental Psychology: Animal Behavior Processes, 6,* 155–174.

Holland, P. C. (1992). Occasion setting in Pavlovian conditioning. In G. Bower (Ed.), *The psychology of learning and motivation* (Vol 28, pp. 69–125). Orlando, FL: Academic Press.

Hollis, K. L. (1982). Pavlovian conditioning of signal-centered action patterns and autonomic behavior: A biological analysis of function. *Advances in the Study of Behavior, 12,* 131–142.

Hollis, K. L. (1997). Contemporary research on Pavlovian conditioning: A "new" functional analysis. *American Psychologist, 52,* 956–965.

Kapp, B. S., Whalen, P. J., Supple, W. F., Jr., & Pascoe, J. P. (1992). Amygdaloid contributions to conditioned arousal and sensory information processing. In J. P. Aggleton (Ed.), *The amygdala: Neurobiological aspects of emotion, memory, and mental dysfunction* (pp. 229–254). New York: Wiley.

Kim, J. A., Siegel, S., & Patenall, V. R. A. (1999). Drug-onset cues as signals: Intraadministration associations and tolerance. *Journal of Experimental Psychology: Animal Behavior Processes, 25,* 491–504.

Kim, J. J., & Fanselow, M. S. (1992). Modality-specific retrograde amnesia of fear. *Science, 256,* 675–677.

Kim, M., Campeau, S., Falls, W. A., & Davis, M. (1993). Infusion of the non-NMDA receptor antagonist CNQX into the amygdala blocks the expression of fear-potentiated startle. *Behavioral and Neural Biology, 59,* 5–8.

Konorski, J. (1967). *Integrative activity of the brain.* Chicago: University of Chicago Press.

Lang, P. J. (1995). The emotion probe: Studies of motivation and attention. *American Psychologist, 50,* 372–385.

LeDoux, J. E. (1996). *The emotional brain: The mysterious underpinnings of emotional life.* New York: Simon & Schuster.

LeDoux, J. E., Iwata, J., Cicchetti, P., & Reis, D. J. (1988). Different projections of the central amygdaloid nucleus mediate autonomic and behavioral correlates of conditioned fear. *Journal of Neuroscience, 8,* 2517–2529.

McNish, K. A., Betts, S. L., Brandon, S. E., & Wagner, A. R. (1997). Divergence of conditioned eyeblink and conditioned fear in backward Pavlovian training. *Animal Learning and Behavior, 25,* 43–52.

Mystkowski, J. L., Mineka, S., Vernon, L. L., & Zinbarg, R. E. (2003). Changes in caffeine states enhance return of fear in spider phobia. *Journal of Consulting and Clinical Psychology, 71,* 243–250.

Nelson, J. B. (2002). Context specificity of excitation and inhibition in ambiguous stimuli. *Learning and Motivation, 33,* 284–310.

Nelson, J. B., & Bouton, M. E. (1997). The effects of a context switch following serial and simultaneous feature-negative discriminations. *Learning and Motivation, 28,* 56–84.

Nelson, J. B., & Bouton, M. E. (2002). Extinction, inhibition, and emotional intelligence. In L. Feldman Barrett & P. Salovey (Eds.), *The wisdom in feeling: Psychological processes in emotional intelligence* (pp. 60–85). New York: Guilford Press.

Öhman, A., & Mineka, S. (2001). Fears, phobias, and preparedness: Toward an evolved module of fear and fear learning. *Psychological Review, 108,* 483–522.

Pain, L., Oberling, P., & Bouton, M. E. (2001). *Effects of interoceptive midazolam context and physical context on extinction and renewal of fear.* Manuscript in preparation.

Pavlov, I. P. (1927). *Conditioned reflexes.* London: Oxford University Press.

Pearce, J. M., & Bouton, M. E. (2001). Theories of associative learning in animals. *Annual Review of Psychology, 52,* 111–139.

Quigley, K. S., & Barrett, L. F. (1999). Emotional learning and mechanisms of intentional psychological change. In J. Brandtstadter & R. M. Lerner (Eds.), *Action and development: Origins and functions of intentional self-development* (pp. 435–464). Thousand Oaks, CA: Sage.

Rescorla, R. A., & Heth, C. D. (1975). Reinstatement of fear to an extinguished conditioned stimulus. *Journal of Experimental Psychology: Animal Behavior Processes, 1,* 8896.

Rescorla, R. A., & Wagner, A. R. (1972). A theory of Pavlovian conditioning: Variations in the effectiveness of reinforcement and nonreinforcement. In A. H. Black & W. F. Prokasy (Eds.), *Classical conditioning II: Current research and theory* (pp. 64–99). New York: Appleton-Century-Crofts.

Schmajuk, N. A., & Holland, P. C. (Eds.). (1998). *Occasion setting: Associative learning and cognition in animals.* Washington, DC: American Psychological Association.

Silva, K. M., & Timberlake, W. (1997). A behavior systems view of response form during long and short CS–US intervals. *Learning and Motivation, 28,* 465–490.

Sokolowska, M., Siegel, S., & Kim, J. A. (2002). Intra-administration associations: Conditional hyperalgesia elicited by morphine onset cues. *Journal of Experimental Psychology: Animal Behavior Processes, 28,* 309–320.

Swerdlow, N. R., Geyer, M. A., Vale, W. W., & Koob, G. F. (1986). Corticotropin-releasing factor potentiates acoustic startle in rats: Blockade by chlordiazepoxide. *Psychopharmacology, 88,* 147–152.

Timberlake, W. (1994). Behavior systems, associationism, and Pavlovian conditioning. *Psychonomic Bulletin and Review, 1,* 405–420.

Timberlake, W. (2001). Motivational modes in behavior systems. In R. R. Mowrer & S. B. Klein (Eds.), *Handbook of contemporary learning theories* (pp. 155–210). Mahwah, NJ: Erlbaum.

Timberlake, W., Wahl, G., & King, D. (1982). Stimulus and response contingencies in the misbehavior of rats. *Journal of Experimental Psychology: Animal Behavior Processes, 8,* 62–85.

Treit, D., Pesold, C., & Rotzinger, S. (1993). Dissociating the anti-fear effects of septal and amygdaloid lesions using two pharmacologically validated models of rat anxiety. *Behavioral Neuroscience, 107,* 770–785.

VanDercar, D. H., & Schneiderman, N. (1967). Interstimulus interval functions in different response systems during classical discrimination conditioning of rabbits. *Psychonomic Science, 9,* 9–10.

Vigorito, M., & Ayres, J. J. B. (1987). Effect of naloxone on conditioned suppression in rats. *Behavioral Neuroscience, 101,* 576–586.

Waddell, J., Morris, R. W., & Bouton, M. E. (submitted for publication). *Effect of bed nucleus of the stria terminalis lesions on aversive conditioning with long-duration conditional stimuli: Anxiety conditioning and reinstatement.*

Wagner, A. R., & Brandon, S. E. (1989). Evolution of a structured connectionist model of Pavlovian conditioning (AESOP). In S. B. Klein & R. R. Mowrer (Eds.), *Contemporary learning theories: Pavlovian conditioning and the status of traditional learning theory* (pp. 149–189). Hillsdale, NJ: Erlbaum.

Walker, D. L., & Davis, M. (1997a). Anxiogenic effects of high illumination levels assessed with the acoustic startle response in rats. *Biological Psychiatry, 42,* 461–471.

Walker, D. L., & Davis, M. (1997b). Double dissociation between the involvement of the bed nucleus of the stria terminals and the central nucleus of the amygdala in startle increases produced by conditioned versus unconditioned fear. *Journal of Neuroscience, 17,* 9375–9383.

Watson, J. B., & Rayner, R. (1920). Conditioned emotional reactions. *Journal of Experimental Psychology, 3,* 1–14.

Weingarten, H. (1983). Conditioned cues elicit feeding in sated rats: A role for learning in meal initiation. *Science, 220,* 431–433.

Wilson, A., Brooks, D. C., & Bouton, M. E. (1995). The role of the rat hippocampal system in several effects of context in extinction. *Behavioral Neuroscience, 109,* 828–836.

Wolpe, J., & Rowan, V. C. (1988). Panic disorder: A product of classical conditioning. *Behaviour Research and Therapy, 26,* 441–450.

Woods, S. C., & Strubbe, J. H. (1994). The psychobiology of meals. *Psychonomic Bulletin and Review, 1,* 141–155.

Zajonc, R. B., & McIntosh, D. N. (1992). Emotions research: Some promising questions and some questionable promises. *Psychological Science, 3,* 70–74.

PART IV

The Experience of Emotion

CHAPTER 10

Emotion Experience and the Indeterminacy of Valence

LOUIS C. CHARLAND

> Words are like the film on deep water.
> —LUDWIG WITTGENSTEIN, *Notebooks*
> (1914–1916, p. 30.5.15)

Many aspects of emotion are said to be valenced and labeled *positive* or *negative*. Indeed, valence is generally considered to be a central feature of emotion. For example, it is probably not an exaggeration to say that "many investigators consider the valence of emotions to be the single most important dimension of affective experience" (Fossum & Barrett, 2000, p. 679). Yet, despite its theoretical proclivity, the philosophical status of valence in emotion science remains largely unexplored. What *is* valence? Is it an objective, intrinsic property of emotion experience, a "given" that is discovered? Or is it instead an outcome of emotion experience, a "product" that is subjectively created in consciousness?

In what follows, emotion experience will be defined rather strictly. Following John Lambie and Anthony Marcel, "emotion experience" is understood as "referring to and including (1) the phenomenological aspect of an emotion state, and (2) second-order awareness of this experience, although the latter is not always present" (Lambie & Marcel, 2002, p. 230). An emotion state, in turn, is defined as "what is common to a certain set of evaluative representations, attitudinal behaviors, and physical states (pp. 229–230). The definition is meant to capture the bare minimum of

1. *What is the scope of your proposed model? When you use the term* emotion, *how do you use it? What do you mean by terms such as* fear, anxiety, *or* happiness?

My discussion deals with emotion valence (the idea that emotions can be classified as positive or negative) and affect valence (the idea that emotional feelings or affects can be classified as positive or negative). The main focus of the discussion is affect valence, although there are implications for emotion valence. The scope of my discussion extends to all studies and theories that rely on the idea that we can classify emotions and emotional feelings or affects as positive and negative.

2. *Define your terms:* conscious, unconscious, awareness. *Or say why you do not use these terms.*

In my chapter emotion experience is understood as "referring to and including (1) the phenomenological aspect of an emotion state, and (2) second-order awareness of this experience, although the latter is not always present" (Lambie & Marcel 2002, p. 230). Emotion state is defined as "what is common to a certain set of evaluative representations, attitudinal behaviors, and physical states (pp. 229–230). This definition is meant to capture the bare minimum of what "people are referring to in mutually understood discourse that uses the term 'emotion' " (p. 230).

3. *Does your model deal with what is conscious, what is unconscious, or their relationship? If you do not address this area specifically, can you speculate on the relationship between what is conscious and unconscious? Or if you do not like the conscious–unconscious distinction, or if you do not think this is a good question to ask, can you say why?*

Following Lambie and Marcel (2002), my account relies on the distinction between first-order phenomenology and second-order awareness in conscious emotion experience. I propose an argument that shows that affect valence is limited to conscious awareness only. This argument makes the notion of unconscious affect valence extremely problematic, and that of nonconscious affect valence impossible. My argument also implies that the attribution of valence to objects and stimuli outside of, or apart from, conscious awareness is metaphorical only. This position creates problems for studies or theories that rely on valence as if it were an objective, reliable property of external objects and stimuli themselves.

what "people are referring to in mutually understood discourse that uses the term 'emotion' " (p. 230). The principal reason for introducing this particular conception of emotion experience is its important distinction between first-order phenomenology and second-order awareness. That distinction plays a central role in our discussion.[1]

Technically stated, the central claim of this chapter is that valence understood as hedonicity (pleasure or displeasure) is not an intrinsic objective property of felt affect in first-order emotion experience. Rather, it is a property of second-order emotion experience that is highly variable and fundamentally indeterminate. Because the scientific literature on valence and affect is so idiosyncratic and complex, explaining and defending this thesis requires considerable background preparation. But intuitively the point should be clear. Very simply, feelings are not intrinsically pleasant or unpleasant in themselves. Their "positive" (pleasant) or "negative" (unpleasant) character is not an objective property that is intrinsic to them. Instead, valence is fixed by the process of attending to feelings in second-order awareness. Some element of "interpretation" appears to be involved (Lambie & Marcel 2002, pp. 220, 244).

The culmination of this argument is called the indeterminacy thesis. According to this thesis, there is no intrinsic objective scientific fact about what the valence of a particular emotional affect or feeling is apart from its elaboration in second-order awareness in emotion experience. Valence is objectively indeterminate because it is impossible to report or measure it without at the same time changing it. The exact character and personal meaning of an emotional feeling is created in second-order awareness by attention. But attention does not create the underlying phenomenology out of which valence is created. Neither does it create the nonconscious mechanisms that underlie valence. Here it is crucial to distinguish between the conscious subjective experience of valence and the nonconscious mechanisms that underlie it.

One important consequence of the indeterminacy thesis is that descriptive structural models of the valence dimension of affect probably fall much shorter of their explanatory goals than is typically thought. This is because the indeterminacy thesis poses serious problems for the idea that *felt* valence is an objective commodity that can be measured reliably. But that is a central assumption of many scientific efforts to explain affect (Carroll, Michelle, Yik, Russell, & Barrett, 1999; Barrett, Chapter 11; Russell, 2003; Watson & Tellegen, 1985).

DESCRIPTIVE STRUCTURAL THEORIES OF AFFECT

To get a clearer grasp of what is at stake in our opening questions, consider the well-known circumplex model of emotion (Russell, 1980; Barrett & Russell, 1998). According to that model, emotion experience is said to include a component of "affect," which informally is referred to as "feeling." Lisa Feldman Barrett probably speaks for many emotion researchers when she says that "self-report represents the most reliable and possibly only window that researchers have on conscious, subjective, emotional experience" (Barrett, 1996, p. 47). She and many others employ self-reports to inquire into valence. The conscious felt subjective experience of valence in these discussions is construed as a component of affect—which, in turn, is considered to be a fundamental constituent of emotion experience (Russell, 2003).

Certainly, much valuable work has been done in mapping the descriptive structure of valence and other components of affect using self-reports (Barrett & Russell, 1998; Cacioppo & Berntson, 1999; Carroll et al., 1999; Larsen & Diener, 1992; Russell, 1980; Watson & Tellegen, 1985). It is interesting that the word *description* is often used in characterizing the epistemological aim of these studies. Thus the aim is to *describe* affect (Carroll et al., 1999, p. 14; Russell & Carroll, 1999, p. 5; Larsen, MacGraw, Meter, & Cacioppo, 2001, p. 692). What is sought is an explanatory model of the "descriptive structure" of affect (Barrett & Russell, 1998, p. 967; Carroll et al., 1999, p. 14).

But how can description capture something that is inherently evaluative? How can we hold valence still, to measure and describe it objectively, without at the same time changing its normative character? Of course, evaluations can sometimes be treated descriptively: thus "*formally*, an evaluation is a valenced (i.e., positive or negative judgment about a stimulus" (Fossum & Barrett, 2000, p. 669; emphasis added). But resorting to evaluative judgments does not solve our problem. The reason is that, in *substance* as opposed to *form*, valence is a very peculiar characteristic of conscious experience. To explain why, it is helpful to distinguish two different but related senses of the term *valence*: (1) a pretheoretical, substantial, experiential one; and (2) an abstract, theoretical, formal one. Note that it is the explanation and description of the *experience* of valence that is at issue here, not the explanation and description of the nonconscious mechanisms which may correspond or contribute to it (Lambie & Marcel, 2002, p. 227; Larsen et al., 2001, p. 686).

On a pretheoretical experiential level, valence is a felt conscious tendency or orientation toward or away from features of experience. This is reflected in the etymology of the term, which signifies a power or capacity to react. It is crucial that valence is not viewed simply as the experience of brute and blind physiological urges. On the contrary, it is laden with personal meaning and is inseparably tied to an experience of the personal significance of what events in the environment mean for us. This personal meaning is what makes valence fundamentally evaluative and interpretive. Through valence, we feel moved toward or away from things, in a manner that is accompanied by an experience of what those things mean to us personally. This pretheoretical conscious felt sense of valence is what the scientific study of valence is meant to explain. It serves as the *explanandum* for many theories of valence. Other starting points are possible. But this one has the notable distinction of starting with the assumption that, paradigmatically, valence is a property of conscious emotion experience. The question then is whether objective descriptive methods that employ self reports can adequately capture the evaluative and interpretive core of this subjective phenomenon. How well can self-report measures succeed in capturing this qualitative aspect of emotion experience, the subjective "qualia" that self-reports are allegedly *about* (Scherer, Chapter 13). How can science capture what it *is* that these reports allegedly *report* (Scherer, Chapter 13)?

We can now restate our opening questions. Is the special felt qualitative tendency in valence, as it is structurally represented in descriptive theories, an intrinsic feature of emotion experience as such; that is, something that exists prior to the self-reports that describe it? Or is it instead created and structured by features of second-order awareness, such as these self-reports? The argument here is that valence is created by attention in second-order awareness. There is nothing scientifically objective or precise that we can *say* about valence apart from its elaboration in second-order awareness. Second-order awareness does not create the underlying phenomenology of emotion experience, but it does shape and articulate what exactly it means to us. This conclusion would appear to threaten the scientific foundation of descriptive theories of affect, because it undermines the objectivity of the phenomenon they claim to study. It also contradicts the driving assumption of several dominant neuroscientific theories of valence, according to which valence is an intrinsic objective property of affective experience.

Affect and *valence* are the central terms involved in our discussion; both have widely variable uses. There are several options available for defining affect, and the matter is partly subject to stipulation (Carroll et al., 1999, p. 21; Russell & Carroll, 1999, p. 7). For present purposes, affect is initially defined as the conscious felt experience of emotion (Berkowitz, 2000, p. 4; Cacioppo & Bernston, 1999, p. 134; Russell & Carroll, 1999, p. 3). Affects, then, are "subjectively experienced feelings" (Buck, 1999, p. 301). In some theories, affect is said to consist of two dimensions; valence and activation; the latter is also sometimes referred to as arousal or activity. This, for example, is how affect is understood in the circumplex model of emotion (Russell, 1980; Feldman, 1995): It treats valence as a component dimension of affect, which in turn is treated as an element of emotion experience.

The circumplex model of emotion and theories like it generally treat valence as a component of *affect*; other approaches treat valence as an attribute of *emotions* (Frijda, 1986; Lazarus, 1991; Ben-Ze'ev, 2000; Prinz, 2004). Accordingly, one of our first tasks is to clarify the distinction between *affect valence* (i.e., valence attributed to individual distinct affects) and *emotion valence* (i.e., valence attributed to individual whole emotions). This distinction will enable us to focus on *affect valence* without, hopefully, inviting too much confusion. It is the valence of the subjective feelings or affects in emotion experience with which we are concerned, not the valence of emotions as such.

DISTINGUISHING EMOTION VALENCE AND AFFECT VALENCE

Valence can be defined as the positive or negative "charge" associated with a particular physical or mental state, or a particular combination of these. The view that individual emotions have valence is widespread in both philosophical and psychological theories of emotion (e.g., Ben-Ze'ev, 2000; Gordon, 1987; Lazarus, 1991; Ortony, Clore, & Collins, 1988; Prinz, 2004). In this case, valence is held to be a property of individual emotions. Thus it is often said that fear is a negative emotion, whereas, joy is a positive one. Call this *emotion valence*. Normally, emotion valence is considered to be an intrinsic objective property of individual whole emotions. A given emotion is simply said to be *positive* or *negative*.

Sometimes it is not individual whole emotions that are said to be positive or negative but, rather, individual affects (e.g., Barrett, 1996; Larsen & Diener, 1992; Russell, 1980; Watson & Tellegen, 1985). In this case, valence is held to be a property of individual affects. Thus it is often said that feeling frightened is a negative affect, whereas feeling joyful is a positive one. Call this *affect valence*. Note that valence can also be attributed to the individual affects in moods. However, in what follows, it is the valenced dimension of affect in emotion experience that concerns us.

To summarize, there are at least two kinds of valence that are sometimes referred to in emotion theory: emotion valence and affect valence.[2] The distinction is helpful exegetically. For example, sometimes individual emotions are said to inherit their emotion valence from the valence of their underlying affective states; that is, affect valence (Russell, 2003). At other times, the valence of individual affects is said to be determined by the valence of their underlying emotion states; that is, emotion valence (Damasio, 2003). There are also cases in which emotion valence is treated as if it were a distinct phenomenon of its own, and affect valence is not mentioned (Gordon, 1987; Lazarus, 1991). Finally, there are cases in which affect valence is the object of study, and emotion valence is not mentioned (Zajonc, 1980).

Evidently, the distinction between emotion valence and affect valence is not trivial, and there are important reasons to respect it. But it is a rather crude distinction. As described, it does not address the various internal components of emotion episodes that might be valenced, such as goals and appraisals. Neither does it address cases in which the cause or object of an emotion is said to be valenced. The point is simply that it is often considered useful to list individual affects or emotions under columns labeled *positive* and *negative*. This practice is what the distinction between emotion valence and affect valence is meant to capture.

PLEASURE AND ITS OPPOSITES

The general definition of valence provided above characterizes it as bivalent; a contrast between two polar opposites. There is a positive "charge," on one hand, and a negative "charge" on the other. The definition is meant to remind us of the chemical connotations of the term but says nothing specific about what valence *is*. The reason is that specific proposals vary considerably. Typical interpretations of the concept of valence in emotion theory include the polarities of good and bad (Kahneman, 1999), hot and cold (Berkowitz, 2000), pleasant and unpleasant (Russell, 1980), pleasure and pain (Frijda, 1986), approach and withdrawal (Davidson, 1992), and joy and sorrow (Damasio, 2003).

When it is defined in terms of pleasure, valence is sometimes referred to as *hedonicity* (Lambie & Marcel, 2002). This is probably the most common understanding of the term. Generally, pleasure and one of its putative opposites are the qualities referred to by the positive and negative "charges" of valence, respectively (e.g., displeasure, unpleasantness, pain, etc.). This is true for both emotion valence and affect valence. Indeed, this usage and its variants are so common that sometimes affect, hedonic quality, and valence, are all used synonymously to denote a pleasant–unpleasant quality, or positive and negative affect, respectively (Barrett, 1996; Russell, 1999). It is, of course, true that affect is often said to have other dimensions, such as activation or arousal. But affectivity, as such, is more closely allied with hedonicity. In the words of John Lambie and Anthony Marcel, "the most markedly affectively valenced aspect of emotion experience is hedonic tone or quality: pleasure and displeasure" (Lambie & Marcel, 2002, p. 343). Lisa Feldman Barrett makes the same point when she states that "the valence dimension typically refers to the hedonic quality of an affective experience (pleasant or unpleasant)" (Barrett, 1996, p. 48).[3]

The distinction between emotion valence and affect valence is fundamental to how pleasure figures into emotional valence. To say that positive *emotions* are associated with pleasure is one thing. To say that positive *affects* are associated with pleasure is another. The supporting theories and arguments are usually quite different. One theory ranges over emotions, the other over affects. As we saw above, it may be that individual emotions inherit their pleasurable characteristics from the pleasurable qualities of their underlying affects (Russell, 2003). An alternative model of the genealogy of valence might be that the pleasurable qualities of affect are derivable from the pleasurable qualities of individual emotions (Damasio, 2003). Both of these proposals involve valence; they simply differ on which aspect of valence is primary in the genealogy of valence. According to the former, affect valence is primary. According to the latter, emotion valence is primary. These two examples should reinforce the reason why it is important to distinguish between emotion valence and affect valence.

To summarize, in the context of emotion theory, valence is generally defined in terms of pleasure and its opposites. This is the most common and central sense of what is meant by the term. In this sense, valence "is an obvious and central feature of emotion" (Lambie & Marcel, 2002, p. 434). An emotion or affect is said to be "positive" because it is associated with pleasure. An emotion or affect is said to be "negative" because it is associated with some opposite of pleasure; perhaps unpleasantness, displeasure, or pain.

One of the most interesting areas of debate in contemporary emotion theory involves affect valence in this hedonic sense. The issue is whether pleasure and its opposites are statistically independent measures, or whether they are linked by correlation (Barrett & Russell, 1998; Russell, 1999; Watson & Tellegen, 1985). This issue is an excellent example of what scientific historian Thomas Kuhn meant by "puzzle-solving" in "normal science" (Kuhn, 1970). There is a widely shared body of experimental practices, or paradigms, and a thriving research industry working on related problems. The association between positive and negative valence, and pleasure and its opposites, is equally popular in discussions of emotion valence. But here we do not find the same focus on sharply defined problems and experimental techniques. Scientific efforts to understand valence therefore tend to be focused in the area of affect valence. The widespread use of the concept of valence in this domain is a prominent feature of the scientific study of emotion. To be sure, there are theorists who downplay or ignore the contribution of valence to emotion (James, 1890/1981; Mandler, 1984; Schacter & Singer, 1962). Nevertheless, when it is combined or identified with hedonicity, valence is fundamental to large segments of emotion theory. Indeed, it is so pervasive that it is hard to imagine emotion theory without it.

WHEN EMOTION VALENCE IS INTRINSIC

In a provocative critique of emotion valence, Robert Solomon and Lori Stone claim that the origins of the concept of valence lie in ethics (Solomon & Stone, 2002, p. 418). This may be true in the case of emotion valence, but it is inaccurate in the case of affect valence, which they hardly mention. In fact, a plausible history of the scientific origins of affect valence can be found in the development of the physiological concept of irritability (Hall, 1975; Pagel, 1967; Temkin, 1964). And certainly many contemporary theories of affect valence do not originate in ethics, although they may have implications for ethics. Solomon and Stone therefore appear to be wrong that the origins of affect valence lie in ethics. But actually their critique of emotion valence ignores affect valence almost entirely. As a result, their discussion of valence is incomplete. However, Solomon and Stone are right in claiming that the concept of emotion valence is more problematic than is commonly realized. In particular, they are right in stating that valence cannot be a fixed *objective* and *intrinsic* feature of emotions.

Very roughly, what Solomon and Stone (2002) argue is that valence is always a matter of interpretation and that interpretation is always relative to a context and a scheme of meaning or evaluation. It therefore makes little sense to say that an emotion is positive or negative, in itself, apart from some scheme of meaning that provides criteria for the application of the "positive" and "negative" valence operators. Hence, it makes little sense to speak of emotion valence as if it were a fixed objective and intrinsic feature of emotion states themselves. It is neither objective nor intrinsic because it is based on interpretation, which involves the assignment of a positive or negative value to those states.

Solomon and Stone (2002) conclude their critique of emotion valence in a rather iconoclastic manner. They write:

> The analysis of emotions in terms of "valence," while it recognizes something essential about emotions (that is, that they involve appraisals and evaluations of the world and are relevant to a life well or ill-lived), is an idea that we should abandon and leave behind. It serves no purpose but confusion and perpetrates the worst old stereotypes about emotion, that these are simple phenomenon unworthy of serious research and analysis. (p. 432)

This certainly is a radical conclusion that would mean the end of large segments of emotion theory as we know it. However, on closer look Solomon and Stone (2002) appear to endorse a more moderate conclusion. They write:

> All emotions involve some positive or negative appraisals (Solomon, 1993). But to collapse all appraisals into a single evaluative polarity, positive-and-negative, is, to put it simply, simple-minded. (p. 427)

What, then, is the correct interpretation of Solomon and Stone's conclusion? The first passage states that we should give up the concept of valence entirely, and the second one denies this. This seems blatantly inconsistent. However, there is a way to resolve the inconsistency. What Solomon and

Stone are really arguing against is the "facile" and "simple-minded" mono-lithic application of the concept of valence to emotions (p. 433). More spe-cifically, they object to emotion valence as a monolithic concept; that is, a concept that is indiscriminately applied to all the various emotions in an attempt to reduce their multifarious evaluative aspects to a single uniform bipolar dimension. As they say, "our argument is not that there is no such thing as valence or no such polarity or contrasts, but rather that there are *many* such polarities and contrasts" (p. 418). To document their case, they list 18 examples of how positive and negative bipolarity is understood in emotion theory (p. 418). They also appeal to Aaron Ben-Ze'ev's rich account of the subtlety of emotion (Ben-Ze'ev, 2000).

So, on closer examination, what Solomon and Stone are against is the "facile" and "simple-minded" monolithic application of the concept of valence to emotions. They do not believe that we should give up the con-cept of valence entirely. Instead, their point is that there are many varieties of emotion valence. This still means doing away with the idea that valence is an intrinsic feature of emotions. That is quite a radical conclusion. As we shall see, the same conclusion applies in the case of affect valence, with equally radical consequences. But here the argument will be quite differ-ent; it is the indeterminacy thesis. The consequences will also be more drastic, since they create doubt over the very possibility of a scientific approach to affect valence.

WHEN AFFECT VALENCE IS INTRINSIC

We have seen that a strong case can be made that valence cannot be an intrinsic objective feature of individual whole emotions. The assignment of valence to individual emotions always depends on interpretation and con-text. What about affect valence? Is the valence of individual conscious feel-ing states ("affects") ever an intrinsic objective feature of those states?

The various descriptive theories of affect discussed earlier all appear to endorse the assumption that valence is an intrinsic objective feature of affect states. An especially vivid expression of that assumption can be found in two recent neuroscientific theories of affect valence (Damasio, 2003; Panksepp, 1998). These proposals share the assumption that valence some-how resides *in* individual affects as an intrinsic objective feature of those states themselves. Thus, in affect valence, subjective affects or feelings are often thought to be positive or negative in themselves. They wear their meanings—their "charges"—on their sleeves. In this view, when we report the valence of an affective state, we uncover and reveal something deter-mined and fixed that is already there. In other words, the assignment of a positive or negative value to that state is verified by the fact that the state *is* positive or negative—prior to being assigned that value. Let us very briefly consider two important examples.

According to Jaak Panksepp, the mammalian brain is genetically predisposed to develop several basic emotion command systems. These natural kinds of emotion embody and reflect values that are fundamental to the survival of the organism. According to Panksepp, there are probably seven basic emotion systems: seeking, rage, fear, panic, play, lust, care (Panksepp, 2001, p. 156; see also Panksepp, 1998). The language of values is important here. What it means is that each basic emotion system provides a distinct kind of evaluative orientation to the world; that is, each system specifies a particular kind of direction the organism may take as it deals with changing features of its environment.

Panksepp's basic emotion systems are all valenced, and, at times, he uses the standard chemical metaphor of positive and negative "charges" to characterize valence (Panksepp, 2001, p. 156, Table 2). But note that in his view, some basic emotions can generate both positive and negative charges, depending on the circumstances. Thus lust can generate erotic feelings, which are pleasurable, and jealous feelings, which are not. And seeking can generate interest, which is pleasurable, and frustration, which is not (p. 156). Clearly, for Panksepp there is sometimes more to valence than simply pleasure and its opposites. However, this does not prevent him from resorting to that simple opposition in order to organize and simplify his overall discussion of affect valence.

Another important example of the view that valence is an intrinsic feature of affective states can be found in the work of Antonio Damasio. He presents a vigorous defense of the idea that valence is an intrinsic and objective feature of affective states themselves. Damasio has a distinct view of the genealogy of affect valence. First, there is the emotion body state. Each basic emotion constitutes an automatic response and particular evaluative orientation to the world and is designed to protect and improve the conditions of the organism (Damasio, 2003, pp. 34–35). Then comes the corresponding affective feeling state, which is the consciousness of that underlying body state. According to Damasio, the feeling state inherits its valence from the underlying emotion state that gives rise to it. In short, "a feeling of emotion is an idea of the body when it is perturbed by the emotion process" (p. 88). This account of the genealogy of affect is accompanied by a thoroughgoing commitment to bivalence. Thus we are told that "all feelings contain some aspect of pain or pleasure" (p. 123). Indeed, in Damasio's view, it is a "well-established" fact that feelings are bivalent:

> There are organism states in which the regulation of life processes becomes efficient, or even optimal, free-flowing and easy. This is a well-established physiological fact. It is not a hypothesis. The feelings that usually accompany

such physiological conducive states are deemed "positive," characterized not simply by the absence of pain but by varieties of pleasure. There also are organism states in which life processes struggle for balance and can even be chaotically out of control. The feelings that usually accompany such states are deemed "negative," characterized not just by absence of pleasure but by varieties of pain. (p. 131)

In a complex series of steps, Damasio extends these observations about the origins of bivalence in bodily regulation and homeostasis to the psychological and social domains. He presents a classification of emotions in which social emotions such as shame and sympathy are labeled as positive or negative, depending on their innate valenced character (p. 156). Damasio actually traces the bivalent character of valence all the way back to the mechanisms of cellular activity. Even the "unbrained paramecium" is capable of emotional reactions, according to him. In this case, valence is characterized as "detection of the presence of an object or event that recommends avoidance and evasion or endorsement and approach" (p. 41).

Like Panksepp, Damasio is a believer in intrinsic valence. In his view, the positive or negative character of the various affective states is not a contextual matter of interpretation requiring comparison with some external standard of meaning. One simply detects and experiences what it is like to be in that state and that's it. The experience of valence is seen as a kind of conscious registration of information. Damasio does insist that consciousness and perception are dynamic. However, in his account of affect valence, the information that a state is valenced is not fundamentally changed or altered by the awareness of it, nor is it altered by the process of becoming conscious of it. It is simply read off as that state.

To conclude, both Panksepp and Damasio appear to endorse some form of the thesis that valence is an intrinsic objective feature of affective states themselves. In this they agree with the defenders of descriptive structural models of affect discussed earlier, who also maintain that valence is an intrinsic objective property of affective states. If our indeterminacy thesis is true, then this assumption must be wrong. To explain why, we turn to John Lambie and Anthony Marcel's novel account of emotion experience. Although they do not defend an indeterminacy thesis, such a thesis can be constructed from their account of emotion experience.

THE HETEROGENEOUS CHARACTER
OF EMOTION EXPERIENCE

In a highly original discussion of emotion experience, John Lambie and Anthony Marcel argue that emotion experience is not single or uniform.

According to them, "emotion experience takes various forms and is hetero-genous" (Lambie & Marcel, 2002, p. 219). They also argue that "there is no one essential type of content of emotion experience" (p. 256). Thus there is a variety of emotion experiences, and the content of emotion experience is both "varied and variable."

There are important lessons in Lambie and Marcel's discussion for our understanding of affect valence. First, their account of the varieties of emo-tion experience poses special problems for the view that affect valence is a single uniform phenomenon. Valence, for Lambie and Marcel, turns out to be multidimensional and multiple. Secondly, their claim that valence is multidimensional and multiple points toward an even more radical thesis—which they, however, do not explore. This thesis is that *affect valence is fun-damentally indeterminate*. However, before this thesis can be stated, it is first necessary to consider more closely Lambie and Marcel's account of emotion experience.

Lambie and Marcel (2002) start by distinguishing two orders of emotion experience, which they refer to as phenomenal experience and awareness (p. 220). These constitute emotion experience, in their sense of the term (p. 230). First-order phenomenal experience is a very basic "what-it's-like" experience. Second-order awareness is normally directed at first-order phe-nomenal experience (p. 230); it is a kind of reflexive knowledge of that first-order phenomenology (p. 228). First-order phenomenology does not have propositional structure (p. 239); it is ineffable, although it is not inexpressible or indescribable (p. 237). Nevertheless, it is significant that "reports of phe-nomenology tend to distort it" (p. 237). Second-order awareness is a kind of knowing directed at first-order phenomenology; its content is created by attending to first-order phenomenal experience, which is logically and temporally prior. Normally, we can only know first-order phenomenology through second-order awareness, "which usually transforms it" (p. 237). Attention is central to second-order awareness. Lambie and Marcel (2002) actually state that "focal attention in particular *creates* awareness" (p. 235).

Lambie and Marcel (2002) cite numerous sources of evidence for their distinction between first- and second-order emotion experience. They illustrate the distinction by arguing that "blindsight is a first-order prob-lem, and Anton's Syndrome, or unawareness of a sensory deficit, is a second-order problem" (p. 228). They also mention the case of people who remember pains or sensations of which they were previously unaware. To make sense of these and other similar phenomena, it is necessary to sup-pose that phenomenal experience can be independent of awareness. This supposition requires something like the distinction between first- and second-order emotion experience.

Phenomenology can be independent of awareness, although usually it is not. Normally, they are linked by focal attention, a mechanism whereby some part of first-order phenomenal experience can become the content of second-order awareness (Lambie & Marcel, 2002, p. 234). Lambie and Marcel are careful to note that even though "phenomenology as such is independent of and prior to focal attention, it is nonetheless subject to two aspects of attention" (p. 234). These are general directedness and attentional mode. *General directedness* addresses whether one's experience is oriented to the self or to the world. *Mode of attention* addresses whether one's stance is analytic or synthetic and/or immersed or detached. An analytic perspective tries to break things down into their component parts. Its opposite is the synthetic perspective, which considers the whole (p. 235). The detached perspective tends to remove the self from the object of attention. Its opposite is the immersed perspective, which puts the self closer to the object of attention (p. 235). With all these factors operating in emotion experience, it is a far more complex and variable affair than is typically supposed. So is the question of the supposed content of emotion experience. The consequences of this line of thinking for the concept of valence are enormous, particularly when valence is understood as hedonicity.

Lambie and Marcel (2002) sometimes distinguish between valence and hedonicity. They limit hedonicity to pleasure and pain and relegate valence to positive and negative evaluation (p. 229). For them, there is a distinction between the evaluation underlying and causing an emotion—namely, valence—and the pain or pleasure of the experience—namely, hedonicity (p. 243). However, as we have seen, many writers on affect valence appear to identify valence with hedonicity. And recall Lambie and Marcel's claim that "the most markedly affectively valenced aspect of emotion experience is hedonic tone or quality: pleasure and displeasure" (p. 343). For our purposes, the central point at issue is the claim that valence is an intrinsic feature of affective states. On that question, Lambie and Marcel also appear to defend a form of the thesis that affect valence is intrinsic. However, somewhat ironically, they also provide good reasons for doubting it. To see why, we need to look closer at the relationship between attention and hedonicity. Recall that, according to Lambie and Marcel, hedonicity is the most "*markedly* affectively valenced aspect of emotion experience" and "an *obvious and central* feature of emotion" (p. 243; emphasis added).

Lambie and Marcel (2002) argue that "hedonicity may be of different kinds" partly because "hedonic tone is not a single simple dimension but differs according to the specific intentionality of the emotion" (p. 244). For example, "the pleasure in relief is different from that in simply satisfying an unhindered concern" (p. 244). Likewise, the "pain of grief is different from that of frustration" (p. 244). In other words, each distinct emotion episode can have its own particular hedonic tone. This pluralistic position on hedonicity appears to be inconsistent with Damasio's theory of affect valence, and others like it. However, the divergence from traditional approaches to valence gets even more pronounced when we add the fact that Lambie and Marcel are not simply saying that each individual emotion episode has its own single hedonic tone. In addition, they also maintain that within a single emotion experience there can be different, sometimes contrasting, varieties of hedonicity. As they put it, "the different sources of hedonics do not contribute to a single hedonic tone but to different hedonic tones coexisting at one moment" (p. 245). Thus the object of love may be experienced as pleasant while the state one is in is not. This means that even within a single emotion experience there can be multiple sources and experiences of hedonicity that range from the appraisal itself, to what is appraised, the result of the appraisal, and the experience of the action tendency associated with that particular emotion state (p. 245).

ATTENTION IN EMOTION EXPERIENCE

So, according to Lambie and Marcel (2002), different hedonic tones can be experienced at a given time; attention determines (1) which one enters awareness, (2) the degree of awareness, and (3) how pleasant or unpleasant it is. The key to all this is the relationship between hedonicity and attention. Hedonicity is determined by mode of attention (p. 243). Focal attention also plays an important role in the generation of hedonicity by selectively focusing consciousness on a particular hedonic tone and making it available for awareness. This formulation sounds very much as if hedonicity were entirely a psychological construction effected by attention. Yet Lambie and Marcel also say that hedonicity is intrinsic: "Hedonicity both is intrinsic to bodily states, movements, and rhythms and depends on the interpretation placed on them" (p. 244). But what really does this statement mean? Is hedonicity somehow *there*, determinate and fixed, temporally and logically prior to its revelation in awareness through attention? And, if so, what is the nature of the theoretical vocabulary used to capture it scientifically?

One way to understand what Lambie and Marcel (2002) mean by the claim that hedonicity is intrinsic is to suppose that the set of hedonic tones one experiences at a given moment is determinate in the sense of being fixed and constrained by the specific nature of the particular emotional episode in question and its attendant circumstances. What varies is the particular hedonic tone that enters awareness and the degree to which the person becomes aware of it (determined by attention). Thus even though there may be variation and fluctuation in awareness of hedonic tone, there is still something fixed and determinate underneath it all: namely, the first-order experience in which multiple hedonic tones are normally present. Yet there are problems making sense of the claim that hedonicity might be intrinsic in this way.

Recall that in Lambie and Marcel's (2002) view, attention affects the hedonic tone of which one is aware. For example, a detached stance can make hedonicity virtually disappear, whereas an immersed stance can allow it to dominate one's being. Attending to the self or to the world brings different features of each into focus while others disappear. And, of course, this happens not only with different emotion experiences; it can also happen within a single ongoing emotion experience. A good example is pain. Lambie and Marcel note that "the more analytically that one attends to a painful sensation, the less its painfulness: The more that one attends to the sensations themselves and the less one's attention encompasses [their] signification, the less is [their] hedonicity" (p. 235). They even go so far as to say that "if one attends to one's bodily sensations in a sufficiently analytic and detached manner, hedonic tone may be distanced, diminished, and disappear" (p. 243). In this way, "the painfulness of the pain is often reduced and sometimes vanishes" (p. 243).

The same mechanisms of attention govern the hedonic character of pleasure, and secondary appraisal can also influence hedonicity. Thus "judging that one can change the situation or that nothing can be done has a large effect" (p. 244). Here Lambie and Marcel (2002) cite the fact that "the pain of torture is increased by knowledge of helplessness" (p. 243).[4] Note that although variations in attention and appraisal may alter the character of hedonicity in second-order emotion experience, they do not create the underlying phenomenology of first-order experience. Nevertheless, as Lambie and Marcel clearly state, the *precise* nature of first-order experience normally eludes us until it is shaped and revealed in attention (p. 228); this is a crucial point. We are now ready to consider the indeterminacy thesis for affect valence.

INDETERMINACY OF AFFECT VALENCE

Lambie and Marcel (2002) tell us that there is something "it is like" to be in a first-order phenomenological emotion state prior to attention. The character of that particular experience may be *expressible* but it is not *reportable* apart from second-order awareness and its mechanisms and processes (p. 229). It is a sort of experience-in-itself that cannot normally be captured except through awareness, which forms and shapes it and therefore changes it. In general, "one's experience is not independent of how one attends to it" (p. 226). Different forms of attention therefore translate into different forms of emotion experience. The "what-it's-like" underneath it all is there but cannot be captured verbally. The problem is that whenever we try to capture, in words, the hedonicity of an emotion state—its hedonic valence—we also change the nature of what is being experienced. The key here is the special subjective evaluative character of the awareness of hedonic valence. Although it may true that the mechanisms underlying first-order emotion experience can be explained scientifically, the first-order subjective evaluative character of that experience—its emotional meaning—cannot. To try and capture the subjective character scientifically is simultaneously to change and transform the nature of what is supposed to be explained. This is the principal reason behind the indeterminacy thesis for affect valence.

The indeterminacy of hedonic valence follows from the fact that valence is semantically and evaluatively permeable to attention. The same is true of affect valence, more generally. Valence cannot be intrinsic to first-order phenomenal emotion experience in the manner Lambie and Marcel (2002) appear to suggest. Neither is it externally created by attention ex nihilo outside first-order phenomenal experience. Rather, it is a dynamic relational evaluative phenomenon that emerges out of the interaction of attention with first-order phenomenology. In other words, affect valence is neither purely intrinsic and "found," nor purely extrinsic and "constructed." It is *enacted* (Varela, 1989). A consequence of this ambiguous ontological status is that to attend to the valence of an affective state is to disrupt and change it. Every act of attention is like a new evaluative baptism. In a nutshell: *Affect valence is indeterminate until it is fixed by attention.*

The perplexing ontological status and indeterminacies of affect valence are reminiscent of early interpretations of quantum mechanics, especially Heinsenberg's uncertainty principle (Heisenberg, 1958). The analogy lies in the fact that to attend to or "measure" affect valence is to disrupt and change the very phenomenon one is attempting to capture. Until hedonic valence is "measured" and becomes fixed and determined through attention, its precise character must therefore remain uncertain and indeterminate. In slogan form, there is no fact about the exact valence of an affective state apart from the act of attention that fixes and determines it.[5] But note again that the act of attention does not create the underlying phenomenology of emotion experience. What attention does is create the form in which the emotion experience reveals itself in awareness; its particular subjective and evaluative meaning—its emotional meaning—for that person.

This leaves the suggestion that hedonicity might be intrinsic in serious trouble. Because hedonicity is typically the main or sole component of affect valence, the same conclusion applies to affect valence more generally. The indeterminacy thesis shows valence is not a subjective evaluative phenomenon with emotional meaning *until it is created and revealed by attention*. For this reason, felt body temperature may not be a good analogy for explicating the nature of "core affect" and affect valence (Russell, 2003), because felt body temperature is subject to the mechanisms of attention just described. "Temperature" in this felt sense falls in the domain of the subjective and evaluative and often has emotional meaning. However, the objective physical temperature recorded by a thermometer is an entirely different matter. Its ontological status is very different: It is not relational in the same way, and it has no subjective meaning. The indeterminacy thesis implies that there is no fact about the valence of felt bodily temperature until that valence is shaped and revealed by attention. To say or assume that the objective temperature recorded by a thermometer is somehow the intrinsic material out of which felt bodily temperature is created therefore seems incorrect. It appears to involve a fallacy of equivocation, because *temperature* means two entirely separate things in both cases. Similar problems with equivocation are likely to arise in attempts to capture first-order phenomenal emotion experience indirectly (Lambie & Marcel, 2002, 237–238).

The above considerations strongly suggest that there is no scientifically defensible sense in which valence can be intrinsic in first-order emotional phenomenal experience. Affect valence is a dynamic enacted, phenomenon that emerges out of the interaction between attention, second-order awareness, and first-order emotion experience. The indeterminacy thesis also shows that there is no scientific fact about the valence of a particular state until that valence is formed and fixed by attention in second-order awareness. Valence, then, is multiple and multidimensional, as Lambie and Marcel (2002) argue. But it apparently cannot be intrinsic in the manner they seem to suggest, and it is subject to a radical indeterminacy they do not anticipate or countenance. In a sense, valence in emotion theory is much like gravity in Newton's *Principia*. It is a "force" we can witness and scientifically describe, up to a certain point; but beyond that point it cannot be scientifically captured and analyzed any further. The fundamental nature of valence must therefore remain a scientific mystery.

CONCLUSION

This discussion began with a definition of affect as the conscious felt dimension of emotion. It follows that affect is invariably conscious. However, the distinction between first- and second-order emotion consciousness complicates this picture. Based on that distinction, the argument was made that affect valence, as such, is solely and entirely a property of second-order emotion experience, because affect valence is created and sustained by second-order awareness, which selects and shapes it through attention. It follows that, strictly speaking, there is no such thing as unconscious or nonconscious affect valence. There is no scientific sense in which valence can be said to reside intrinsically in mental or physical states that fall outside of the active range of attention. Hence, to speak of first-order phenomenology or stimuli as valenced makes the character of first-order emotion experience even more problematic than it already is. Lambie and Marcel (2002) are certainly right that it is a crucial aspect of emotion experience. They may, however, have overestimated what can be known about it scientifically.

The indeterminacy thesis also contends that the nature of affect valence within second-order experience is problematic. The ontological and semantic vagaries of indeterminacy seriously undermine attempts to generalize about valence as a uniform scientific phenomenon. In particular, indeterminacy makes the concept of core affect particularly problematic and the status of experimental studies that employ it precarious (Barrett, Chapter 11; Russell, 2003). The reason is that there is no verifiable fact underneath it all, nor can there be, because once one tries objectively to isolate and identify a subjectively valenced conscious state, one has simultaneously changed it.

Admittedly, the indeterminacy thesis is hard to reconcile with the fact that there appear to be fixed and determinate unconscious affective processes in emotion experience (Winkielman, Berridge, & Wilbarger, Chapter 14; Clore, Storbeck, Robinson, & Centerbar, Chapter 16). These processes are perhaps best conceptualized as a sort of proto-valence but not valence itself. There is also the problem of modularity. The indeterminacy thesis explains the plasticity of affective experience, which would appear to be important for evolutionary success. Yet there is also convincing evidence that fixed modular affective processes exist and are equally important for evolutionary success. So perhaps not all aspects of affect valence are equally permeable to attention; some may be relatively fixed and modular (Charland, 1995; Zajonc, 1980). Finally, there is the question of animal affect. Homology in underlying neurobiological mechanisms suggests that, like humans, many animals probably have some experience of subjective valence and affect (Panksepp, 1998). But just what that experience consists of may be scientifically impossible to identify. Recall Wittgenstein's dictum that even if a lion could talk, we would not understand it. All of these facts and findings do seem hard to square with the indeterminacy thesis. But it is also hard to see how they could constitute a total refutation of that thesis, which has strong independent supporting reasons of its own. This is probably a good place for philosophy to step aside and invite the relevant sciences to the challenge.

PHILOSOPHICAL POSTSCRIPT

It might be thought that the perplexities of affect valence outlined here are of the same kind as those associated with the qualia problem discussed by contemporary philosophers (Chalmers, 1996; McGinn, 1999). That would be an error. The qualia problem, at least as it is typically discussed by philosophers, has more to do with the descriptive nature of the felt conscious quality of experience. Touch and vision are the paradigmatic sensory modalities discussed, although pain is also often mentioned. But, in fact, pain is a very different kind of phenomenon that has more to do with emotional meaning and valence, which is an evaluative and normative matter. The difference is crucial.

Standard philosophical qualia are typically considered to be descriptive phenomena that inform us about the state of the world and the body. Not surprisingly, these are the paradigmatically favored qualia of "cognitive" science. However, the valenced qualia in emotion are vastly different: They are evaluative and normative phenomena that address the way the world or the body *should* be. Their primary function is to orient and move us. These are the paradigmatically favored qualia of "affective" science.

So there appear to be two quite different kinds of qualia in our "phenomenological garden" (Dennett, 1991, pp. 43–65). There are qualia that *inform* us and qualia that *move* us. The valenced qualia in emotion pull and push us in a way that standard sensory qualia do not. Those valenced qualia involve concern, orientation, and personal meaning of a sort that is very different, and is usually absent, from standard sensory qualia. *Valence* is what makes the difference. There may also be mixed qualia that somehow combine informative and motivational functions (Millikan, 1996). But the possibility of mixed qualia does not annul the fact that, in mammals at least, cognitive and affective qualia are distinguishable. Indeed, they appear to be under the control of relatively distinct neurobiological systems (Panksepp, 2003; see also Panksepp, 1998, p. 62). This neurobiological distinction constitutes an important strand for the hypothesis that emotion is a special *normative* natural kind of its own, distinct from cognition (Charland, 1997, 2002; Griffiths, 2003).

To sum up the importance of this philosophical postscript: The significance of the distinction between the cognitive qualia that inform us and the emotional qualia that move us may be reflected in what can be scientifically known about them. Even if we could solve the famous "hard problem" for standard cognitive qualia, we would not have explained the mysteries and perplexities of affect valence. The difficulties posed by the scientific explanation of affect valence appear to be of a different order. This is not simply a hard problem for the science of mind. It may constitute a genuine *inexplicable* mystery.

ACKNOWLEDGMENTS

Thanks to Aaron Ben-Ze'ev, Sylvia Berryman, John Lambie, Anthony Marcel, Harold Merskey, Jim Russell, Robert Solomon, and Evan Thompson for helpful comments on earlier drafts of this chapter.

NOTES

1. See Buck (1999, p. 304) for an interesting but different variant of this distinction, which he traces to Bertrand Russell's famous discussion of "knowledge-by-acquaintance" and "knowledge-by-description" (Russell, 1912).
2. Different aspects of valence can be stressed in different contexts. For example, Fossum and Barrett (2000) allude to emotion valence when they state that "the valence of an *emotion* term refers to both its hedonic tone and evaluative connotation" (p. 670; emphasis added). However, in another context, Barrett alludes to affect valence when she states that "the valence dimension of the circumplex refers to the hedonic tone of the *mood*" (Barrett, 1996, p. 49; emphasis added). One can also treat *affect* as the "conscious subjective aspect of an *emotion*" (Cacioppo & Berntson, 1999, p. 134; emphasis added). The circumplex model can sometimes be interpreted this way (e.g., Barrett, 1998; Russell, 2003).
3. Note that the valence of an affective state in this sense is quite different from its desirability (Barrett, 1996). The "positively" valenced affect allegedly referred to by the statement "I feel good" is different from the "positively" evaluated affect reported by the statement "This is a good feeling to have" (p. 49). However, this does not imply that the valence dimension of affective states is not inherently evaluative. This is precisely what makes valence so special and important.
4. I leave open the question of whether affect valence is so permeable and mutable that a painful affect can be completely transformed into a pleasurable one that is in no way unpleasant. In a fascinating discussion of masochism, psychiatrist Harold Merskey considers the question whether "'pain' is ever solely pleasant" (Merskey & Spear, 1967, p. 122). He states that "it is possible, although it is disputed, that in some cases 'pain' is pleasant and in no way unpleasant" (p. 121). Noting that the issues may be semantic as well as clinical, he concludes that the question "must remain open to investigation" (p. 122). I agree. The issue is important, because it bears directly on the validity of the

definition of pain. According to the International Association for the Study of Pain, pain is defined as "an unpleasant sensory and emotional experience associated with actual or potential tissue damage, or described in such terms" (Merskey & Bodguk, 1994, p. 210). In this definition "pain is always subjective" (p. 210). The paradoxical possibility of pains that are not subjectively experienced as unpleasant is therefore extremely theoretically significant. As Merskey notes, "if it should prove to be the case that something called 'pain' by masochists is experienced without any quality of unpleasantness the definition [of pain] would need revision" (p. 122).

5. The indeterminacy thesis for affect valence is partly inspired by Quine's (1960) argument for the indeterminacy of translation. Another inspiration is Amelie Rorty's (1986) argument that emotional states are dynamic and permeable. Finally, a third inspiration is the problem of indeterminacy in quantum mechanics. William Reddy (2001) appears to defend a related thesis. According to him, emotions are a kind of performative utterance, since they "do something to the world" (Reddy, 2001, p. 111). But they are different from performatives, because of the special way in which "they are both self explorative and self-altering" (Reddy, 2001, p. 122; see also pp. 104–111). Reddy makes use of Quine's principle of the indeterminacy of translation to argue that there is an unavoidable indeterminacy to emotional experience (pp. 78–96, 320, 332).

REFERENCES

Barrett, L. F. (1996). Hedonic tone, perceived arousal, and item desirability: Three components of self-reported mood. *Cognition and Emotion, 10*(1), 47–68.

Barrett, L. F., Russell, J. A. (1998). Independence and bipolarity in the structure of affect. *Journal of Personality and Social Psychology, 17*(4), 967–984.

Ben-Ze'ev, A. (2000) *The subtlety of emotions.* Cambridge, MA: MIT Press.

Berkowitz, L. (2000). *Causes and consequences of feelings.* Cambridge, UK: Cambridge University Press.

Buck, R. (1999). The biological affects: A typology. *Psychological Review, 106*(2), 301–336.

Cacioppo, J. T., & Berntson, G. G. (1999). The affect system: Architecture and operating characteristics. *Current Directions in Psychological Science, 8*(5), 133–137.

Cacioppo, J. T., & Berntson, G. G. (1994). Relationships between attitudes and evaluative space. *Psychological Bulletin, 115,* 401–423.

Carroll, J., Michelle, M., Yik, S. M., Russell, J., & Barrett, L. F. (1999). On the psychometric principles of affect. *Review of General Psychology, 3*(1), 14–22.

Chalmers, D. J. (1996). *The conscious mind.* New York: Oxford University Press.

Charland, L. C. (1995). Feeling and representing: Computational theory and the modularity of affect. *Synthese, 105,* 273–301.

Charland, L. C. (1997). Reconciling cognitive and perceptual theories of emotion. *Philosophy of Science, 64,* 555–579.

Charland, L. C. (2002). The natural kind status of emotion. *British Journal for the Philosophy of Science, 53,* 511–537.

Damasio, A. (2003). *Looking for Spinoza: Joy, sorrow, and the feeling brain.* New York: Harcourt.

Davidson, R. J. (1992). Emotion and affective style. *Psychological Science, 3,* 39–43.

Dennett, D. (1991). *Consciousness explained.* Boston: Little, Brown.

Feldman, L. (1995). Valence focus and arousal focus: Individual differences in the structure of affective experience. *Journal of Personality and Social Psychology, 69,* 153–166.

Fossum, T. A., & Barrett, L. (2000). Distinguishing evaluation from description in the personality–emotion relationship. *Personality and Social Psychology Bulletin, 26*(6), 669–678.

James, W. (1981). *Principles of psychology* (2 Vols.). Cambridge, MA: Harvard University Press. (Original work published 1890)

Frijda, N. (1986). *The emotions.* Cambridge, UK: Cambridge University Press.

Gordon, R. M. (1987). *The cognitive structure of the emotions.* Cambridge, UK: Cambridge University Press.

Griffiths, P. E. (2003). *Emotions as natural and normative kinds.* Paper presented at the Philosophy of Science Association 18th biennial meeting,

Hall, T. S. (1975). *History of general physiology.* Chicago: University of Chicago Press.

Heisenberg, W. (1958). *Physics and philosophy: The revolution in modern science.* New York: Harper.

Kahneman, D. (1999). Objective happiness. In D. Kahneman, E. Diener, & N. Schwartz (Eds.), *Well-being: The foundations of hedonic psychology* (pp. 3–25). New York: Russell Sage Foundation.

Kuhn, T. S. (1970). *The structure of scientific revolutions* (2nd ed.). Chicago: University of Chicago Press.

Lambie, J. A., & Marcel, A. A. (2002). Consciousness and the varieties of emotion experience: A theoretical framework. *Psychological Review, 109*(2), 219–259.

Larsen, J. T., MacGraw, M. A., & Cacioppo, J. T. (2001). Can people feel happy and sad at the same time? *Journal of Personality and Social Psychology, 81*(4), 684–696.

Larsen, R. J., & Diener, E. (1992). Problems with the circumplex model of emotion. *Review of Personality and Social Psychology, 13,* 25–59.

Lazarus, R. (1991). *Emotion and adaptation.* Oxford, UK: Oxford University Press.

Mandler, G. (1984). *Mind and body: The psychology of emotion and stress.* New York: Norton.

McGinn, C. (1999). *The mysterious flame: Conscious minds in a material world.* New York: Basic Books.

Merskey, H., & Bodguk, N. (1994). *Classification of chronic pain* (2nd ed.). Seattle: IASP Press.

Merskey, H., & Spear, F. G. (1967). *Pain: Psychological and psychiatric aspects.* London: Balliere, Tindall & Cassell.

Millikan, R. (1996). Pushmepullyou representations. In L. May & M. Friedman (Eds.), *Mind and morals* (pp. 145–161). Cambridge, MA: MIT Press.

Ortony, A., Clore, A. C., & Colins, A. (1988). *The cognitive structure of emotions.* New York: Cambridge University Press.

Pagel, Walter. (1967). Harvey and Glisson on irritability with a note on Van Helmont. *Bulletin of the History of Medicine*, *41*, 497–551.

Panksepp, J. (1998). *Affective neuroscience*. Oxford, UK: Oxford University Press.

Panksepp, J. (2001). The neuro-evolutionary cusp between emotions and cognitions. *Evolution and Emotion*, *7*(2), 141–163.

Panksepp, J. (2003). At the interface of affective, behavioural, and cognitive neurosciences: Decoding the emotional feelings of the brain. *Brain and Cognition*, *52*, 4–14.

Prinz, J. (2004). *Gut reactions*. Oxford, UK: Oxford University Press.

Quine, W. V. O. (1960). *Word and object*. Cambridge, MA: MIT Press.

Reddy, W. M. (2001). *The navigation of feeling: A framework for the history of emotions*. Cambridge, UK: Cambridge University Press.

Rorty, A. (1986). The historicity of psychological attitudes: Love is not love which alters when it alteration finds. *Midwest Studies in Philosophy*, *10*, 399–412.

Russell, B. (1912). *The problems of philosophy*. New York: Simon & Schuster.

Russell, J. A. (1980). A circumplex order of affect. *Journal of Personality and Social Psychology*, *39*, 1161–1178.

Russell, J. A. (1999). On the bipolarity of positive and negative affect. *Psychological Bulletin*, *125*(1), 3–30.

Russell, J. A. (2003). Core affect and the psychological construction of emotion. *Psychological Review*, *110*(1), 145–172.

Russell, J. A., & Carroll, J. M. (1999). On the bipolarity of positive and negative affect. *Psychological Bulletin*, *125*, 3–30.

Schacter, S., & Singer, J. (1962). Cognitive, social and physiological determinants of emotional state. *Psychological Review*, *69*, 379–399.

Solomon, R. C. (1993). *The passions: Emotions and the meaning of life*. Indianapolis: Hackett.

Solomon, R. C. (2003). *Not passion's slave*. Oxford, UK: Oxford University Press.

Solomon, R. C., & Stone, L. D. (2002). On "positive" and "negative" emotions. *Journal for the Theory of Social Behavior*, *32*, 417–436.

Temkin, O. (1964). The classical roots of Glisson's doctrine of irritation. *Bulletin of the History of Medicine*, *38*, 297–328.

Varela, F. (1989). *Connaître, les sciences cognitives: Tendances et perspectives*. Paris: Editions du Seuil.

Watson, D., & Tellegen, A. (1985). Toward a consensual structure of mood. *Psychological Bulletin*, *98*, 219–235.

Zajonc, R. (1980). Feeling and thinking: Preferences need no inferences. *American Psychologist*, *35*, 151–175.

CHAPTER 11

Feeling Is Perceiving

Core Affect and Conceptualization in the Experience of Emotion

Lisa Feldman Barrett

What is the experience of emotion? This question fascinates friends and family members, novelists and poets, psychologists and philosophers alike. In this culture we ask and answer questions pertaining to feelings many times each day. Over coffee, we gossip about the emotions of others and speculate about why they reacted as they did. We pay large sums of money to psychotherapists to help us understand why we feel the way we do, and to grapple with ways of changing those feelings. Poets and novelists attempt to capture the indescribable nature of what emotion feels like, bringing its richness and complexity to life. In psychological science, questions about feelings are ubiquitous. Whether to explain, predict, or control for feelings, scientists ask participants how they feel, and participants easily answer. Scientists debate whether or not feelings lie at the heart of emotion, but presumably no one would deny that the experience of emotion is something important to understand in its own right. Many people, both in the scientific study of emotion and in everyday life, often presuppose a theory of emotion experience that goes unexamined: We experience emotion because we have "emotions"—internal causal mechanisms that, when triggered, leave measurable traces of their existence.

1. *What is the scope of your proposed model? When you use the term* emotion, *how do you use it? What do you mean by terms such as* fear, anxiety, *or* happiness?

Emotions are not causal entities. They are not a set of facial movements, a vocal signal, changes in peripheral physiology, and some voluntary action that are coordinated in time and correlated in intensity. In this chapter, emotions are defined as perceptions. A state of anger (fear, etc.) is the categorization of a core affect state, which itself is the neurophysiological state that results from the process of evaluation.

2. *Define your terms:* conscious, unconscious, awareness. *Or say why you do not use these terms.*

The distinction between conscious and unconscious processes is more phenomenological than mechanistic (see Barrett, Tugade, & Engle, 2004). The idea of endogenous (stimulus-driven) and exogenous (goal-driven) forms of attention is more relevant to the ideas presented in this chapter. Also, the definitions of experience and awareness used in this chapter follow the spirit of Lambie and Marcel's (2002) discussion of these concepts.

3. *Does your model deal with what is conscious, what is unconscious, or their relationship? If you do not address this area specifically, can you speculate on the relationship between what is conscious and unconscious? Or if you do not like the conscious–unconscious distinction, or if you think this is not a good question to ask, can you say why?*

In this chapter I suggest that core affect can influence behavior in a way that is driven by both exogenous (or stimulus-driven) and endogenous (or goal-driven) forms of attention, and that this can happen outside of awareness (and can therefore result in unconscious affective behavior). I also suggest that core affect (and its resulting behaviors) have sensory–motor consequences that are available to be consciously represented and felt (although they need not be).

In this chapter I challenge the view that emotions are entities causing experience, and offer an equally plausible model to account for the experience of emotion. This account involves the recently defined scientific concept of core affect (i.e., the affective state that results from the process of evaluation; Russell, 2003; Russell & Barrett, 1999), ideas and evidence from the social-psychological literature on "person perception," and work on embodied conceptual knowledge in cognitive science. Specifically, I pursue the idea that we experience an emotion when we categorize an instance of core affective feeling. From this perspective, the experience of emotion is a perceptual act, guided by conceptual knowledge about emotion.

EMOTIONS AS CAUSAL ENTITIES

Many contemporary models of emotion assume that emotions have onto-logical status as causal entities—that is, emotions are believed to exist in the brain or body and cause changes in sensory, perceptual, motor, and physiological outputs. Each emotion, in this view, can be characterized by a set of recognizable behavioral and physiological outcomes (including a set of facial movements, a vocal signal, changes in peripheral physiology, and some voluntary action) that are coordinated in time, correlated in intensity, and constitute the components of an emotional response. These aspects of emotional responding are thought to give evidence that kinds of emotions exist. Although not all scientific models of emotion expound this view (e.g., Mandler, 1975; Ochsner & Barrett, 2001; Russell, 2003), the idea of emotions as causal entities characterizes both popular (e.g., Goleman, 1995) and scientific models (e.g., Lundqvist & Öhman, Chapter 5; Scherer, Chapter 13; for a review, see Barrett, 2004a; Barrett, Ochsner, & Gross, 2004). Even when emotion models are more complex, they often continue to assume that traditional emotion categories exist as real entities in nature, whether nature is defined as residing in the brain, body, or the deep structure of the situation (depending on the preferred level of description). The general idea is that the category *emotion* is a natural kind, unlike other psychological phenomenon (say, cognition or attention; e.g., see Charland, Chapter 10), and each category of "basic" emotion, referred to by such English words as *anger*, *sadness*, and *fear*, is a natural kind (Barrett, 2005).

The Experience of Emotion

A correspondingly simple perspective on the experience of emotion falls out from the natural kind view of emotion: the experience of an emotion is the simple, veridical sensory detection of the causal mechanism (or, in some models, the detection of the other outputs, such as facial muscle movements). The emotion is an object of consciousness, like a table or a chair. Some models make additional assumptions about the attentional processes involved in becoming aware of an emotion experience (e.g., Lambie & Marcel, 2002; Prinz, Chapter 15), but the fundamental assumption remains the same: emotion mechanisms (e.g., an anger mechanism) trigger an emotion state (e.g., a state of anger), producing the experience of an emotion (a feeling of anger). From the emoter's perspective, the awareness of this experience is taken as clear evidence that the causal mechanism—the emotion—has been triggered. Feeling angry is evidence that the anger mechanism has fired.[1]

The idea of emotions as causal mechanisms produces an easy answer to questions about emotions and consciousness. Emotions (i.e., the causal mechanisms) are unconscious and can cause us to behave in ways of which we are not aware. To be sure, there is considerable evidence that unconscious affect exists and that affective behaviors occur without awareness (e.g., Niedenthal, Barsalou, Ric, & Krauth-Gruber, Chapter 2; Winkielman, Berridge, & Wilbarger, Chapter 14). But the question is whether this is really evidence of "unconscious emotion" (i.e., an inescapable, involuntary, and automated set of synchronized changes in response systems that produces a signature emotional response; e.g., Scherer, Chapter 13). According to several emotion models (e.g., Charland, Chapter 10; Scherer, Chapter 13; Prinz, Chapter 15), the answer to that question is yes. And when the resulting sensations register, the experience of emotion results. The sensory and perceptual processes involved are typically thought to occur unconsciously, although deliberate introspection can also take place (and might be better thought of as emotion regulation, because it usually involves language). The endpoint—the feeling—is conscious, by definition, although it may not be a focal point for attention (e.g., Lambie & Marcel, 2002; Schooler, 2002).

EVALUATING THE IDEA OF EMOTIONS AS CAUSAL ENTITIES

The assumption that emotions are entities that cause behavior and experience has been valuable in the scientific study of emotion. It has helped define emotion as a topic worthy of study in its own right, and it has generally organized scientific inquiry for several decades. The idea of emotions as causal entities has several strengths as a scientific view. It is simple to state: Emotions cause behavior and experience. It explains why our own feelings of anger, fear, etc., have a given quality. We experience feelings as erupting or "happening to us" because the causal entity—the emotion—hijacks our mind and body and sometimes causes us to behave in ways that we would rather not (i.e., ways that interfere with the more reasoned responses that we identify as part of human selves). The idea of emotions as causal entities is also consistent with a variety of scientific assumptions that guide psychological theorizing and measurement (for a discussion, see Barrett, 2005).

Much to everyone's surprise, however, research has not established a strong evidentiary basis for the idea that anger, sadness, fear, and so on, constitute natural kinds of emotion that cause behavior or experience. Thus far, researchers have yet to identify patterns of observable behaviors that consistently distinguish among types of emotion, nor have they identified clear and consistent evidence for distinct neural systems corresponding to each kind of emotion. Most importantly, they have not observed the kind of response clusters within categories that would confirm their status of emotions as natural kinds (for a more detailed review of evidence, see Barrett, 2005). It is instructive to review this evidence briefly before considering what it means for the scientific study of emotion experience.

The Evidence

Perhaps the most compelling idea in the psychology of emotion is that emotional states have specific and unique patterns of somatovisceral changes. Although individual studies sometimes report distinct autonomic correlates for different emotion categories (e.g., Christie & Friedman, 2004; Ekman, Levenson, & Friesen, 1983; Levenson, Ekman, & Friesen, 1990), meta-analytic summaries generally fail to find distinct patterns of peripheral nervous-system responses for each discrete emotion (Cacioppo, Berntson, Larsen, Poehlmann, & Ito, 2000). Peripheral nervous-system responses configure for conditions of threat and challenge (Quigley, Barrett, & Weinstein, 2002; Tomaka et al., 1993; Tomaka, Blascovich, Kibler, & Ernst, 1997), and for pleasant versus unpleasant affect (Cacioppo et al., 2000; Lang, Greenwald, Bradley, & Hamm, 1993), but do not robustly distinguish between traditional emotion categories.

Evidence from studies of facial behavior has yielded the same result. Facial electromyography measurements coordinate around positive versus negative affect (Cacioppo et al., 2000) or intensity of affect (Messinger, 2002), rather than discrete emotion categories. Participants can assign posed facial configurations to discrete emotion categories with some reliability, but these findings are open to alternative explanations (e.g., Russell, 1994; Russell, Bachorowski, & Fernandez-Dols, 2003), including that perceivers are imposing, rather than detecting, categorical distinctions in the facial configurations that they rate (I return to this point later).

Evidence from studies of instrumental behavior is similar. Instrumental behavioral responses such as flight or fight correspond to situational demands (Bouton, Chapter 9), rather than to specific categories of emotion. Behaviors are specific, context-bound attempts to deal with a situation (Cacioppo et al., 2000; Lang, Bradley, & Cuthbert, 1990). Functional demands vary with situations, making it likely that instances of the same emotion can be associated with a range of behaviors. For example, Lang et al. (1990) note that the behaviors associated with fear can range from freezing to vigilance to flight. Not only are different behaviors associated with the same emotion category, but also one type of behavior can be associated with many categories. For example, there are several types of aggressive behavior, such as defensive, offensive, or predatory, each of which is assumed to be associated with a different type of stimulus situation caused by different neural circuitry (Blanchard & Blanchard, 2003).

Many theorists assume that kinds of emotion have specific neural essences (e.g., Buck, 1999; Damasio, 1999; Dolan, 2002; Ekman, 1992; Izard, 1993; LeDoux, 1996; Panksepp, 1998). Yet two recent meta-analyses of neuroimaging studies (Murphy, Nimmo-Smith, & Lawrence, 2003; Phan, Wager, Taylor, & Liberzon, 2002) failed to find consistent evidence of particular neural correlates for anger, sadness, disgust, and happiness. A fear–amygdala correspondence was noted across both analyses, but can be accounted for by alternative explanations (see Phan et al., 2002). Although there are a number of methodological and theoretical factors that presently limit our ability to draw inferences about the neural bases of emotional responses, the failure to find neural signatures for distinct emotions thus far is consistent with the behavioral evidence. Furthermore, although there is good evidence that specific behaviors (e.g., freezing) may depend upon specific brainstem and subcortical nuclei (e.g., Panksepp, 1998), there is little evidence to suggest that each behavior can be uniquely associated with any single emotion category (although we can effortlessly assign behaviors to categories).

Just as behavioral and biological findings have not produced strong evidence for "kinds" of emotions, there is no clear evidence for qualitatively different "kinds" of experiences. Self-reports of experienced emotion take on a circumplex shape, rather than a simple structure configuration (with one factor or cluster for the report of each emotion; e.g., Barrett, 2004; Feldman, 1995a, 1995b; Russell, 1980). A circumplex shape indicates that reports of anger, sadness, fear, and so on, can be broken down into more elemental properties. Although there is some debate about the content of those properties, valence (hedonic tone) and arousal (feelings of activation and deactivation) are prime candidates (Russell, 2003; Russell & Barrett, 1999). It has been argued that the valence and arousal properties observed in self-reports of emotion experience reflect (1) people's beliefs about what they feel (Dennett, 1991), (2) the contaminating influence of emotion language (i.e., the words used in the rating process; e.g., Frijda, Markam, Sako, & Wiers, 1995), or (3) evaluative processes that occur subsequent to the experience of emotion (Charland, Chapter 10). Evidence is accumulating against these alternative explanations, however (Barrett, 2004; Barrett, Quigley, Bliss-Moreau, & Aronson, 2004; Barrett & Niedenthal, 2004).

Most importantly, physiological, behavioral, and experiential outputs for each emotion category are not highly intercorrelated (Bradley & Lang, 2000; Lang, 1968; Mandler, Mandler, Kremen, & Sholiton, 1961), undermining the claim that the various aspects of emotional responding emanate from a single common cause. Although no single study has yet measured all possible outputs simultaneously, even two or three response channels fail to correlate when researchers induce anger, sadness, fear, and so on. Enough evidence has accumulated for some theorists to conclude that the lack of coherence within each category of emotion is empirically the rule rather than the exception (Bradley & Lang, 2000; Russell, 2003; Shweder, 1994).

Although the instrument-based data do not cohere to reveal categories of emotion, they do show more consistency when measuring pleasant and unpleasant affects. Judgments of facial behaviors (for a recent review, see Russell et al., 2003), electromyographic (EMG) recordings of facial movements (for a meta-analytic review, see Cacioppo et al., 2000), autonomic physiology (for a meta-analytic review, see Cacioppo et al., 2000), and expressive behavior (for a review, see Cacioppo & Gardner, 1999) can all be described in terms of valence–arousal combinations. Emotion data are only confusing when scientists search for evidence of coordinated response profiles for anger, sadness, fear, and so on. Of course, it is always possible to postulate inhibitory and modulating factors that interfere with coordinated outputs. Alternatively, it is possible to consider other plausible ways to account for the failure to observe the kind of response clusters that would confirm the existence of natural kinds of emotion.

Implications for Understanding the Experience of Emotion

Despite its intuitive appeal, research has not produced a strong evidentiary basis for the idea that there are kinds of emotion. A brief review indicates that after almost a century of searching, scientists still do not have strong, consistent evidence to support the idea that emotions have causal status and produce the substrates for the experience of anger, sadness, fear, and so on. The only place scientists observe strong evidence for the existence of these emotion categories is in perceiver reports. People automatically and effortlessly assign anger, sadness fear, and so on to others on the basis of their behaviors, and they identify these emotions in themselves. How can scientists understand the experience of anger, sadness, fear, and so on, if there are no real emotion mechanisms producing distinct experiences? For the remainder of the chapter, I suggest one possible answer to this question.

THE EXPERIENCE OF EMOTION
AS A PERCEPTUAL ACT

As people, we rely on our experiences to tell us about the world. Because immediate experience is so compelling, and because we do not have access to its generation, we believe that our experiences faithfully reveal things as they actually are. We conduct ourselves as if experience gives us direct access to the world around us, on the assumption that the world as we feel (hear, taste, see, or smell) it is identical to the physical world that exists apart from us. We see (at least, in Western cultures) anger, sadness, fear, and so on, in people's behavior, and experience it in ourselves, leading us to assume that those emotions are actual causal entities lurking somewhere within the brain or body. Yet it is possible that we are naïve realists (Asch, 1952/1957; Jones & Nisbett, 1971) when it comes to emotion—we believe that our experiences of emotion reveal an unbiased, internal reality but they may not. Careful study has determined that we rarely experience things as they actually are. Perception is constructive, even at the most basic sensory level (Ramachandran, 1992, 1993). We cannot discern the causes of behavior from our experience, even though we believe that we can (Nisbett & Wilson, 1977). Our knowledge of people and situations unconsciously shapes what we "see" people doing and gives rise to how we explain that behavior (for a review, see Gilbert, 1998). Perhaps the same is true for emotion. In the pages that follow, I develop this idea, suggesting that emotions are perceptions (where perception is defined as assigning objects to meaningful categories so that we "see" an instance of a category). I suggest that the experience of emotion is a perceptual act, or an instance of categorization that involves what we know about emotion.

As an analogy, consider the experience of color. Although the light spectrum is a continuum of wavelengths, color perception is categorical. The English words *red*, *green*, *blue*, and so on, correspond to sets of wavelengths that are experienced as qualitatively different categories. There are some embodiment constraints on color categorization, because at a sensory level, the human visual system constrains and shapes how we perceive and experience the light spectrum. We *sense* light at a particular wavelength in a way that is constrained by how the retina registers sensory information and the low-level visual processing that takes place. In the end, we experience some color corresponding to that wavelength, and that color is influenced by our conceptual knowledge of color (Davidoff, Davies, & Roberson, 1999; Özgen & Davies, 2002; Roberson, Davies, & Davidoff, 2000). In this culture people have knowledge about what constitutes the category *red*, including knowledge of different hues, what objects have them, what colors match, and so on. There is variability in this knowledge (both across individuals and across cultures), so the way I categorize the experience of a certain wavelength may differ from someone else. For example, when my husband and I look at a pillow in our front parlor, we both take in the same wavelengths of light that are bouncing off the pillow (and the rest of the room), and we both detect that wavelength as dictated by what our visual system produces in its early stages of sensory processing.

Our experience of that pillow as red, or pink, or rose, depends on what we know about those colors and how we use what we know as we categorize the pillow's color. Behavior toward this pillow, such as deciding what other objects we might match it with, is driven by our experience of its color. Furthermore, as we learn more about color (e.g., by taking an interior design course), the way we experience and act on the pillow, or other red-like objects, will change (Özgen & Davies, 2002).

I propose that something similar happens with the experience of emotion. At a sensory level, a continuous stream of homeostatic feedback from the body delivers affective information about each individual's current relationship to the world. It is not a specific interoceptive readout of autonomic activity or anything so precise. Rather, it is a core affective state that gives rise to feelings of displeasure (or pleasure) and activation (or deactivation) that results from ongoing automatic evaluations or primary appraisals of the world. This information is available to be felt or experienced. The way that people perceive this feeling will depend on the conceptual knowledge about emotion that they bring to bear when they categorize their affective state. A person might experience his or her core affective state as sadness, anger, or nervousness. In this view, emotion experience depends, in part, on what knowledge the person brings to bear at the moment of experience. Although the person's initial behavior might be a function of his or her affective state, what comes next (how the person acts to change his or her current state) will depend, at times, on what is known about emotion and how that knowledge is used.

The basic premise is that the experience of emotion begins with effortless, automatic perception—a perception of affect through the lens of category knowledge about emotion. It is not interoception—the simple sensory detection of an internal event. Instead, it is, as William James (1884, 1890/1950, 1894/1994) suggested, a self-perception. To be more specific, the experience of emotion is the categorization of core affect. The perceptual process proceeds according to the general principles of behavior identification that can be found in the social-psychological literature on person perception. The category knowledge brought to bear does not consist of symbolic representations but of sensory–motor representations that involve the body and are designed for action. So, like several other contributors to this volume (Niedenthal et al., Chapter 2; Atkinson & Adolphs, Chapter 7; Prinz, Chapter 15), I suggest that conceptual knowledge about emotion involves sensory, somatovisceral, and motor states, and that people use this knowledge both when perceiving someone else's emotion and when perceiving their own feelings. Unlike those contributors, however, I assume that there is nothing privileged about such knowledge. We do not learn about *anger* and *sadness* and *fear* because they are real categories in nature.

We learn about them the way we learn about other abstract concepts, and we integrate sensory and motor states into basic-level emotion categories based on the language that we speak.

Self-Perception

In the field of psychology the idea that emotion is a perception began with William James. In the most general terms, James (1884, 1890/1950, 1894/1994) suggested that the experience of emotion (which he merely called *emotion*) results from the self-perception of automatic processes. He focused primarily on the ways in which the peripheral nervous system acts on somatovisceral and voluntary muscle activation. A number of modern accounts are inspired by the idea that the experience of emotion is a self-perception (e.g., Damasio, 1994; Dolan, 2002; Laird & Bresler, 1992; Russell, 2003), although they vary in the type and specificity of processes proposed.

A strict interoceptive account of the self-perception of emotion, such as that proposed by James and later by Schachter and Singer (1962), is untenable for several scientific reasons (Barrett, Quigley, et al., 2004). People do not have automatic, immediate, and explicit access to autonomic and somatic activity, and there is considerable variation (both across persons and across contexts) in the ability to accurately perceive somatovisceral information. Moreover, and perhaps more important for the view being developed here, different categories of emotion are not associated with signature visceral sensations, suggesting that feelings of anger, fear, and so on, do not derive uniqueness from interoceptive readouts of somatovisceral activity.

Nonetheless, James's general idea—that the experience of emotion results from the self-perception of automatic processes—has some merit. I suggest here that when we experience an emotion, we are perceiving our core affective state at a given instance in time. Core affect is the ongoing, neurophysiological state that results from evaluations of the (internal and external) environment (Russell, 2003; Russell & Barrett, 1999). Core affect causes us to feel moved, compelled, or generally emotional. It can be characterized as having hedonic (pleasant or unpleasant) and arousal (activation and deactivation) properties, which are associated with the value of a stimulus situation (whether something is good or bad for us), as well as with the predictive certainty of this value (whether or not active coping or more information is required; but for an alternative view, see Charland, Chapter 10). Core affect alone does not produce feelings of anger, sadness, fear, and so on, but it is where these experiences begin. Perceiving core affect at a given moment in time is the first step to experiencing an emotion.

Core Affect

All the neural processes by which an organism judges, represents, and responds to the value of objects in the world are central to what I mean when I say something involves affect (see also Cardinal, Parkinson, Hall, & Everitt, 2002). Organisms continually and automatically evaluate situations and objects for their relevance and value—that is, whether or not their properties signify something important to well-being (see Bargh & Ferguson, 2000, but for a contrasting view see Clore, Storbeck, Robinson, & Centerbar, Chapter 16; Storbeck & Robinson, 2004). An object is valuable when it is potentially important to survival (Davis & Whalen, 2001), salient and meaningful (Phan et al., 2002), or relevant to immediate goals (Smith & Kirby, 2001). Objects rarely have intrinsic value or meaning (i.e., they rarely act directly on the nervous systems without involving prior learning; see Owren, Rendell, & Bachorowski, Chapter 8). Typically, meaning is determined by a particular person in a particular context at a particular point in time. This is the basic point made by appraisal models of emotion (e.g., Scherer, Chapter 13; Clore et al., Chapter 16). The result of this evaluative processing has a pervasive influence on a person's core affective state at any given point in time.

There is a distributed network within the brain that performs evaluation, computes value, and produces changes in core affect. The amygdala is the centerpiece of this system. The evaluation of a stimulus begins when sensory information from the world reaches the amygdala (e.g., Lundqvist & Öhman, Chapter 5; de Gelder, Chapter 6; Atkinson & Adolphs, Chapter 7). According to work by Whalen and colleagues (Kim, Somerville, Johnstone, Alexander, & Whalen, 2003; Whalen, 1998; Whalen, Shin, McInerney, Fischer, Wright, & Rauch, 2001), the ventral lateral aspect of the amygdala (corresponding to the lateral nucleus) computes a quick, initial assessment of a stimulus's predictive value (i.e., to what extent it will predict a subsequent threat). When a stimulus has a high predictive value (i.e., its threat value is certain), information is sent directly to various output systems so that the organism can respond appropriately. Potentially, this process allows a person to produce simple, evolutionarily tuned behaviors to deal with threat or reward (see Phelps, Chapter 3). Given the world in which humans live, it is rare to encounter stimuli with a certain predictive value, so that other processes are usually engaged to help determine the meaning of a stimulus when its predictive value is uncertain. The ventral amygdala can disinhibit the dorsal amygdala (corresponding to the central nucleus) to marshal attention and other output systems to gather more information to better assess the predictive value of the stimulus (and to allow the person to better predict its stimulus value the next time it is encountered).

In addition, value prediction can be improved by identifying that an object is present and recognizing what it is, both of which involve perceptual processing. The available sensory information is extracted and matched with stored unimodal representations in perceptual memory. This process involves primary, secondary, and association areas of sensory cortex that are connected to the ventral region of the amygdala. When viewing a snake, for example, bottom-up (or stimulus-driven) processes extract information about perceptual features of the object. These features constrain one another during a matching process, leading to stimulus recognition, and the stimulus is recognized as familiar or not. Although the object is not yet named or identified as belonging to a specific category, this perceptual information contributes to predicting its value and helps the person to respond accordingly.

Evaluations can also be influenced by information from the later stages of perceptual processing when an object is interpreted. This is when conceptual knowledge begins to play a role in affective processing (involving left-inferior prefrontal areas). The stimulus is assigned to a category (e.g., the object is categorized as an instance of *snake*), can be named (e.g., "that is a snake"), although it need not be, and an action plan is generated to deal with it (e.g., the perceiver prepares to walk in the other direction).

Finally, when the predictive value of a stimulus is uncertain, information from the lateral nucleus of the amygdala is forwarded to the ventral medial aspect of the amygdala (corresponding to the basal nucleus), where information is combined with context-relevant information coming from the orbitofrontal and medial prefrontal cortices. Although some researchers consider this a form of regulation, I think of it as a later processing component of evaluation, in that contextual information can be brought to bear to determine whether or not a stimulus is threatening in a particular circumstance (as in extinction and other forms of contextual conditioning; see Bouton, Chapter 9). So, although I would act on my propensity to walk away from the snake if it is across my path when I am hiking in the forest, I might actually approach the snake if I were visiting a zoo and the snake was behind glass. My 5-year-old daughter, on the other hand, would likely approach the snake regardless, because she is very curious about snakes. In this way, evaluations can also be influenced by more complex conceptual processing, which can alter the behavioral plan.

The neural consequences of evaluation have a neuromodulatory effect on a wide array of output systems, from those that are typically associated with emotional responding (e.g., autonomic and endocrine changes, voluntary behavior, facial movements) to those that are not (e.g., selective attention, memory). These output response systems are influenced by non-affective processes as well (e.g., autonomic changes occur with simple changes in posture, endocrine changes occur after eating, facial movements occur for social communication), such that there is no specific class of "emotional behaviors," no specific "action tendency," facial "expression," nor autonomic nervous system "patterning" that is unique to each kind of emotion. The output of any given response system (behavior, attention, facial movements) is multiply determined and can be considered more or less affectively infused in a given instant, depending on the extent to which it is constrained by evaluation. Furthermore, the extent to which behavior can be thought of as "affective" versus "emotional" depends on the kind of conceptual knowledge that is brought to bear during evaluation (a point to which I return later). As a consequence, freezing may be an innate behavior, and it may be part of the Western script for *fear* such that we automatically categorize freezing as an instance of fear, but this is not evidence, in and of itself, that freezing behavior is caused by some module of fear responding or gives evidence of fear.

A person's core affective state is an accounting of how events and objects are influencing the state of the organism at a given moment in time (cf. Russell, 2003). It is similar to what Lambie and Marcel (2002) refer to as "emotion state." In a sense, core affect is a neurophysiological barometer of the individual's relationship to an environment. Core affect, at a given moment in time, can be influenced by automatic evaluations of what is in the focus of attention, as well as what is in the periphery (one's background environment; Russell & Snodgrass, 1987; see evidence on background conditioning, Phillips & LeDoux, 1994). Everything that has been said about "emotion" may be true of core affect. The hardwiring to support core affect is present at birth (Bridges, 1932; Emde, Gaensbauer, & Harmon, 1976; Spitz, 1965; Sroufe, 1979). It can be acquired and modified by associative learning (e.g., Cardinal et al., 2002), although the original learning is indelible, and newer learning is controlled by the context (Bouton, Chapter 9). Core affect (i.e., the neurophysiological state) can exist and influence behavior without being labeled or interpreted, and can therefore function unconsciously (e.g., Berridge & Winkielman, 2003; Winkielman, Berridge, & Wilbarger, Chapter 14). Core affect (and corresponding behavioral responses) can exist alone or can be represented and reported as a feeling.

Whether because of extreme changes that capture attention or deliberate introspection (such as when a person is asked to report a feeling), people verbally represent core affect as feelings of valence (pleasure or displeasure) and activation (feeling sleepy or excited). When people are asked directly about feelings of pleasure or displeasure, activation or deactivation, they can report them (e.g., Russell, Weiss, & Mendelsohn, 1989). When people are asked about their experiences of emotion, they also communicate their core affective feelings (Feldman, 1995b; Russell, 1980; for a review, see Barrett & Russell, 1999). In fact, core affective feelings are implicitly communicated in self-reports of emotion experience. The extent to which a conscious feeling is characterized by one or the other property varies within a person over time (Barrett, in press), across people (Feldman, 1995a; Barrett, 1998, 2004b), and across cultures (Mesquita, 2003).

Indeed, people most often report core affective feelings as part of an emotional episode—a short-lived response that corresponds to the collo-quial idea of "having an emotion." Although emotion is experienced as a discrete act, core affect is in constant flow and flux. People are continuously in some state of core affect, constantly moving their faces and their bodies. The possibility pursued here is that the ebb and flow of core affect is parsed into discrete events during the process of perception, and it becomes per-ceptually bound to the object that is believe to have caused the feeling in the first place. As a result, a person becomes angry *with* someone, afraid *of* something, sad *about* something. I suggest that we perceive emotion in our-selves in a way that is similar to the way we perceive the behaviors of oth-ers, termed *person perception* or *ordinary personology*. The general idea is that people emit a stream of actions (perhaps facial actions that are caused by evaluative processing and associated with core affective states). Cate-gory knowledge shapes those actions into the perception of an emotional event in others—emotion identification, if you will. Similarly, I argue here that we engage in emotion identification when we use category knowledge about emotion in the perception of our own core affective states, producing the experience of emotion.

How Is Emotion Perception Achieved?

Social psychology has accumulated a large and nuanced body of research on how people perceive one another's behavior and infer causes (for review of this literature, see Gilbert, 1998). Originally, it was believed that people, like physical objects (or emotions, for that matter), had real properties that could be observed, so that it was possible to quantify the accuracy of per-ceptions of those properties (Brunswick, 1947). Very quickly, however, the field shifted away from questions about accuracy because it was discovered that the person properties under investigation—traits—defied simple mea-surement and clear definition. Instead, researchers became interested in understanding how people infer the properties of others—in particular, why people see certain behaviors and how they come to understand what caused them (Heider, 1944). In a sense, ordinary personology is the study of theory of mind—how people attribute mental states to self and others in order to explain and predict the behavior that is perceived in others. It might prove helpful to follow a path set by attribution theorists almost half a century ago to focus on the judgment process as a way of understanding how people perceive an emotion in themselves—and therefore experience that emotion.

Person Perception

Person perception involves three processes (for a review, see Gilbert, 1998), but for the purposes of this chapter we are most concerned with the process of behavior identification—how an observer perceives what a target person is doing. People are constantly moving and doing things (such as moving their facial muscles). Somehow, we partition that continuous movement into recognizable, meaningful, discrete acts (such as a facial expression). Bob is contracting his facial muscles, and water is coming out of his eyes; we recognize this movement as the behavioral act of crying. Bob is moving his feet heavily as he walks; we recognize this movement as the behavioral act of stomping. Inferring an intention is part of the behavior identification stage because observers prefer to identify behavioral acts in terms of the target's intentions (cf. Gilbert, 1998). The inference of intention gives meaning to the behavioral act. If Bob is stomping, then he is behaving angrily. He is in an intentional state (i.e., his behavior is caused). Because his anger mechanism is triggered, Bob is angry at this moment in time. We have categorized an instance of anger in Bob.

It is a well-known finding in social and cognitive psychology that prior information structures incoming information. This dynamic is very clearly the case in person perception, where the knowledge that is active in our minds influences what behaviors we see and what causes we infer, often without our awareness. Person perception researchers have focused their investigations on how category knowledge about persons (based on their prior behavior, group membership, etc.) influences behavior identification. Just as stereotypes about people shape our perceptions of what they do and why, category knowledge about emotion may act like "emotion stereotypes" to shape our perceptions of emotion in others and in ourselves. The argument, then, is that self-perception is an act of person perception when the target of perception is the self.

Emotion Perception

Just as behavior identification is shaped by category knowledge about persons, emotion identification may be shaped by category knowledge about emotion. Behavior identification involves parsing a stream of actions into discrete bits by assigning them an intention to render them meaningful. Similarly, emotion identification (the act of emotion perception) may involve parsing the stream of core affect—whether the internal state (accessible to the emoter) or its behavioral consequence (accessible to the observer)—into discrete emotional bits by assigning an intention to render it meaningful. Just as we interpret or imbue behavioral actions with intention when we parse them into a discrete behavioral act, so we imbue core affect with intention or emotional "aboutness" when we parse it into discrete acts of feeling. When a person identifies his or her core affect as being about something, it becomes intentional, and the experience of emotion begins.

There is evidence that conceptual knowledge about emotion seamlessly shapes the perception of emotion in others. Some of the initial research on behavior identification examined how emotion category information influenced the identification of emotion in photographs of facial configurations and in verbal descriptions of emotional reactions (Trope, 1986). Additional studies have replicated and extended these findings (Bouhuys, Bloem, & Groothuis, 1995; Carroll & Russell, 1996; Halberstadt & Niedenthal, 2001; Trope & Cohen, 1989). If processes that enable us to know one another also allow us to know ourselves, then conceptual knowledge about emotion may quickly and unconsciously shape our identification of our own emotions in much the same way that it serves to shape our perceptions of emotion in others. Early perceptual processing may extract sensory information from the internal context in much the same way that sensory information is extracted from the external stimulus environment during object recognition (to determine whether or not there is an object present). For example, in much the same way as bottom-up (or stimulus-driven) processes extract information about perceptual features of the face during face recognition, processing of the somatovisceral information (constituting a person's core affective state at a particular moment in time) may allow people to recognize that a shift in core affect has occurred. Shifts in core affect are then available to be identified in a manner that is similar to object identification. Just as conceptual knowledge is necessary to categorize a set of facial behaviors as an instance of *anger*, so too this knowledge may influence the categorization of our own core affective state during a process of emotion identification. It is possible that the categorization process can also be the result of more deliberative processing, either during introspection or when core affect is intense enough to be represented in awareness (in a manner reminiscent of Mandler, 1975, or Schachter & Singer, 1962). The reason that our experiences of emotion have a given quality is that emotion identification occurs outside of our awareness the majority of the time.

The conceptual system might shape the categorization of core affect into the experience of emotion with several consequences. These ideas were inspired by Barsalou's (1999, 2003) discussion of the ways in which conceptual information supports perceptual inferences. First, to the extent that conceptual knowledge performs some sort of figure–ground segregation, the experience of an emotion will "pop out" as separate from the ebb and flow in ongoing core affect. Second, once an instance of core affect is categorized, a rich set of inferences is available that constitutes expertise about how to deal with the world (including our feelings) at that instant in time. Third, conceptual knowledge of emotion can help us anticipate other aspects of the emotional response that are (whether correctly or erroneously) expected, either speeding their perception or going beyond the information present to fill them in at a given perceptual instance. This part of the process can, perhaps, result in illusory correlations between response outputs (helping to explain why researchers continue to search for coordinated autonomic, behavioral, and experiential aspects of an emotional response). Fourth, conceptual knowledge about emotion allows us to go beyond the information given in another way, in that it guides us to assume what happened before the instance of core affect and what will happen next—we fit what we see into a script so as to better predict our own behavior. In the next section, I consider how conceptual knowledge about emotion might achieve these effects.

Conceptual Knowledge and Categorization

Whenever we selectively attend, with some consistency, to components of experience, knowledge of a category develops (cf. Schynn, Goldstone, & Thibaut, 1998). The human conceptual system contains a collection of category knowledge, including knowledge about kinds of emotion. Children acquire emotion concepts over time (Widen & Russell, 2003). Each time a parent labels a child's behavior with an emotion term, or a child hears the emotion term being used to label someone else's behavior, the child extracts information about that instance and integrates it with past information associated with the same term that is stored in memory. In this way, children acquire emotion categories that conform to their culture.

In most discussions of emotion categories, the basic unit of knowledge is an emotion concept. A concept of a particular emotion, say, *anger*, is thought to contain a feature list that includes what triggers an instance of anger, what it feels like to be angry, what relational theme is likely to be present, physiological changes to be expected, what voluntary movements, vocal cues, and facial movements are typically involved, and what are the social rules for expressing the emotion. To know the script for *anger* in your culture is to know what *anger* is (Fehr & Russell, 1984). In the past, researchers have argued over the structure and format of these conceptual representations (e.g., Russell, 1991; Clore & Ortony, 1991), but most have agreed that concepts are part of the semantic memory system—decontextualized distillations of invariant properties that are extracted from previous instances of the category. These representations are termed *amodal* because they are abstracted from sensory–motor events and stored in some sort of propositional form, such as in an encyclopedia (Barsalou, 2003). They are thought to be nomothetically and idiographically stable. For a given emotion category, different people within a culture share roughly the same representation, and the same person uses the same representation on different occasions. All cognitive processes operate on these redescriptions, as the original sensory–motor representations are no longer needed.

More recently, Barsalou and his colleagues (Barsalou, 1999, 2003, in press; Barsalou, Simmons, et al., 2003) have challenged these ideas, suggesting that static entities called *concepts* do not exist. Instead of viewing categories as represented by invariant concepts that can be retrieved intact from long-term memory, each category is represented by a large number of specific instances, called *situated conceptualizations*. These situated conceptualizations are not amodal, abstract exemplars; rather, they are partial reenactments or simulations of the sensory–motor states that occurred with previous instances of the category. No single situated conceptualization need give a complete account of the category. An instance of a category involves the sensory, motor, and introspective states that come together in working memory in a way that is tailored to the current situation. Niedenthal and colleagues (e.g., Chapter 2) have reinterpreted existing evidence from research on attitudes, social perception, and emotion to support the idea that social knowledge is grounded in sensory–motor representations. Most important for the position advanced here is their suggestion that emotion categories, as situated conceptualizations, are implicated in emotion perception.

A situated conceptualization (i.e., an instance of conceptualizing a category) is produced by a simulator (or set of simulators). As discussed in Niedenthal et al. (Chapter 2), a simulator for a category of knowledge, such as *anger*, develops as sensory–motor and somatovisceral sources of information are encoded during instances when words for *anger* are used. Sensory information about the objects (e.g., people) that are seen as causing *anger*, motor programs for dealing with *anger*, the coincident interoceptive states (such as those associated with core affect or cognitive operations), the broader stimulus situation or context are all integrated into the simulator. Extending this view, it is possible that an instance of core affect (i.e., the person's current homeostatic state resulting from evaluation), along with representations of concurrent objects in the focus of attention, actions taken, the relational context, the emotion label provided by others, and so on, bind together to form an instance of *anger*. Because core affect is a category of experience, it may have its own simulator or be represented by its own collection of simulations that is embedded in emotion category simulators (see Barsalou, Niedenthal, Barbey, & Ruppert, 2003, for a discussion of embedded simulators). Properties that are pointed out by parents (or other speakers) or those that are functionally relevant in everyday activities will bind with core affect to represent *anger* in that instance. As these instances accumulate, knowledge about *anger* develops as a distributed neural system that involves both modality-specific and association areas. These establish the conceptual content for the basic-level category *anger* and can be retrieved for later simulations of *anger* when needed. As a result, a situated conceptualization view of emotion knowledge is consistent with the view that core affect is a necessary part of every instance of emotion.

At the simplest level, the central hypothesis outlined in this chapter— that conceptual knowledge shapes the identification of core affective events—becomes more plausible if emotion knowledge is simulated. Category representations are characterized as sensory–motor events. Core affect consists of sensory–motor information. Since the two share a representational format, they could be seamlessly integrated during an instance of perception. This integration may be especially likely because emotion categories are abstract, and introspective state information is particularly important to abstract concepts (Barsalou & Wiemer-Hastings, in press).

Furthermore, situated conceptualizations have several distinctive properties (for a detailed discussion, see Barsalou, 1999, 2003, in press) that allow for specific predictions about how emotion perception should proceed, as well as its consequences for the experience of emotion. First, and most importantly, *the situation will influence what is felt*. A situated conceptualization (e.g., an instance of conceptualizing *anger*) is inherently bound to a particular context (Yeh & Barsalou, 2002). Context is particularly important to conceptualizations of abstract categories (Barsalou & Wiemer-Hastings, in press) such as emotion. Information about the relational context (Lazarus, 1991) or a situation's meaning to a person at a particular point in time (Clore & Ortony, 2000) may constitute some of the background information contained in situated conceptualizations of an emotion category that, like objects, may serve to launch a simulation. An experience of emotion, then, may be shaped by the situation, such that the experience of a given emotion, such as anger, will show great heterogeneity across instances within a person and across people. There are a multitude of sensory–motor simulations that belong to *anger*, each one producing a distinct feeling state. This view is similar to what James (1884) proposed but is clearly different from Damasio's (1994) somatic marker hypothesis, which

states that there are specific somatic markers for particular emotion categories (Damasio et al., 2000).

Second, *language can intrinsically influence the experience of emotion.*
To the extent that language drives category acquisition, words will determine which simulations are available for use during emotion identification.
Language might also shape experience via production of novel simulations
(i.e., representations of things that have never been encountered together;
Barsalou, 2003). People may integrate in LTM two representations from the
same emotion category, even when their surface similarities differ (see
Barsalou et al., 2003), because the label for the emotion links them in memory (see Gelman & Markman, 1987). Highly different instances for the
same category can become integrated over time and become available for
simulation during emotion identification. As a result, people can simulate
and experience new combinations that will add to the range of emotion
experience. This generative feature of situated conceptualizations may help
to explain why people perceive prototypical emotion episodes, even though
those episodes seem impossible to capture with the use of scientific instruments.

Third, *experience may shape subsequent behavior.* Situated conceptualizations contain inferences about situated action (i.e., the actions needed
in a given situation). Although some of the behavior that we typically think
of as "emotional" may result from core affective processes, it is possible,
even likely, that once conceptual knowledge about emotion is activated, it
can direct subsequent behavioral responses. Across varied situations, different situated conceptualizations of a given emotion category arise, each
designed to optimize one particular type of situated action associated with
that category. For example, you may have learned a host of different actions
associated with the category *anger.* Sometimes it works to yell, sometimes
to pound your fist, sometimes to cry or walk away, sometimes to hit. During
a given act of conceptualizing, you are most likely to simulate whatever
action will allow you to achieve yours goals for the given situation. As a
result, situated conceptualizations deliver highly specific inferences tailored to particular situations regarding what actions to take.

Fourth, *experiencing an emotion, like conceptualizing in general, may
be a skill.* Some people may be better than others at tailoring conceptual
knowledge to meet the needs of situated action (Barsalou, 2003). The people who are better at tailoring their simulations to the needs of the particular situation will be more functionally effective than those who are less able
to do so. Similarly, constructing such an emotion experience may also be a
skill. Presumably, there is no single experience of *anger,* but many, dependent on the content of the simulation. It is a skill to simulate the most
appropriate or effective representation, or even to know when to inhibit a

simulated conceptualization that has been incidentally primed (Barrett et al., 2004).

Finally, *the importance of situated action in situated conceptualizations may help explain why people perceive a prototypical emotional episode* (i.e., what most people consider the clearest cases of emotion characterized as having all the necessary component parts; Russell, 2003; Russell & Barrett, 1999), even though such episodes are quite rare. Barsalou (2003) has argued that people are goal achievers who organize knowledge in categories to support acting in the most functionally effective way. Over time, goal-directed categories become well established in memory (Barsalou & Ross, 1986), such that the most typical members of the category are those that maximize goal achievement (not those that are most frequently encountered). If emotion categories are goal-directed categories, then the most typical instances of a category will not contain properties that appear most commonly as instances of the category, but those that represent the ideal form of the category—that is, whatever is ideal for meeting the goal around which the category is organized. This may be one reason that scientists typically theorize about and focus their empirical efforts on, prototypical emotional episodes, even though the nonprototypical cases are more frequent in our everyday lives.

WHAT IS THE EXPERIENCE OF EMOTION?

In this chapter I have argued that the dominant scientific paradigm for explaining the experience of emotion assumes that there are natural kinds of emotion mechanisms that cause behavior and experience. Despite the lack of strong, compelling instrument-based evidence, many scholars continue to hold this view, believing that there are real behaviors that can be called *angry, fearful, sad,* and so on. As a challenge to this view, I have outlined the equally plausible model that to experience an emotion is to perceive it. In this view, emotions are not causal entities. They, themselves, are caused. Emotions do not explain anything. They are the things to be explained. My model of emotion experience involves three propositions. First, I proposed that core affect, as the neurophysiological state resulting from assessing the predictive value of a stimulus, is one basic substrate of experience. Core affect is available to be felt, although it need not be felt in any given instance. Second, I argued that the experience of emotion is psychologically constructed via the same processes with which we experience color, and each other. Knowledge of emotion categories shapes the perception of core affect into an experience of emotion in much the same way that knowledge of color categories shapes the experience of a continuous wavelength light spectrum, or how category knowledge about people shapes our perceptions of other people's behavioral actions into meaningful acts. Third, I have suggested that the content and structure of category knowledge about emotion determines which emotion is perceived and, potentially, even what we feel. Because conceptualizing involves sensory–motor representations, conceptual knowledge about emotion can seamlessly shape the perception of core affect into the experience of an emotion.

The model that I have proposed clearly builds on key ideas from the psychological literature on emotion. Most clearly, my view owes a debt to social-constructivist models in which emotional states are culture-bound descriptions that are differentiated, defined, and labeled via schemas or mental representations of emotion concepts (e.g., Averill, 1980; Harre, 1986; White, 1993). It bears some resemblance to Schachter and Singer's (1962) two-factor theory and to Scherer's (e.g., Chapter 13) level of processing view, although there are notable differences. It is also broadly consistent with an appraisal perspective on emotion, in which appraisals are not so much a set of processes for generating emotion but the rules for describing which emotions are felt when (Clore et al., Chapter 16). My view also is clearly inspired by William James, who, contrary to popular belief, did not argue that anger, sadness, and so on, have specific and unique patterns of somatovisceral changes in the entitive sense; rather, he argued for the heterogeneity of instances within each emotion category. According to James, there can be variable sets of bodily symptoms associated with a single category of emotion, making each a distinct feeling state and therefore a distinct emotion. By the term *emotion,* James was referring to particular instances of feeling, not to discrete emotion categories. What differentiates my model from these other perspectives is the emphasis on categorization processes as a core mechanism driving emotion experience.

It also seems important to point out that the view of embodied emotion knowledge discussed here can in principle be consistent with the idea of emotions as causal entities. People may have situated conceptualizations, not because they acquired emotion categories through language and labeling, but because they learned about emotion mechanisms that already exist in the brain and body. Even the idea that emotion knowledge allows people to know emotions in others can be consistent with the idea that emotions exist as causal entities. Ontology is not identical to epistemology. Anger, sadness, fear, and so on, may be real mechanisms that cause behavior and experience, and people may perceive them accurately or inaccurately. Of course, this position assumes that there is some clear empirical criterion for judging the accuracy of emotion perceptions, which currently there is not. At best, the empirical glass is half full.

Of course, the value of the perspective that I have outlined in this chapter will rest or fall with empirical evidence. Undoubtedly, a major research initiative is required to test these ideas. For now, it is reasonable to point out that there is scientific precedent for taking this point of view. Many psychological constructs that scientists once thought of as fixed, unitary causal entities with an identifiable essence (e.g., memory, personality, concepts, attitudes) are now thought of as emergent properties or byproducts of distinct but interacting systems (Barsalou et al., 2003; Johnson, 1992; Johnson & Hirst, 1993; Mischel, 1984; Mischel & Shoda, 1995; Schacter, 1996). Furthermore, there is recent evidence from artificial intelligence research indicating that language shapes the acquisition of category knowledge (Steels & Belpaeme, in press). People come to know what the color *blue* is because other people (parents, other adults, etc.) teach them, as children, to associate objects that reflect particular wavelengths with words for *blue*. Recent research on the categorical perception of color (Özgen, 2004; Özgen & Davies, 2002) suggests that language influences perception by shaping the boundaries of specific color categories. There is also good scientific evidence for the idea that conceptual knowledge influences perception, whether about physical objects (e.g., Palmer, 1975), phenomenal contents such as color (Davidoff, 2001), or people (Gilbert, 1998). And then there is evidence that conceptual knowledge is embodied (Barsalou, 1999; Barsalou et al., 2003), that emotion knowledge, in particular, may be embodied (see Niedenthal et al., Chapter 2) and have a role in shaping perception (for a review, see Niedenthal & Halberstadt, 2003). If conceptual knowledge has pervasive effects on perception, then perhaps it is involved with perceiving emotion in the self and others. Why should we assume that the perception of emotion is different from the perception of anything else?

ACKNOWLEDGMENTS

Many thanks to Larry Barsalou, Paula Niedenthal, and Piotr Winkielman for their helpful comments on an earlier draft of this chapter. Preparation of this chapter was supported by National Science Foundation Grant Nos. SBR-9727896, BCS 0074688, and BCS 0092224, and by National Institute of Mental Health Grant No. K02 MH001981.

NOTES

1. Feeling does not necessarily serve as evidence of the causal mechanism to observers, however. For the observer (observing the emoter), an emotion is revealed by expressive behavior, over and above anything else (including the emoter's verbal report).
2. Admittedly, the neural systems involved in early sensory processing of faces and

core affective information would be somewhat different, however. Early perceptual processing of somatovisceral information associated with core affective state may involve posterior aspects of the insula. This information is re-represented in the anterior insular cortex and other parts of a larger system (including anterior cingulate cortex, limbic motor areas, and orbital frontal cortex) thought to be responsible for the subjective experience of feelings in humans (Craig, 2002).

REFERENCES

Asch, S. E. (1987). *Social psychology*. New York: Oxford University Press. (Original work published 1952)

Averill, J. R. (1980). A constructivist view of emotion. In R. Plutchik & H. Kellerman (Eds.), *Theories of emotion* (pp. 339–368). New York: Plenum Press.

Bargh, J. A., & Ferguson, M. J. (2000). Beyond behaviorism: On the automaticity of higher mental processes. *Psychological Bulletin, 126*, 925–945.

Barrett, L. F. (1998). Discrete emotions or dimensions? The role of valence focus and arousal focus. *Cognition and Emotion, 12*, 579–599.

Barrett, L. F. (2004). Feelings or words? Understanding the content in self-report ratings of experienced emotion. *Journal of Personality and Social Psychology, 87*, 266–281.

Barrett, L. F. (2005). *Emotions as natural kinds: Commonsense or reality?* Manuscript submitted for publication.

Barrett, L. F. (in press). Valence as a basic building block of emotional life. *Journal of Research in Personality*.

Barrett, L. F., & Niedenthal, P. M. (2004). Valence focus and the perception of facial affect. *Emotion, 4*, 266–274.

Barrett, L. F., Ochsner, K. N., & Gross, J. J. (in press). Beyond automaticity: A course correction for emotion research. In J. Bargh (Ed.), *Automatic processes in social thinking and behavior*. New York: Psychology Press.

Barrett, L. F., Quigley, K., Bliss-Moreau, E., & Aronson, K. R. (2004). Arousal focus and interoceptive sensitivity. *Journal of Personality and Social Psychology, 87*, 684–697.

Barrett, L. F., & Russell, J. A. (2004c). *Has neuroimaging revealed the essence of emotion?* Manuscript submitted for publication.

Barrett, L. F., Tugade, M. M., & Engle, R. W. (2004). Individual differences in working memory capacity and dual-process theories of the mind. *Psychological Bulletin, 130*, 553–573.

Barsalou, L. W. (1999). Perceptual symbol systems. *Behavioral and Brain Sciences, 22*, 577–609.

Barsalou, L. W. (2003). Situated simulation in the human conceptual system. *Language and Cognitive Processes, 18*, 513–562.

Barsalou, L. W. (in press). Abstraction as dynamic interpretation in perceptual symbol systems. In L. Gershkoff-Stowe & D. Rakison (Eds.), *Building object categories* (Carnegie Cognition Series). Mahwah, NJ: Erlbaum.

Barsalou, L. W., Niedenthal, P. M., Barbey, A., & Ruppert, J. (2003). Social embodiment. In B. Ross (Ed.), *The psychology of learning and motivation* (Vol. 43, pp. 43–92). San Diego, CA: Academic Press.

Barsalou, L. W., & Ross, B. H. (1986). The roles of automatic and strategic processing in sensitivity to superordinate and property frequency. *Journal of Experimental Psychology: Learning, Memory, and Cognition, 12,* 116–134.

Barsalou, L. W., Simmons, W. K., Barbey, A. K., & Wilson, C. D. (2003). Grounding conceptual knowledge in modality-specific systems. *Trends in Cognitive Sciences, 7,* 84–91.

Barsalou, L. W., & Wiemer-Hastings, K. (in press). Situating abstract concepts. In D. Pecher & R. Zwaan (Eds.), *Grounding cognition: The role of perception and action in memory, language, and thought.* New York: Cambridge University Press.

Berridge, K. C., & Winkielman, P. (2003). What is unconscious emotion? *Cognition and Emotion, 17,* 181–211.

Blanchard, R. J., & Blanchard, D. C. (2003). What can animal aggression research tell us about human aggression? *Hormones and Behavior, 44,* 171–177.

Bouhuys, A. L., Bloem, G. M., & Groothuis, T. G. G. (1995). Induction of depressed and elated mood by music influences the perception of facial emotional expressions in healthy subjects. *Journal of Affective Disorders, 33,* 215–226.

Bradley, M. M., & Lang, P. J. (2000). Measuring emotion: Behavior, feeling, and physiology. In R. D. Lane & L. Nadel (Eds.), *Cognitive neuroscience of emotion* (pp. 242–76). New York: Oxford University Press.

Bridges, K. M. B. (1932). Emotional development in early infancy. *Child Development, 3,* 324–334.

Brunswick, E. (1947). *Systematic and representative design in psychological experiments.* Berkeley: University of California Press.

Buck, R. (1999). The biological affects: A typology. *Psychological Review, 106*(2), 301–336.

Cacioppo, J. T., Berntson, G. G., Larsen, J. T., Poehlmann, K. M., & Ito, T. A. (2000). The psychophysiology of emotion. In M. Lewis & J. M. Haviland-Jones (Eds.), *Handbook of emotions* (2nd ed., pp. 173–191). New York: Guilford Press.

Cacioppo, J. T., & Gardner, W. L. (1999). Emotion. *Annual Review of Psychology, 50,* 191–214.

Cardinal, R. N., Parkinson, J. A., Hall, J., & Everitt, B. J. (2002). Emotion and motivation: The role of the amygdala, ventral striatum, and prefrontal cortex. *Neuroscience and Behavior Reviews, 26*(3), 321–352.

Carroll, J. M., & Russell, J. A. (1996). Do facial expressions express specific emotions? Judging emotion from the face in context. *Journal of Personality and Social Psychology, 70,* 205–218.

Christie, I. C., & Friedman, B. H. (2004). Autonomic specificity of discrete emotion and dimensions of affective space: A multivariate approach. *International Journal of Psychophysiology, 51,* 143–153.

Clore, G. L., & Ortony, A. (1991). What more is there to emotion concepts than prototypes? *Journal of Personality and Social Psychology, 60,* 48–50.

Clore, G. L., & Ortony, A. (2000). Cognition in emotion: Always, sometimes, or never? In L. Nadel, R. Lane, & G. L. Ahern (Eds.), *The cognitive neuroscience of emotion* (pp. 24–61). New York: Oxford University Press.

Damasio, A. R. (1994). *Descartes' error: Emotion, reason and the human brain.* New York: Grosset/Putnam.

Damasio, A. R. (1999). *The feeling of what happens: Body and emotion in the making of consciousness.* New York: Harcourt Brace.

Damasio, A. R., Grabowski, T. J., Bechara, A., Damasio, H., Ponto, L. L., Parvizi, J., & Hichwa, R. D. (2000). Subcortical and cortical brain activity during the feeling of self-generated emotions. *Nature Neuroscience, 3,* 1049–1056.

Davidoff, J. (2001). Language and perceptual categories. *Trends in Cognitive Science, 5,* 382–387.

Davidoff, J., Davies, I. R. L., & Roberson, D. (1999). Is colour categorisation universal? New evidence from a Stone-Age culture. *Nature, 398,* 203–204.

Davis, M., & Whalen P. J. (2001). The amygdala: Vigilance and emotion. *Molecular Psychiatry, 6,* 13–34.

Dennett, D. (1991). *Consciousness explained.* Boston: Little, Brown.

Dolan, R. J. (2002). Emotion, cognition and behavior. *Science, 298,* 1191–1194.

Ekman, P. (1992). An argument for basic emotions. *Cognition and Emotion, 6,* 169–200.

Ekman, P., Levenson, R. W., & Friesen, W. V. (1983). Autonomic nervous system activity distinguishes between emotions. *Science, 221,* 1208–1210.

Emde, R. N., Gaensbauer, T., & Harmon, R. (1976). Emotional expression in infancy: A biobehavioral study. *Psychological Issues, 10*(1, Whole No. 37).

Fehr, B., & Russell, J. A. (1984). Concept of emotion viewed from a prototype perspective. *Journal of Experimental Psychology: General, 113,* 464–486.

Feldman, L. A. (1995a). Valence focus and arousal focus: Individual differences in the structure of affective experience. *Journal of Personality and Social Psychology, 69,* 153–166.

Feldman, L. A. (1995b). Variations in the circumplex structure of emotion. *Personality and Social Psychology Bulletin, 21,* 806–817.

Frijda, N. H., Markam, S., Sato, K., & Wiers, R. (1995). Emotion and emotion words. In J. A. Russell, J. M. Fernández-Dols, A. S. R. Manstead, & J. C. Wellenkamp (Eds.), *Everyday conceptions of emotion: An introduction to the psychology, anthropology, and linguistics of emotion* (pp. 121–143). Netherlands: Kluwer.

Gelman, S. A., & Markman, E. M. (1987). Young children's inductions from natural kinds: The role of categories and appearances. *Child Development, 8,* 157–167.

Gilbert, D. T. (1998). Ordinary personology. In D. T. Gilbert, S. T. Fiske, & G. Lindzey (Eds.), *The handbook of social psychology* (4th ed.). New York: McGraw Hill.

Goleman, D. (1995). *Emotional intelligence: Why it can matter more than IQ.* New York: Bantam.

Halberstadt, J., & Niedenthal, P. M. (2001). Effects of emotion concepts on perceptual memory for emotional expressions. *Journal of Personality and Social Psychology, 81,* 587–598.

Harre, R. (Ed.). (1986). *The social construction of emotions.* Oxford, UK: Blackwell.

Heider, F. (1944). Social perception and phenomenal causality. *Psychological Review, 51,* 358–374.

Hochberg, J. (Ed.). (1998). *Perception and cognition at centuries end: Handbook of perception and cognition* (2nd ed.). San Diego CA: Academic Press.

Izard, C. E. (1993). Four systems for emotion activation: Cognitive and noncognitive processes. *Psychological Review, 100,* 68–90.

James, W. (1884). What is an emotion? *Mind, 9,* 188–205.

James, W. (1950). *The principles of psychology, Volume II, Chapter 25: The emotions* (pp. 442–485). New York: Dover. (Original work published 1890)

James, W. (1894). The physical basis of emotion. *Psychological Review, 1,* 516–529.

Johnson, M. K. (1992). MEM: Mechanisms of recollection. *Journal of Cognitive Neuroscience, 4,* 268–280.

Johnson, M. K., & Hirst, W. (1993). MEM: Memory subsystems as processes. In A. F. Collins, S. E. Gathercole, M. A. Conway, & P. E. Morris (Eds.), *Theories of memory* (pp. 241–286). East Sussex, UK: Erlbaum.

Jones, E. E., & Nisbett, R. E. (1971). *The actor and the observer: Divergent perceptions of the causes of behavior.* New York: General Learning Press.

Kim, H., Somerville, L. H., Johnstone, T., Alexander, A., Whalen, P. J. (2003). Inverse amygdala and medial prefrontal cortex responses to surprised faces. *NeuroReport, 14,* 2317–2322.

Laird, J. D., & Bresler, C. (1992). The process of emotional feeling: A self-perception theory. In M. Clark (Ed.), *Emotion: Review of personality and social psychology* (Vol 13, pp. 223–234). Newbury Park, CA: Sage.

Lambie, J. A., & Marcel, A. J. (2002). Consciousness and emotion experience: A theoretical framework. *Psychological Review, 109,* 219–259.

Lang, P. J. (1968). Fear reduction and fear behavior: Problems in treating a construct. In J. M. Schlien (Ed.), *Research in psychotherapy* (Vol. 3, pp. 90–103). Washington, DC: American Psychological Association.

Lang, P. J., Bradley, M. M., & Cuthbert, B. N. (1990). Emotion, attention, and the startle reflex. *Psychological Review, 97,* 377–398.

Lang, P. J., Greenwald, M. K., Bradley, M. M., & Hamm, A. O. (1993). Looking at pictures: Affective, facial, visceral, and behavioral reactions. *Psychophysiology, 30,* 261–273.

Lazarus, R. S. (1991). *Emotion and adaptation.* New York: Oxford University Press.

LeDoux, J. E. (1996). *The emotional brain: The mysterious underpinnings of emotional life.* New York: Simon & Schuster.

Levenson, R. W., Ekman, P., & Friesen, W. V. (1990). Voluntary facial action generates emotion specific autonomic nervous system activity. *Psychophysiology, 27,* 363–384.

Mandler, G. (1975). *Mind and emotion.* New York: Wiley.

Mandler, G., Mandler, J. M., Kremen, I., & Sholiton, R. (1961). The response to threat: Relations among verbal and physiological indices. *Psychological Monographs, 75*(No. 513).

Mesquita, B. (2003). Emotions as dynamic cultural phenomena. In R. J. Davidson, K. R. Scherer, & H. H. Goldsmith (Eds.), *Handbook of affective sciences* (pp. 871–890). London: Oxford University Press.

Messinger, D. S. (2002). Positive and negative: Infant facial expressions and emotions. *Current Directions in Psychological Science, 11*, 1–6.

Mischel, W. (1984). Convergences and challenges in the search for consistency. *American Psychologist, 39*, 351–364.

Mischel, W., & Shoda, Y. (1995). A cognitive–affective system theory of personality: Reconceptualizing situations, dispositions, dynamics, and invariance in personality structure. *Psychological Review, 102*, 246–268.

Murphy, F. C., Nimmo-Smith, I., & Lawrence, A. D. (2003). Functional neuroanatomy of emotion: A meta-analysis. *Cognitive, Affective, and Behavioral Neuroscience, 3*, 207–233.

Niedenthal, P. M., Barsalou, L. W., Winkielman, P., Krauth-Gruber, S., & Ric, F. (in press). Embodiment in attitudes, social perception, and emotion. *Personality and Social Psychology Review.*

Niedenthal, P. M., & Halberstadt, J. B. (2003). Top-down influences in social perception. In W. Stroebe & M. Hewstone (Eds.), *The European Review of Social Psychology* (Vol. 14, pp. 49–76). London: Wiley.

Nisbett, R. E., & Wilson, T. D. (1977). Telling more than we can know: Verbal reports on mental processes. *Psychological Review, 84*, 231–259.

Ochsner, K. N., & Barrett, L. F. (2001). A multiprocess perspective on the neuroscience of emotion. In T. J. Mayne & G. Bonnano (Eds.), *Emotion: Current issues and future directions* (pp. 38–81). New York: Guilford Press.

Özgen, E. (2004). Language, learning, and color perception. *Current Directions in Psychological Science, 13*(3), 95–98.

Özgen, E., & Davies, I. R. L. (2002). Acquisition of categorical color perception: A perceptual learning approach to the linguistic relativity hypothesis. *Journal of Experimental Psychology: General, 131*(4), 477–493.

Palmer, S. E. (1975). The effects of contextual scenes on the identification of objects. *Memory and Cognition, 3*, 519–526.

Panksepp, J. (1998). *Affective neuroscience: The foundations of human and animal emotions.* New York: Oxford University Press.

Phan, K. L., Wager, T. D., Taylor, S. F., & Liberzon, I. (2002). Functional neuroanatomy of emotion: A meta-analysis of emotion activation studies in PET and fMRI. *Neuroimage, 16*, 331–348.

Phillips, R. G., & LeDoux, J. E. (1994). Lesions of the dorsal hippocampal formation interfere with background but not foreground contextual fear conditioning. *Learning and Memory, 1*, 34–44.

Quigley, K. S., Barrett, L.F., & Weinstein, S. (2002). Cardiovascular patterns associated with threat and challenge appraisals: Individual responses across time. *Psychophysiology, 39*, 1–11.

Ramachandran, V. S. (1992). Filling in gaps in perception: Part I. *Current Directions in Psychological Science, 1*, 199–205.

Ramachandran, V. S. (1993). Filling in gaps in perception: Part II: Scotomas and phantom limbs. *Current Directions in Psychological Science, 2,* 56–65.

Roberson, D., Davies, I., & Davidoff, J. (2000). Color categories are not universal: Replications and new evidence from a Stone-Age culture. *Journal of Experimental Psychology: General, 129,* 369–398.

Rolls, E. T. (1999). *The brain and emotion.* New York: Oxford University Press.

Russell, J. A. (1980). A circumplex model of affect. *Journal of Personality and Social Psychology, 39,* 1161–1178.

Russell, J. A. (1991). Culture and the categorization of emotion. *Psychological Bulletin, 110,* 426–450.

Russell, J. A. (1994). Is there universal recognition of emotion from facial expression?: A review of the cross-cultural studies. *Psychological Bulletin, 115,* 102–141.

Russell, J. A. (2003). Core affect and the psychological construction of emotion. *Psychological Review, 110,* 145–172

Russell, J. A., Bachorowski, J.-A., & Fernandez-Dols, J.-M. (2003). Facial and vocal expressions of emotion. *Annual Review of Psychology, 54,* 329–349.

Russell, J. A., & Barrett, L. F. (1999). Core affect, prototypical emotional episodes, and other things called emotion: Dissecting the elephant. *Journal of Personality and Social Psychology, 76,* 805–819.

Russell, J. A., & Snodgrass, J. (1987). Emotion and the environment. In D. Stokols & I. Altman (Eds.), *Handbook of environmental psychology* (pp. 245–280). New York: Wiley.

Russell, J. A., Weiss, A., & Mendelsohn, G. A. (1989). Affect grid: A single-item scale of pleasure and arousal. *Journal of Personality and Social Psychology, 57,* 493–502.

Schacter, D. L. (1996). *Searching for memory: The brain, the mind, and the past.* New York: Basic Books.

Schachter, S., & Singer, J. E. (1962). Cognitive, social, and physiological determinants of emotional state. *Psychological Review, 69,* 379–399.

Schooler, J. W. (2002). Re-representing consciousness: Dissociations between experience and meta-consciousness. *Trends in Cognitive Science, 6,* 339–344.

Schyns, P. G., Goldstone, R. L.,& Thibaut, J. P. (1998). The development of features in object concepts. *Behavioral and Brain Sciences, 21,* 1–54.

Shweder, A. (1994). "You're not sick, you're just in love": Emotion as an interpretive system. In P. Ekman & R. J. Davidson (Eds.), *The nature of emotion: Fundamental questions* (pp. 32–44). New York: Oxford University Press.

Smith, C. A., & Kirby, L. D. (2001). Breaking the tautology: Toward delivering on the promise of appraisal theory. In K. Scherer, A. Schorr, & T. Johnstone (Eds.), *Appraisal theories of emotion* (pp. 121–138). Oxford: Oxford University Press.

Spitz, R. A. (1965). *The first year of life.* New York: International Universities Press.

Sroufe, L. A. (1979). Socioemotional development. In J. D. Osofsky (Ed.), *Handbook of infant development* (pp. 462–516). New York: Wiley.

Steels, L., & Belpaeme, T. (in press). Coordinating perceptually grounded categories through language: A case study for color. *Behavioral and Brain Sciences.*

Storbeck, J., & Robinson, M. D. (2004). Preferences and inferences in encoding visual objects: A systematic comparison of semantic and affective priming. *Personality and Social Psychology Bulletin, 30,* 81–93.

Tomaka, J., Blascovich, J., Kelsey, R. M., & Leitten, C. L. (1993). Subjective, physiological, and behavioral effects of threat and challenge appraisal. *Journal of Personality and Social Psychology, 65,* 248–260.

Tomaka, J., Blascovich, J., Kibler, J., & Ernst, J. M. (1997). Cognitive and physiological antecedents of threat and challenge appraisal. *Journal of Personality and Social Psychology, 73,* 63–72.

Trope, J., & Cohen, O. (1989). Perceptual and inferential determinants of behavior-correspondent attributions. *Journal of Experimental Social Psychology, 25,* 142–158.

Trope, Y. (1986). Identification and inferential processes in dispositional attribution. *Psychological Review, 93,* 239–257.

Whalen, P. J. (1998). Fear, vigilance, and ambiguity: Initial neuroimaging studies of the human amygdala. *Current Directions in Psychological Science, 7,* 177–188.

Whalen, P. J., Shin, L. M., McInerney, S. C., Fischer, H., Wright, C. I., & Rauch, S. L. (2001). A functional MRI study of human amygdala responses to facial expressions of fear vs. anger. *Emotion, 1,* 70–83.

White, G. M. (1993). Emotions inside out: The anthropology of affect. In M. Lewis & J. M. Haviland (Eds.), *Handbook of emotions* (pp. 29–39). New York: Guilford Press.

Widen, S. C., & Russell, J. A. (2003). A closer look at preschoolers' freely produced labels for facial expressions. *Developmental Psychology, 39,* 114–128.

Yeh, W., & Barsalou, L. W. (2005). *The situated character of concepts.* Manuscript submitted for publication.

PART V

Perspectives on the Conscious–Unconscious Debate

CHAPTER 12

Emotion Processes Considered from the Perspective of Dual-Process Models

Eliot R. Smith
Roland Neumann

For at least two millennia, people seeking to explain their own and others' behavior have resorted to explanations in terms of two distinct and often conflicting inner mechanisms. For example, St. Paul, in his Epistle to the Romans, lamented:

> I can will what is right, but I cannot do it. For I do not do the good I want, but the evil I do not want is what I do. Now if I do what I do not want, it is no lon- ger I that do it, but sin which dwells within me. . . . I see in my members another law at war with the law of my mind and making me captive to the law of sin which dwells in my members. (Rom. 7:15–23)

This same core insight—that our thoughts and behavior are driven by two separate and often conflicting mechanisms—has recently become part of social-psychological theories of phenomena as diverse as stereotyping (Devine, 1989), attitude–behavior relations (Fazio, 1986), and persuasion (Petty & Cacioppo, 1986). These dual-process models, of course, do not use labels such as "the law of sin" and "the law of my mind," but refer to the two processes as heuristic and systematic (e.g., Chaiken, 1980) or associative

1. *What is the scope of your proposed model? When you use the term* emotion, *how do you use it? What do you mean by terms such as* fear, anxiety, *or* happiness?

Emotion refers to a bundle of loosely related processes (involving appraisal, affect, motivation, expressive behaviors, activation and use of semantic knowledge, subjective feelings, and self-regulation), not to a single "thing." In paradigm cases all these processes may unfold in parallel in reaction to the same event, but dissociations among the processes are also common (because each process has many potential causes). This definition is similar to the one we would give for cognition, which also refers to a bundle of loosely coupled processes involving information transformation, representation, etc., rather than to a single conceptual entity.

2. *Define your terms:* conscious, unconscious, awareness. *Or say why you do not use these terms.*

A useful and at least somewhat precise term is *preconscious,* which refers to processes that are (a) generally automatic, given relevant stimulus input, and (b) whose results are accessible to conscious awareness. Examples are recognizing a familiar face or accessing the meaning of a written word in one's native language, which are automatic in that one cannot simply decide not to perform these processes. Preconscious processes constitute our subjective experience, allowing us to see a world of meaningful objects and events. In contrast, fully conscious processes involve effortful, controlled search for and use of relevant or appropriate information, with the process itself as well as its result being available to awareness.

3. *Does your model deal with what is conscious, what is unconscious, or their relationship? If you do not address this area specifically, can you speculate on the relationship between what is conscious and unconscious? Or if you do not like the conscious–unconscious distinction, or if you do not think this is a good question to ask, can you say why?*

Our theory deals with two types of processing (which we term *associative* and *rule based*) that are correlated with, but not identical to, the preconscious–conscious distinction.

and rule based (Sloman, 1996). Recently, Smith and DeCoster (2000) reviewed a number of such dual-process models that have been formulated in different topic areas, making the argument that despite differences in detail, they all essentially rest on the same distinction between two basic processing systems. They adopted Sloman's (1996) labels, *associative* and *rule based,* for the systems. Since Smith and DeCoster's review, still other models sharing the same family resemblance have appeared (Strack & Deutsch, 2004; Lieberman, Gaunt, Gilbert, & Trope, 2002). Except for a few who adhere to single-process models (e.g., Kruglanski, Thompson, &

Spiegel, 1999), it seems that dual-process models represent mainstream thinking within wide areas of social psychology, particularly social cognition, today.

However, although emotion theorists have addressed several related ideas, explicit application of dual-process models to the processes involved in the elicitation and control of emotion is only beginning. This chapter begins by summarizing the general features of existing dual-process models, including brief comments on the two recent ones just referenced. Like Smith and DeCoster (2000), we emphasize their similarities rather than their points of difference. The core of the chapter then describes thoughts and hypotheses about how emotion fits into the general dual-process framework. We conclude with comments on a number of implications arising from this way of thinking.

DUAL-PROCESS MODELS

Review of Dual-Process Models

In their review and integration, Smith and DeCoster (2000) draw on evidence from cognitive and neuropsychological sources as well as from existing dual-process models in social psychology. Their starting point is dual-memory-system models, discussed by numerous theorists in recent decades (e.g., Tulving, 1983; Sherry & Schacter, 1987; McClelland, McNaughton, & O'Reilly, 1995). These models hold that humans have two interacting but separate memory systems. The rationale for a dual-system model is that the adaptive demands on memory inherently conflict and are difficult or impossible to satisfy within a single memory system. One demand is to record information incrementally, slowly building up representations based on a large sample of experiences, so that stable knowledge and expectancies about the environment can be recorded in an enduring fashion. A conflicting demand is to record information quickly, so that events that occur only once can be recorded and used to direct adaptive action in the future. But if each passing event leaves a strong and lasting trace in memory, the resulting disruption will make it impossible to build up a stable record based on a multitude of experiences. This conflict has been termed the "stability/plasticity dilemma."

This logical argument about the conflicting demands of slow and rapid learning is paralleled by neuropsychological evidence (reviewed in McClelland et al., 1995) that points to the existence of two memory systems that serve these adaptive demands. A slow-learning system (based in cortical regions) records information slowly and subserves learning of cognitive skills based on extensive practice, as well as learning of general regularities, covariations, or associations in input stimuli, possibly across many sensory modalities. After they are learned, these regularities are used to generate expectations and fill in unobserved details in new input information, a function that has often been termed *schematic processing* in cognitive and social psychology. A fast-learning system, mediated by the hippocampal region of the brain, records episodic memories of events that occur only once. Probably the strongest evidence for the independence of the two memory systems is that the latter system is selectively impaired by hippocampal lesions that leave the slow-learning system relatively unimpaired (e.g., Squire, 1992). Because the fast-learning system requires attention and other cognitive resources for its operation, it can be disrupted by distraction, competing task demands, etc.

Two processing modes depend on the respective properties of the two memory systems, according to Smith and DeCoster (2000). *Associative* processing is based on the properties of the slow-learning system. When new stimulus information is encountered, this type of processing uses knowledge that has been acquired from a large number of previous experiences to fill in information that is unobserved in the current situation, quickly and automatically. The process can be aptly characterized as a preconscious "pattern completion" mechanism (see Niedenthal, Barsalou, Ric, & Krauth-Gruber, Chapter 2). That is, suppose one has encountered dogs on many occasions, leading to the development of a multimodal representation in the slow-learning memory system that involves dogs' visual appearance, barking sounds, their typical behaviors, the sound of the word for *dog*, as well as one's typical affective and behavioral responses to the presence of a dog (whether fearful withdrawal or joyful playfulness). This entire representation can be reactivated (i.e., the pattern can be completed via memory retrieval) by an encounter with any sufficiently distinctive subpart—such as the sound of a bark. Importantly, distinct representations could be built up for dogs encountered in separate contexts (e.g., household pets vs. dogs running wild outside) or for separate types of dogs (e.g., large German shepherds vs. small poodles), and then the context-specific version could be reactivated on a future occasion, depending on the perceptual cues. Associative processing is shared with nonhuman animals, for it does not depend on linguistic or other abilities that are unique to humans. There is little or no conscious awareness of the retrieval or pattern-completion process, only of its results (thus the process is termed *preconscious*).

In contrast, *rule-based* processing uses symbolically represented knowledge (such as logical inference rules) to direct processing. For example, suppose someone from a different culture treats one in a way that seems disrespectful. An immediate (associative) response may be anger. But an attributional search involving effortful consideration of all the surrounding circumstances may lead to the conclusion that the offense was inadvertent, caused by the person's ignorance of local cultural norms. This conclusion might dissolve the anger. Rule-based processing is unique to humans (and, perhaps, a few of our closest primate cousins). Rules may be stored in either memory system, depending on whether they have been encountered only a few times or many times over an extensive period (in which case they could be stored in the slow-learning system). Rule-based processing is more effortful and less automatic than associative processing, so it can be selectively disrupted by distraction, cognitive load, and the like. Rule-based processing is also generally available to conscious awareness at each step of the processing (e.g., each potential attribution for a person's behavior that is considered), not only the final result.

One of the key points emphasized by Smith and DeCoster (2000) is that the two processing modes draw on partially independent memory systems or "databases" of stored knowledge. Associative processing depends on associations, built up by repeated experiences over time, through which a person might form a representation (for example) linking yellow-striped insects and painful stings. Such a representation may not be verbalizable or accessible as explicit knowledge. Smith and DeCoster describe how associative learning and pattern completion can be accomplished by a connectionist network.[1] In contrast, rule-based processing depends on linguistically encoded propositions, structured by logical relations rather than by simple repeated co-occurrence. Such a rule could be learned from a single exposure. Interestingly, associative and rule-based knowledge might conflict. In fact, social-psychological studies using dual-process approaches have often focused on exactly that issue. For example, dual-process models have been widely applied to help understand stereotyping processes. Researchers assume that many people have learned associations of stereotypic traits to various social and ethnic groups (based on a long history of exposure to cultural stereotypes in the media, etc.) but also maintain explicit propositional beliefs that reject those stereotypes (e.g., Devine, 1989). Given adequate time and attentional capacity, people may be able to use their explicit beliefs to override the automatically (associatively) activated stereotypic information.

Most of the dual-process models that have been formulated within specific topic areas in social psychology (e.g., Fazio, 1986; Petty & Cacioppo, 1986; Chaiken, 1980; Brewer, 1988) and in cognitive psychology (e.g., Sloman, 1996) fit quite well within this general framework. The models use different terminology, of course, and they differ in some details, notably regarding whether the two types of processing proceed in parallel or sequentially (associative followed by rule based)—Smith and DeCoster (2000) hold that processing is parallel. But all the reviewed models share the general theme that one processing mode operates automatically and preconsciously to structure people's conscious experience, with little dependence on attention or cognitive resources. For example, people may evaluate a persuasive message without much explicit thought if easily noticed features (e.g., its length or the attractiveness of the communicator) are associated with positive or negative evaluations; such an association allows the perceiver to arrive at a quick favorable or unfavorable impression. Or people may respond negatively to an individual who is a member of a particular group if negative stereotypic features associated with that group are automatically activated upon encountering the individual. The second processing mode operates optionally, uses more powerful inferential means, and requires attention and subjective effort. Using this mode, people may scrutinize the persuasive arguments in a message in detail, comparing them to their general knowledge to arrive at a reasoned judgment about the message. Or they may examine the individual's personal attributes, effortfully seeking to go beyond the simple group-membership information (and associated stereotypes) to determine the individual's true characteristics.

Newer Dual-Process Models

Strack and Deutsch (2004) recently advanced a new dual-process model that has some innovative features but also shares the same general assumptions. Briefly, Strack and Deutsch distinguish an impulsive system (similar to the associative system discussed above) from a reflective system (similar to rule based). Their discussion emphasizes the role of the two systems in governing overt behavior, such as approach or avoidance of an object, and not just processing within the head. They also propose that the reflective system, as part of its ability to process propositional representations, can represent and use negations, whereas the impulsive system cannot do so. In fact, a frequently encountered negation (e.g., "Nixon is not a crook") may lead to an association between the concepts and therefore the automatic activation of *crook* whenever *Nixon* is encountered—despite the fact that the propositionally based reflective system can produce judgments or behavior indicating correct comprehension of the negation.

Lieberman et al. (2002) also recently advanced a dual-process model that again fits the same general outline. Their terms are *reflexive* (x) for the associative system and *reflective* (c) for the rule-based system. Like Smith and DeCoster (2000), they hold that the reflexive system rests directly on the properties of a connectionist memory system that slowly builds up associations over time and uses them as a pattern-completion mechanism. Their unique contribution is to emphasize the way the reflexive system structures our conscious experiences of the world, whereas the operation of the reflective system is experienced as our reflections, thoughts, or reactions to the perceived world. They also devote attention to the "alarm" functions that call the reflective system into activity when the more automatic (but less powerful) reflexive system gets into trouble or reaches an impasse. Finally, they hypothesize linkages of the distinct processing systems to separate brain structures. They follow McClelland et al. (1995), on whom Smith and DeCoster (2000) also rely, in linking the reflective system to hippocampal areas (see also Phelps, Chapter 3), as well as to the anterior cingulate and prefrontal cortices.

Despite these differences in emphasis, overall, the processing modes described by Strack and Deutsch and Lieberman et al. seem to be readily identifiable with those of the other models discussed in Smith and DeCoster's (2000) review.

EMOTION PROCESSES FROM THE PERSPECTIVE OF DUAL-PROCESS MODELS

Our main purpose in this chapter is to discuss processes involved in the elicitation and control of emotion within this dual-process conceptual framework. Several emotion theorists have advanced ideas that can be directly related to this framework, and we briefly review these before discussing a conceptual integration in more general terms. We begin, though, by noting that important classes of emotion models have not explicitly incorporated the notion that humans possess two distinct modes of mental processing.

Ambiguity of the Term *Appraisal*

Highly influential approaches to emotion, such as appraisal models and related theories (e.g., Weiner's attributional model of emotion, 1986) sought to specify the cognitive processes that determine the quality and the intensity of emotions. However, these approaches were often unclear on whether appraisals are conscious/reflective or not. Some researchers explicitly proposed that appraisal processes are relatively automatic and inflexible, whereas others suggested (either explicitly or by implication) that appraisal processes that have more of a flavor of reflective reasoning might be responsible for eliciting emotions (e.g., Weiner, 1986).

From the dual-process perspective, it appears that the term *appraisal* has been used to label fundamentally different types of information that are processed in fundamentally different ways. (In a similar way, the term *infer-*

ence has been used to refer to both automatic/associative and reflective forms of processing, despite their different properties; see Lieberman et al., 2002). Many emotion theorists have recognized this point (e.g., Smith & Kirby, 2001; Scherer, 2001), which was also central in the "affective primacy" debate between Zajonc and Lazarus (see Schorr, 2001, for a summary). Appraisals can include relatively low-level perceptual features (e.g., an object rapidly looming in the field of vision) that produce affective reactions. But equally, high-level conceptual features resulting from sophisticated reasoning and inferential processes, such as attributional inferences, can also produce emotional responses. In summary, the widespread use of the single term *appraisal* in these very different ways may have subtly discouraged application of dual-process thinking in the area of emotion processes.

Dual-Process Ideas in Emotion Theory

Several emotion theorists have advanced ideas that overlap in important ways with dual-process models of the sort reviewed above. Keltner and Haidt (2001) distinguish two classes of emotions. *Primordial* emotions are universal, biologically based patterns of appraisals and responses observed across species and cultures, whereas *elaborated* emotions are packages of meanings, social practices, and norms that are built up around emotions in a particular culture. The authors emphasize that the elaboration process loosens the link between a primordial emotion and its original evolutionary function. For example, the primordial emotion of disgust, originally serving to compel the organism to avoid ingestion of contaminated food, comes to be applied to norm violators or holders of unpopular ideas, who might metaphorically contaminate the social group. The distinction drawn by Keltner and Haidt has obvious relevance to dual-process ideas, but with two important caveats. First, we would refer to distinct *processes* (i.e., associative vs. rule based) that give rise to emotion, rather than distinct *classes of emotion*. In other words, and consistent with some of these authors' own points, a given emotion such as disgust may, at times, be produced by one type of process and, at times, by another, so it seems imprecise to talk of two classes of emotions. According to our point of view, a similar outcome (e.g., a simple affective response or a fully self-aware emotional experience) may be produced by either type of process (Nisbett & Wilson, 1977). Second, we would emphasize that elaborated emotions (as well as primordial ones) could be experienced frequently enough over time that they too could come to be elicited through associative processes, given a relevant situation.

Ochsner and Barrett (2000) describe emotion as resulting from interactions between automatic, nonconscious processes and more deliberative processes, using an overall framework that has much in common with social-psychological dual-process models. Automatic bottom-up processes classify events or objects as positive or negative in valence and initiate general affective responses and preparations for generic bodily actions such as approach or avoidance. Top-down reflective processes can operate flexibly, directing attention to specific aspects of an event, regulating or inhibiting overt actions, or applying complex knowledge (including general knowledge about emotions), often in the service of self-understanding or self-regulatory goals. For these writers, a consciously experienced emotion occurs only when both types of processes are engaged and produce an affective response that is accompanied by the activation of semantic knowledge, including a verbal label for the emotion. We would add that an emotion label (such as fear) may become associated with a particular situation (the sight of a large dog) and affective responses (negative arousal), so that the entire package of responses, including not only affective changes but also activation of a verbal label, may be generated fairly automatically by associative pattern-completion processes.

Leventhal and Scherer (1987) distinguished three forms of information processing that can lead to affective responses, two automatic and one more deliberate. On a first level of information processing, sensory–motor processes can lead to affective responses. For example, loud and abrupt sounds can trigger fear responses. Second, learned associations (such as that between weapons and aggression; Berkowitz, 1993) mean that an encounter with such a cue (a weapon) can activate schematic representations that in turn elicit affect (see Teasdale, 1999, for a similar idea). Both of these more automatic and inflexible forms of information processing are examples of associative processes, in our view. Leventhal and Scherer (1987) distinguish these two automatic forms of processing from conceptual processing, a more deliberate form of information processing that involves propositionally organized memory structures (similar to our rule-based processing).

Clore and Ortony (2000) use the same terms as Smith and DeCoster (2000), associative and rule based, to describe two processing modes that can result in emotion elicitation. Associative processing is regarded as a form of memory retrieval in which a prior affective response to an object is reactivated or reconstructed, in a fast and automatic but relatively inflexible way, when the object is encountered again. Rule-based processing, in contrast, is driven more by sensory inputs and "computes" an appropriate affective response, taking more time but allowing great flexibility of responding. These theorists differ from Keltner and Haidt (2001) in postulating two types of processes that can produce the same set of emotions, rather than two distinct sets of emotions. Overall this view is similar to our own.

Similar emphases are evident in the discussion by Matthews and Wells (1999) of automatic and controlled processes in emotion. Focusing on negative stimuli, they postulate that a stimulus-driven network automatically generates affective responses to threat stimuli. A separate supervisory system maintains and regulates processing with regard to specific goals. The authors emphasize that the attention-demanding quality of negative stimuli may result from either type of processing: automatic attentional demands arising from the lower-level system, or the activation in the supervisory system of specific goals leading to attentional focusing (on the self or on the environment, monitoring for threats), which lead to rumination or worry.

LeDoux (e.g., 1996) provides a broadly similar analysis, but with the addition of significant neurophysiological detail (see also Teasdale, 1999). Focusing on threat-related stimuli, LeDoux notes that cognitive analyses (of what the stimulus is) are distinct from affective analyses (of what the stimulus means for the individual's safety). These affective computations are generally performed in the amygdala, which receives inputs from many different areas of the sensory cortex, and lead to multiple behavioral and autonomic responses (e.g., increased heart rate, preparation for flight). Other inputs flow to the amygdala from the hippocampus, facilitating affective responses based on episodic memories of previously experienced events—in other words, associative reactivation of an affective response. These latter pathways also allow for the cognitive modulation of amygdala activity based on larger situational contexts, such as the recognition that a specific stimulus poses a threat in one class of situations but not in another. However, the ability to carry out such modulations requires repeated practice; one cannot simply cognitively "decide" not to be afraid of a given type of stimulus and have that decision become immediately effective. In our model this requirement of considerable repetitions marks the "cognitive modulation" process as part of the associative processing mode.

Toward Conceptual Integration

A paradigm example of the application of dual-process thinking in social cognition involves the stereotyping processes. Upon encountering a member of a stereotyped group, well-learned stereotypic attributes are automatically activated through associative processes in the perceiver. If the perceiver is processing minimally, the stereotype will likely control behavior (leading, e.g., to avoidance of the target). In contrast, given time and cognitive capacity, the perceiver can effortfully call to mind more symbolically represented beliefs and personal standards against using stereotypes and try, in various ways and with varying degrees of success, to control or override the effect of the automatically activated material on judgments and behavior.

Applying similar thinking to a central example of emotion processing, phobias, we would say that upon encountering a trigger stimulus (perhaps a snake or a large dog) that has frequently been associated with fear in the past, affective responses are automatically reactivated in the phobic person. If the perceiver is processing minimally, the affective response will control behavior. In contrast, with time and cognitive capacity the perceiver can remind him- or herself that the stimulus is not actually dangerous and try, in various ways, to control or override the effects of the automatically activated feelings. These efforts may be more or less successful (Gross, 1998).

Associative Processes in the Elicitation of Emotions

To flesh out different aspects of the overall similarities between these accounts, we begin by discussing the associative activation of emotion. In standard dual-process models several points are similar to the associative processing mode. First, frequent pairing in the past of a specific stimulus with an emotional response (as with a social stereotype) leads to the development of an association, which can reactivate the response when the stimulus is again encountered. Thus a child who has been burned by a fire several times may come to fear the sight or sound of a fire even if no heat can be felt. In the development of panic disorders, it is assumed that exposure to panic attacks causes the conditioning of anxiety to exteroceptive and interoceptive cues (Bouton, Mineka, & Barlow, 2001). The resulting network of associations allows the cues to activate the whole network, including the different emotional components. This formulation explains why behavioral responses such as emotional expressions can influence emotions (for an overview, see Adelman & Zajonc, 1989). In a similar vein, for an individual suffering from a posttraumatic stress disorder (PTSD), a single cue such as a smell or the shape of an object can reactivate the whole pattern of associations, which in turn trigger the emotional response. The operation of the pattern-completion mechanism explains why a degradation of the perceptual input can nevertheless activate the same response. Evidence for such a mechanism comes from a study by Bradley, Codispoti, Cuthbert, and Lang (2001). In this study pictures generated essentially the same affective responses—both self-reported emotion and physiological reactions—whether they were presented in color or black and white. Thus a reduced version of the presented information might nevertheless be sufficient to elicit affective responses. According to Dimberg, Thunberg, and Elmehed (2000), subliminal exposure to facial expressions elicits congruent facial responses. Lundqvist and Öhman (Chapter 5) suggest that this effect might be due to some specific patterns of facial features, such as the eyebrows.

In sum, it has been shown that many different types of cues have the potential to activate various experiential, physiological, and behavioral aspects of emotion. We emphasize that this is (in our view) due to the operation of an associative pattern-completion mechanism. Once an entire pattern involving multiple components is experienced many times, any one of the components becomes capable of reactivating the entire pattern. One implication of this perspective is that arguments about the "true" causal sequence between different components of emotion (e.g., appraisals and subjective experience, or experience and expressive behaviors) are pointless, because any of these components can be causally effective in reactivating any other.

Second, the associative reactivation of a well-learned pattern is fast and automatic in the sense that a simple cognitive decision cannot prevent it (i.e., deciding that the dog is not dangerous or that the stereotype is incorrect). In other words, associative responses are not "cognitively penetrable." For example, Rozin, Millman, and Nemeroff (1986) reported that people exhibited disgust at the sight of chocolate in the shape of feces, despite their knowledge that the material was simply chocolate. The speed of an associative response might be adaptive, but on the other hand, it makes this process relatively inflexible.

Third, associative reactivation can occur without conscious awareness of the stimulus that triggers the reactivation. This point has been amply established in many studies demonstrating that subliminal stimuli (of which the perceiver is not consciously aware) influence both social–cognitive judgments and affective responses (Bargh, Chen, & Burrows, 1996; Murphy & Zajonc, 1993). For example, Öhman and Soares (1994) showed that people with phobias experience elevated skin conductance responses to subliminally presented pictures of spiders or snakes. Aside from laboratory presentations of stimuli in highly controlled brief flashes, this process may have much relevance in everyday life. An affectively laden past experience may be reactivated by a stimulus that receives little conscious attention (perhaps because it is but one element in a crowded scene), leading to a "mood" for which the perceiver is unable to assign a cause.

Despite these similarities, one salient point regarding associative processes and emotion differs from other areas in which dual-process models have been applied. In general such models have assumed that frequent cooccurrences are necessary to build up an association between a stimulus and response. However, it is well known that specific stimuli are orders of magnitude easier to associate with particular affective responses (e.g., snakes with phobic responses) compared to arbitrary stimuli. One or a few experiences with such a biologically relevant stimulus may suffice to create an association that would otherwise take much repetition to develop.

A major component of such quick associative responses may be the creation of simple linkages between the fundamental dimension of evaluation and various other responses, including behavioral approach or avoidance. Evaluation has been shown to influence many types of responses, early in processing. For example, smiles can be generated faster in response to positive words and frowns faster for negative words (Neumann, Hess, Schulz, & Alpers, in press). Not only facial expressions but also approach and avoidance movements are closely linked to the processing of valence (Strack & Deutsch, in press; Neumann, Foerster, & Strack, 2003; Winkielman, Berridge, & Wilbarger, Chapter 14). For example, bodily movements interpreted as avoidance are faster in response to negative words, whereas movements interpreted as approach are faster in response to positive words (Chen & Bargh, 1999).[2] It is likely that a few experiences suffice to create an association between the valence of an object and the representation of behavioral approach or avoidance responses. Of course, it is possible to engage in action that is opposite to these automatic behavioral tendencies, but only by exercising effortful control.

Rule-Based Processes in the Elicitation of Emotions

Emotion can be elicited by thoughtful, reflective processing. For example, anxiety can result from thinking about what other people might think of me (reflective or rule-based processing) as well as by the mere perception of a snake (associative processing). Disgust can be elicited not only by the visual qualities of an object (as just mentioned) but by what one explicitly knows about the object—for example, by the knowledge that an insect had crawled over tasty-looking food (Rozin et al., 1986). Fear can be elicited by actual exposure to a fearful object or by the anticipation of threats in the future. Anger can be induced by aversive stimuli such as cold or hot temperatures or by considering whether someone deliberately violated a norm (Berkowitz, 1993).

Thus rule-based processing allows for a more flexible activation of emotional response, in ways that are more sensitive to the social context. For example, foods that are eaten with gusto in some cultures are viewed as disgusting in others. Similarly, cultural norms can influence the situations and events that elicit emotions such as shame or pride (Mesquita, 2001; Neumann & Steinhäuser, 2003). However, this higher sensitivity of rule-based emotional responses to potentially shifting circumstances and cultural norms has its price: Reflective or rule-based processes are more effortful and can thus be undermined by a lack of cognitive resources. Therefore, distraction is sometimes successful in regulating emotions. For example, anger can be generated by an effortful analysis of the motives behind another person's action. In such cases counting to 10 might be a successful (distraction) strategy to prevent socially inappropriate behavior because it redirects one's attention, thereby (ideally) preventing the attributional analysis that gave rise to the angry feelings.

Emotion Regulation

Rule-based processing is important not only in the initial evocation of emotion but also when people attempt to control or regulate emotions. The examples that opened this section both dealt with intentional control (of activated stereotypes or of an affective response viewed as inappropriate). It seems clear that the very automaticity of associatively generated responses makes their direct suppression difficult and costly at best, and ineffective at worst (stereotypes: Macrae, Bodenhausen, & Milne, 1995; emotions: Richards & Gross, 2000). Under what conditions can associatively driven responses be controlled or overridden by more reflective processes?

According to the approach presented in this chapter, rule-based control should be successful to the extent that an event or situation has not already triggered associative processes. Recent research has shown that smiles can be produced faster in response to pleasant words, whereas frowns are faster in response to unpleasant words (Neumann et al., in press). This finding suggests that although one can exert voluntary control over one's emotional expression (e.g., smiling when processing negative information), associative processes are faster in supplying a congruent response than an incongruent response.[3] Moreover, suppression of already activated responses requires cognitive resources and may therefore impair other processes essential for social interaction and memory encoding (Butler et al., 2003; Richards & Gross, 2000).

More successful control uses one of three strategies. One can attempt to reinterpret or recategorize the original stimuli—in other words, to think of them in new ways (i.e., reappraisal strategies; Gross, 1998). Whether this strategy is possible when the emotion is due to associative processing is currently unclear. One can direct attention to different (less affectively evocative) aspects of the overall stimulus situation (analogous to directing one's attention to a stereotyped target's unique individual attributes rather than to the target's group membership). However, this approach might not be feasible in highly evocative circumstances: for example, the would-be ski-jumper who suffers from fear of height, or a tunnel-phobic person confronted with spelunking.

Finally, in a longer-range sense, control is possible by repeatedly pairing the stimulus with a different, incompatible affective response. This approach recognizes that a single experience cannot have much impact on the slow-learning memory system on which associative processing is based, but that repeated experiences can build up new representations over time. Thus, in the treatment of phobias, people are exposed to the nondangerous stimulus time after time, without experiencing any harm. As an effect of the frequency of exposure, the phobic response gradually weakens (Bouton, Chapter 9; Bouton et al., 2001; Foa & Kozak, 1986; Quigley & Barrett, 1999). In a similar way, the sight of blood or saliva evokes disgust in most people. It is therefore an important part in the training of physicians to overcome their immediate emotional response toward these classes of stimuli. From the perspective of the dual-process model, the need for repeated exposures is clear evidence that these emotional responses are due to associative processing rather than to reflective processing. In contrast, an emotional response that hinges on rule-based processing, such as fear in response to hearing that a dangerous criminal is on the loose in one's neighborhood, should evaporate immediately upon learning that the criminal has been captured by the police.

Relation to Core Affect Theory

For insights into the ways that associative and rule-based or reflective processing interact to shape an entire emotion episode, we turn to core affect theory. Russell (2003; Barrett & Russell, 1999) recently advanced this integrative model of emotion. In this model, affect states that are describable within a two-dimensional space whose axes are *pleasantness* and *arousal*, are at the core of all emotions (as well as moods). Core affect changes in response to many types of external stimuli as well as internal processes (such as diurnal rhythms) and is assumed to be subjectively perceptible (leading to a sense of feeling good, bad, energized, tired, etc.). A change in core affect that is consciously experienced and attributed to some cause constitutes the beginning of an emotional episode. This attribution marks the transition between feeling an amorphous, unpleasant activation and feeling that way *because of* a snake, or between feeling vaguely unpleasantly deenergized and feeling that way *about* a just-ended relationship. As Russell (2003, p. 149) writes, "Sometimes the cause is obvious; sometimes a search is required; sometimes mistakes are made." The attribution is functional in directing attention and behavior with regard to the object that is responsible for the emotion.

In the next stage of the core affect model various components of the emotional episode, including the core affect and the perceived cause, as well as situational factors, overt behaviors, and bodily experiences (such as physiological changes), form input to a perceptual process that gives rise to the experience of emotion (Barrett, Chapter 11), or to what Russell

(2003) terms "emotional meta-experience." In effect, the person consciously notices or recognizes that he or she is afraid, sad, guilty, or experiencing any of numerous other emotions. Thus the perception of emotions is composed of many different inputs, and the mechanisms involved are analogous to those that have been well studied in the area of person perception (Barrett, Chapter 11).

Note that the core affect model inverts the causal ordering assumed in the naïve or common-sense model of emotion, which says that some event (e.g., danger) causes an emotion (fear) that is assumed to be a unique inner state, which then causes subjective feelings (being afraid), nonverbal expressions, autonomic changes, and instrumental actions. This idea implies that all these types of changes should generally covary, contrary to the findings of emotion researchers (Russell, 2003; Barrett, Chapter 11). In core affect theory, as noted earlier, these various factors are used to categorize the emotion perceptually based on the extent of resemblance between these factors and a mental representation of a given emotion's prototype.

How does the core affect model fit with the dual-process framework? Quite well. We assume that the changes in core affect caused by some external events may be hardwired (e.g., fear at the visual appearance of great height) or learned from previous encounters (e.g., fear at the sight or smell of a fire). Other reactions closely linked to core affect (such as expressive nonverbal behaviors or increases in physiological action readiness) may also occur automatically. Automatic responses take place within the associative processing mode, without any necessary participation by rule-based or reflective processing (Barrett, Chapter 11). Notably, these processes can occur in nonhuman species as well. The identification of a cause may also often be automatic and associative: The sight of a snake triggers both the affective reaction and the recollection of previous encounters with frightening snakes.

Other processes within the core affect model invoke the type of symbolic/propositional reasoning that is a uniquely human power. Sometimes this is the case for causal identification. Identifying the cause may require an effortful, intentional search, and occasionally misattributions are made. A person may come home and snap at his or her spouse, not realizing that the true cause of the annoyed feelings is an abrasive encounter with a coworker that occurred earlier in the day. Similarly, Neumann, Seibt, and Strack (2001) showed that positive feedback about one's performance in an intelligence test leads to stronger feelings of pride if a positive rather than a negative mood state was unobtrusively induced previously. Apparently, participants in a positive mood identified the positive feedback as the source of their feeling state, although their feelings stemmed, in part, from the prior mood induction. Thus, whenever feelings are induced in quick succession, which might be common in everyday life, much more effort is needed to identify with precision the contribution of each emotion-eliciting event.

Sometimes reflective processing can help people identify the true cause of the emotion in such cases. And "emotional meta-experience," the categorical knowledge that one is experiencing a discrete emotion (e.g., annoyance, guilt, anxiety), is clearly in the province of reflective thought (for an alternative view, see the section on "Functional Modularity of Emotion" in Barrett, Tugade, & Engle, 2004). Moreover, core affect can be input to reflective processing and thereby form the basis for conscious decisions—in effect, affective states can inform the individual about significant events (Keltner & Haidt, 1999; Schwarz & Clore, 1983). Reflective processing about one's emotions can also lead to meta-emotions, such as shame at feeling angry.

These linkages to dual-process thinking yield testable predictions. Dual-process models in other areas of social psychology have often been tested by manipulating cognitive load or distraction, which is believed to selectively impair rule-based processing while having little impact on associative processing (see Barrett et al., 2004). In the area of emotional processes, cognitive load or distraction ought to make it more difficult for people to identify which emotion they are experiencing (meta-experience), even though it should not greatly reduce the core affect changes. Load or distraction also should interfere with people's ability to accurately identify the cause of the emotion, at least in cases where it is not overwhelmingly obvious. Tentative support for this assumption comes from a study by Siemer and Reisenzein (1998). Consistent with the mood-as-information approach (Schwarz & Clore, 1983), in this study moods were more likely to affect subsequent judgments when participants were under time pressure or when their processing capacity was reduced by a secondary task. This study suggests that cognitive load indeed interferes with the ability to identify the cause of a core affect state, making it more likely for the affect to be misattributed to irrelevant sources. Importantly, however, and consistent with our predictions, the core affect state itself (the mood state) was not influenced by the secondary task. However, further research is needed to explore whether reduced processing capacity exerts similar influences on the ability to identify the causes of emotions.

IMPLICATIONS

Several interesting implications arise from the distinction between the associative and rule-based or reflective processes that underlie emotions.

Modes of Emotion Regulation

Whereas emotions that are due to reflective processes might be changed by a reconsideration or reappraisal of the situation, emotions that are due to associative processes are likely to change only if the stimulus input is interrupted—because they are more or less automatically activated by perception of the stimulus. This proposition has implications for emotion control. In order to avoid perceptual input that elicits fear, people might try to avoid the whole situation or shut their eyes (as a child might do at a scary part of a movie). On the other hand, distraction might be appropriate to control, for example, fear of public speaking.

Selective Effects of Misattribution

The core affect model leaves open the possibility of misattribution (i.e., being mistaken about the cause of an emotion) and also of misidentifying the specific emotion that one is experiencing. This aspect of the model reflects the well-known idea that people have access to their experiences but not to the causes and processes underlying these experiences (Nisbett & Wilson, 1977). Especially if distinct emotions are evoked in quick succession, it is likely that affective responses may carry over from one event to the next, making it more difficult to identify the correct causes of one's emotion. Research has shown that, in principle, people are able to correct judgments about their emotion (Neumann et al., 2001). However, despite efforts to correct for unwanted influences (e.g., persuading oneself that the current feeling of anger is not due to the remark of one's partner but rather to a prior frustration), behavioral responses such as facial expression nevertheless reflect these influences (e.g., more frowning toward the partner). The facial component of an emotion may be more influenced by associative processing and less by conscious (rule-based) control (Neumann et al., 2001). In other words, although one can make efforts to find out the correct cause of all emotion, one's feelings and facial expression might nevertheless reflect the influence of prior events.

Dissociations from Cognitive Beliefs

Dissociations can occur when the associative system produces a specific emotion that the reflective system views as inappropriate. As Sloman (1996) emphasized in his discussion of dual-process models, perceptual illusions such as the Müller–Lyer illusion persist and are subjectively compelling even though one explicitly knows they are false in appearance (e.g., the arrows are the same length). Blascovich (personal communication, August, 2002) reports that people often are afraid to walk over a "pit" they can see in virtual reality goggles, even though they know they are on a safe, stable floor. Russell (2003) captured this same type of dissociation in his "virtual reality" principle, which says that people will experience emotions in response to fictional accounts, movie portrayals, etc., even if they know that the depicted events are untrue. This is an interesting finding, given that some emotion researchers (Frijda, 1988; Ortony, Clore, & Collins, 1988) argue that the object of an emotion needs to be construed as real before it can elicit emotional responses. No doubt, knowing that the object of one's emotion is real can intensify emotional responses, and the belief that the object is not real dampens emotional responses (Gross, 1998; Lazarus & Alfert, 1964). We suggest, however, that this pattern should be true only to the extent that the emotion is evoked by reflective process. Knowing that a pit that visually appears before one's feet is unreal should have little impact on the affective response, assuming that it is generated by associative processes.

Dissociations Due to Input Stimuli

The associative and rule-based systems are most effectively activated by different types of input. Associative processes can be most directly activated by visual or other actual sensory inputs (e.g., the sight of a charging bear) (see Lundqvist & Öhman, Chapter 5; de Gelder, Chapter 6; Atkinson & Adolphs, Chapter 7). Rule-based processes, with their heavy linguistic component, are directly activated by symbolic input (e.g., reading "The bear charges at you"). This point has many implications (see Lieberman et al., 2002). One is methodological: Researchers often use verbal or symbolic stimuli for their convenience, but should understand that results may not be equivalent to those resulting from images, movies, etc. Nevertheless it is obvious that people can respond emotionally to words. How does this response occur? One potential route is that people can transform symbolic stimuli into vivid images that, in turn, trigger emotion through associative processing. Consistent with this suggestion, Lang (1977) has shown that good imagers are more likely to respond affectively to degraded input (short phrases) than poor imagers. In short, the experiential quality of the internal representation influences whether the associative mode of processing is activated (see also Niedenthal, Barsalou, Ric, & Krauth-Gruber, Chapter 2, for a related view).

Implications of Emotions for Dual-Process Theories

We have been discussing implications of dual-process thinking for understanding processes relevant to emotion, but emotions also have implications for dual-process models. As Lieberman et al. (2002) explain, one function of negative emotions is as an alarm or wake-up call for the reflective system, indicating that more automatic (associative mode) regulatory processes have failed. Berkowitz (1993) demonstrates that negative affect can be automatically elicited by a variety of different factors (e.g., heat, foul odors, loud noises). The evoked negative feeling might, in turn, activate the reflective system to understand whether and why the individual's goals are blocked. If the resulting causal search identifies another person's actions as the source of the negative situation, subjectively experienced anger may result. Accordingly, ruminative thoughts might be able to transform a mild shudder into a full-blown panic attack (Bouton, Chapter 9; Martin & Tesser, 1989). Thus the two processing modes can have parallel effects in emotional responses.

Attributions for Emotional Responses

We advance one more speculative suggestion concerning the way in which emotional reactions are subjectively experienced. Processing in the associative mode is automatic and preconscious, becoming subjectively part of the experience of the perceived object itself, as Lieberman et al. (2002) emphasize. For this reason, emotions based on the associative processing system may be seen as intrinsic to the object itself: The fire or the storm cloud is experienced as inherently frightening (for a similar point, see Barrett, Chapter 11). In contrast, responses generated by rule-based or reflective processes are subjectively experienced as one's own thoughts or reactions to events (Lieberman et al., 2002) rather than as inherent in the object. We may say "I feel upset" or "I feel guilty," attributing the emotional response to ourselves, rather than assuming that the emotion is inherent in the object and that everyone else would feel the same in the same situation. Still, the determinants of the outward or inward "focus" of emotions are multiple and complex (see Lambie & Marcel, 2002), and this hypothesis based on the properties of dual-processing modes is speculative and requires further elaboration and empirical test.

CONCLUSIONS

Dual-process approaches have become common in many topic areas across social and cognitive psychology (Smith & DeCoster, 2000). In this chapter we have attempted to sketch the outlines of a dual-process approach to processes involved in the elicitation and control of emotion, and to review some of the implications of such a model. In general, we believe that this integrative theoretical effort makes good sense. Our dual-process approach makes sense of facts such as the following: (1) some affective responses are evidently shared by nonhumans, whereas others rest on types of verbal/propositional reasoning that are more uniquely human; (2) some emotions are easily altered by changing high-order knowledge or beliefs, whereas others are recalcitrant and cannot be changed by beliefs (e.g., disgust felt at a disgusting-looking object that one knows is a wholesome food); (3) emotions can be misattributed (linked to an incorrect cause) and misidentified (given an incorrect label), suggesting that the more automatic processes that generate the emotion are distinct from the more thoughtful processes involved in causal search and emotion labeling; (4) sometimes emotions are generated by preconscious processes, so that we are conscious only of a sudden onset of affect, and sometimes by conscious processes, in which we are aware of each step in a chain of reasoning that leads us to an emotionally evocative conclusion. The success and empirical fruitfulness of dual-process thinking in other domains suggest that as this approach to emotion processes is carried further, it may well lead to important conceptual and empirical insights.

NOTES

1. A connectionist network is a large number of simple yet richly interconnected processing units (loosely analogous to neurons), in which a flow of signals across the connections allows the network to perform the basic functions of information transformation and representation. Each experience leads to small changes in the strengths of the connections between units. The result of many such changes is that the network becomes able to reconstruct patterns that it had previously generated in response to similar patterns of inputs.
2. Recent research suggests that it is not the movement direction that is associated with the processing of valence but rather the increase (withdrawal) or decrease (approach) of distance between the self and an object (Neumann, Seibt, & Levy-Sadot, 2004). Thus, if the reference point of a movement is the self, pushing a lever away is executed faster (increasing the distance to the self). However, if the reference point is the object, moving the hand away from the object is executed faster (increasing the distance to the object).
3. From that point of view it might not be surprising that the timing of facial responses seems to be a critical variable in lie detection (Ekman, 1986).

REFERENCES

Adelmann, P. K., & Zajonc, R. B. (1989). Facial efference and the experience of emotion. *Annual Review of Psychology, 40,* 249–280.
Bargh, J. A., Chen, M., & Burrows, L. (1996). Automaticity of social behavior:

Direct effects of trait construct and stereotype activation on action. *Journal of Personality and Social Psychology, 71,* 230–244.

Barrett, L. F., & Russell, J. A. (1999). The structure of current affect: Controversies and emerging consensus. *Current Directions in Psychological Science, 8,* 10–14.

Barrett, L. F., Tugade, M. M., & Engle, R. W. (2004). Individual differences in working memory capacity and dual process theories of the mind. *Psychological Bulletin, 130,* 553–573.

Berkowitz, L. (1993). *Aggression: Its causes, consequences, and control.* New York: McGraw-Hill.

Bouton, M. E., Mineka, S., & Barlow, D. H. (2001). A modern learning theory perspective on the etiology of panic disorder. *Psychological Review, 108,* 4–32.

Bradley, M. M., Codispoti, M., Cuthbert, B. N., & Lang, P. J. (2001). Emotion and motivation: I. Defensive and appetitive reactions in picture processing. *Emotion, 1,* 276–298.

Brewer, M. B. (1988). A dual process model of impression formation. In R. S. Wyer & T. K. Srull (Eds.), *Advances in social cognition* (Vol. 1, pp. 1–36). Hillsdale, NJ: Erlbaum.

Butler, E. A., Egloff, B., Wilhelm, F. H., Smith, N. C., Erickson, E. A., & Gross, J. J. (2003). The social consequences of expressive suppression. *Emotion, 3,* 48–67.

Chen, M., & Bargh, J. A. (1999). Consequences of automatic evaluation: Immediate behavioral predispositions to approach or avoid the stimulus. *Personality and Social Psychology Bulletin, 25,* 215224.

Chaiken, S. (1980). Heuristic versus systematic information processing and the use of source versus message cues in persuasion. *Journal of Personality and Social Psychology, 39,* 752–766.

Clore, G. L., & Ortony, A. (2000). Cognition in emotion: Always, sometimes, or never? In R. D. Lane, L. Nadel, G. L. Ahern, J. J. B. Allen, A. W. Kaszniak, S. Z. Rapcsak, & G. E. Schwartz (Eds.), *Cognitive neuroscience of emotion* (pp. 24–61). New York: Oxford University Press.

Devine, P. G. (1989). Stereotypes and prejudice: Their automatic and controlled components. *Journal of Personality and Social Psychology, 56,* 5–18.

Dimberg, U., Thunberg, M., & Elmehed, K. (2000). Unconscious facial reactions to emotional facial expressions. *Psychological Science, 11,* 86–89.

Ekman, P. (1986). *Telling lies.* New York: Berkeley.

Fazio, R. H. (1986). How do attitudes guide behavior? In R. M. Sorrentino & E. T. Higgins (Eds.), *Handbook of motivation and cognition, Vol. 1. Foundations of social behavior* (pp. 204–243). New York: Guilford Press.

Foa, E. B., & Kozak, M.J. (1986). Emotional processing of fear: Exposure to corrective information. *Psychological Bulletin, 99,* 20–35.

Frijda, N. (1988). The laws of emotion. *American Psychologist, 43,* 349–358.

Gross, J. J. (1998). Antecedent- and response-focused emotion regulation: Divergent consequences for experience, expression, and physiology. *Journal of Personality and Social Psychology, 74,* 224–237.

Keltner, D., & Haidt, J. (2001). Social functions of emotions. In T. J. Mayne & G. A. Bonanno (Eds.), *Emotions: Current issues and future directions* (pp. 192–213). New York: Guilford Press.

Kruglanski, A. W., Thompson, E. P., & Spiegel, S. (1999). Separate or equal? Bimodal notions of persuasion and a single-process "unimodel." In S. Chaiken & Y. Trope (Eds.), *Dual-process theories in social psychology* (pp. 293–313). New York: Guilford Press.

Lambie, J. A., & Marcel, A. J. (2002). Consciousness and the varieties of emotion experience: A theoretical framework. *Psychological Review, 109,* 219–259.

Lang, P. J. (1977). Imagery in therapy: An informational-processing analysis of fear. *Behavior Therapy, 8,* 862–886.

Lazarus, R. S., & Alfert, E. (1964). Short-circuiting of threat by experimentally altering cognitive appraisal. *Journal of Abnormal and Social Psychology, 69,* 195–205.

LeDoux, J. (1996). *The emotional brain: The mysterious underpinnings of emotional life.* New York: Simon & Schuster.

Leventhal, H., & Scherer, K. R. (1987). The relationship of emotion and cognition: A functional approach to a semantic controversy. *Cognition and Emotion, 1,* 3–28.

Lieberman, M. D., Gaunt, R., Gilbert, D. T., & Trope, Y. (2002). Reflexion and reflection: A social cognitive neuroscience approach to attributional inference. *Advances in Experimental Social Psychology, 34,* 199–249.

Macrae, C. N., Bodenhausen, G. V., & Milne, A. B. (1995). The dissection of selection in person perception: Inhibitory processes in social stereotyping. *Journal of Personality and Social Psychology, 69,* 397–407.

Martin, L.L., & Tesser, A. (1989). Toward a motivational and structural theory of ruminative thought. In J.S. Uleman & J.A. Bargh (Eds.), *Unintended thought* (pp. 306–326). New York: Guilford Press.

Matthews, G., & Wells, A. (1999). The cognitive science of attention and emotion. In T. Dalgleish (Ed.), *Handbook of cognition and emotion* (pp. 171–192). West Sussex, UK: Wiley.

Mesquita, B. (2001). Emotions in collectivist and individualist context. *Journal of Personality and Social Psychology, 80,* 68–74.

Murphy, S. T., & Zajonc, R. B. (1993). Affect, cognition, and awareness: Affective priming with optimal and suboptimal stimulus exposures. *Journal of Personality and Social Psychology, 64,* 723–739.

Neumann, R., Foerster, J., & Strack, F. (2003). Motor compatibility: The bidirectional link between behavior and evaluation. In J. Musch & K. C. Klauer (Eds.), *The psychology of evaluation: Affective processes in cognition and emotion* (pp. 762–768). Mahwah, NJ: Erlbaum.

Neumann, R., Hess, M., Schulz, S., & Alpers, G. (in press). Automatic behavioral responses to valence: Evidence that facial action is facilitated by evaluative processing. *Cognition and Emotion.*

Neumann, R., Seibt, B., & Levy-Sadot, R. (2004). *The malleability of automatic approach and avoidance movements: Self and object as reference points.* Unpublished manuscript, University of Würzburg, Germany.

Neumann, R., Seibt, B., & Strack, F. (2001). The influence of global mood on emotions: Disentangling feeling and knowing. *Cognition and Emotion, 15,* 725–747.

Neumann, R., & Steinhäuser, N. (2003). *How self-construal shapes emotion: Cul-*

tural differences in the feeling of pride. Unpublished Manuscript. University of Würzburg.

Nisbett, R. E., & Wilson, T. D. (1977). Telling more than we know: Verbal reports on mental processes. *Psychological Review, 84,* 231–259.

Ochsner, K., & Barrett, L. F. (2000). The neuroscience of emotion. In T. J. Mayne & G. A. Bonnano (Eds.), *Emotions: Current issues and future directions* (pp. 38–81). New York: Guilford Press.

Öhman, A., & Soares, J. J. F. (1994). "Unconscious anxiety": Phobic responses to masked stimuli. *Journal of Abnormal Psychology, 103,* 231–240.

Ortony, A., Clore, G. L., & Collins, A. (1988). *The cognitive structure of emotions.* New York: Cambridge University Press.

Petty, R. E., & Cacioppo, J. T. (1986). The Elaboration Likelihood Model of persuasion. In L. Berkowitz (Ed.), *Advances in experimental social psychology* (Vol. 19, pp. 123–205). New York: Academic Press.

Quigley, K. S., & Barrett, L. F. (1999). Emotional learning and mechanisms of intentional psychological change. In J. Brandtstädter & R. M. Lerner (Eds.), *Action and self-development: Theory and research through the lifespan* (pp. 435–464). Thousand Oaks, CA: Sage.

Richards, J. M., & Gross, J. J. (2000). Emotion regulation and memory: The cognitive costs of keeping one's cool. *Journal of Personality and Social Psychology, 79,* 410–424.

Rozin, P., Millman, L., & Nemeroff, C. (1986). Operation of the laws of sympathetic magic in disgust and other domains. *Journal of Personality and Social Psychology, 50,* 703–712.

Russell, J. A. (2003). Core affect and the psychological construction of emotion. *Psychological Review, 110,* 145–172.

Scherer, K. R. (2001). Appraisal considered as a process of multi-level sequential checking. In K. R. Scherer, A. Schorr, & T. Johnstone (Eds.). *Appraisal processes in emotion: Theory, methods, research* (pp. 92–120). New York: Oxford University Press.

Schorr, A. (2001). Appraisal: The evolution of an idea. In K. R. Scherer, A. Schorr, & T. Johnstone (Eds.). *Appraisal processes in emotion: Theory, methods, research* (pp. 20–34). New York: Oxford University Press.

Schwarz, N., & Clore, G. (1983). Mood, misattribution, and judgments of well-being: Informative and directive functions of affective states. *Journal of Personality and Social Psychology, 45,* 513–523.

Sherry, D. F., & Schacter, D. L. (1987). The evolution of multiple memory systems. *Psychological Review, 94,* 439–454.

Siemer, M., & Reisenzein, R. (1998). Effects of mood on evaluative judgments: Influence of reduced processing capacity on mood salience. *Cognition and Emotion, 12,* 783–805.

Sloman, S. A. (1996). The empirical case for two systems of reasoning. *Psychological Bulletin, 119,* 3–22.

Smith, C. A., & Kirby, L. D. (2001). Affect and cognitive appraisal: From content to process models. In: J. Forgas (Ed.), *Handbook of affect and social cognition* (pp. 75–92). Hillsdale. NJ: Erlbaum.

Smith, E. R., & DeCoster, J. (2000). Dual process models in social and cognitive psychology: Conceptual integration and links to underlying memory systems. *Personality and Social Psychology Review, 4,* 108–131.

Squire, L. R. (1992). Memory and the hippocampus: A synthesis from findings with rats, monkeys, and humans. *Psychological Review, 99,* 195–231.

Strack, F., & Deutsch, R. (2004). Reflective and impulsive determinants of social behavior. *Personality and Social Psychology Review, 8,* 220–247.

Teasdale, J. D. (1999). Emotional processing, three modes of mind, and the prevention of relapse in depression. *Behaviour Research and Therapy, 37*(Suppl. 1), S53–S77.

Tulving, E. (1983). *Elements of episodic memory.* Oxford, UK: Clarendon Press.

Weiner, B. (1986). Attribution, emotion, and action. In R. M. Sorrentino & E. T. Higgins (Eds.), *Handbook of motivation and cognition, Vol. 1: Foundations of social behavior* (pp. 281–312). New York: Guilford Press.

CHAPTER 13

Unconscious Processes in Emotion
The Bulk of the Iceberg

Klaus R. Scherer

This chapter reviews some of the central emotion processes and the respective role of consciousness (or its absence). Contrary to what seems to be current practice, I attempt to refrain from classifying phenomena into conscious and unconscious, which implies a divide between two separate categories. Rather, I assume that a large majority of emotion processes functions in an unconscious mode and that only some of these processes (or their outcomes) will emerge into consciousness for some periods of time. I like Freud's metaphor of an iceberg, the bulk of which is invisible (the unconscious) with only a small tip above the surface (the conscious). If we assume that the fluid in which the emotion iceberg floats (the mental soup) can vary in consistency, buoyancy will determine the degree of emergence (the buoyant force is equal to the weight of the liquid that the object displaces. If the liquid is denser, the buoyant force is greater. Steel sinks in water but floats in mercury). Similarly, increases in density of mental processing may result in a greater emergence of processing into consciousness.

The major purpose of this chapter is to analyze theoretically the conscious and unconscious processes in emotion elicitation and differentiation. Specific research is cited as illustration, but no coherent, let alone exhaustive, review is intended. To identify contrasting positions and to stimulate

1. *What is the scope of your proposed model? When you use the term* emotion, *how do you use it? What do you mean by terms such as* fear, anxiety, *or* happiness?

In this chapter, I present a comprehensive component process model of emotion that defines emotion as an episode of interrelated, synchronized changes in the states of all or most of five organismic subsystems (cognition, neurophysiological support, motivation, motor expression, subjective feeling) in response to the evaluation of an external or internal stimulus event as relevant to major concerns of the organism. Emotion-constituent evaluation is described as recursive sequences of appraisal at several levels of processing (sensory–motor, schematic, conceptual) based on a set of universal criteria. This account allows for an almost unlimited number of differentiated emotional qualities to emerge, depending on the respective appraisal profile and sequence (for further details, see Scherer, 2001a, 2004a). Verbal labels such as fear, joy, or anger are seen as language-based categories for modal emotions, i.e., frequently and universally occurring events and situations that generate similar appraisal profiles (Scherer, 1994).

2. *Define your terms:* conscious, unconscious, awareness. *Or say why you do not use these terms.*

It would be inappropriate to attempt to define "consciousness," given the extraordinary multiplicity of definitions currently in existence. Thus, a generic core of understanding of consciousness and unconsciousness is presupposed. However, I suggest separating these notions from assumptions made about the nature of cognitive processing, such as automatic, effortful, or implicit.

3. *Does your theory model with what is conscious, what is unconscious, or their relationship? If you do not address this area specifically, can you speculate on the relationship between what is conscious and unconscious? Or if you do not like the conscious–unconscious distinction, or if you do not think this is a good question to ask, can you say why?*

Importantly, it is assumed that a large majority of emotion processes function in an unconscious mode and that only some of these processes (or their outcomes) will emerge into consciousness for some periods of time. This process is seen as linked to the degree of synchronization between organismic subsystems produced by emotion elicitation and the attention generated by a monitoring system. A process whereby parts of an integrated representation of the underlying component processes emerge into consciousness, as a prerequisite for verbal labeling and communication, is suggested and illustrated in this chapter (see Scherer, 2004a, for further details).

debate, some issues are presented in an exaggerated fashion. Most important, the spirit in which the chapter is written is exploratory, as is appropriate for the vast and largely uncharted territory of the conscious and the unconscious in emotion.

Given the rampant terminological confusion in the area of emotion theorizing and research, it may be useful to start with a definition of emotion. I have suggested seven different types of affective states in the form of a design feature analysis (see Figure 13.1), with examples of each: Preferences, utilitarian emotions, aesthetic emotions, mood, interpersonal stances, attitudes, and affective personality traits. These different constructs are compared on the basis of a set of design features (see Scherer, 2004b) that includes (1) typical intensity, (2) duration, (3) the degree of synchronization or coordination of different organismic systems during the state, (4) the extent to which the change in state is triggered by, or focused on, an event or a situation, (5 and 6) the extent to which the differentiated nature of the state is due to a process of antecedent appraisal or evaluation (either intrinsic, i.e., determined by the object, or transactional, i.e., determined by the object in interaction with the needs/goals of the appraiser), (7) the rapidity of change in the nature of the state, (8) the degree to which the state affects behavior, and (9) the relative importance for emotion induction via art or music. Specifically, emotion is defined as *an episode of massive, synchronous recruitment of mental and somatic resources to adapt to, or cope with, a stimulus event that is subjectively appraised as being highly pertinent to the needs, goals, and values of the individual.*

In this chapter, I focus on three major processes directly determined by the reactive nature of emotion that commonly occur during an emotion episode: (1) the detection and evaluation of the significance of a stimulus event for the individual; (2) the preparation of response tendencies; and (3) the integration of evaluative and proprioceptive information, resulting in subjective feeling states. A number of issues pertinent to consciousness and elaboration is explored for each of these processes. Researchers working on unconscious phenomena in affect and emotion have their preferred terms to distinguish conscious and unconscious processes in a larger sense. This is not the place for a detailed historical overview and assignment of responsibility for the definition and use of certain terms via conscientious citation. Even a cursory overview of the literature in this domain (Bargh, 1994; Bargh & Ferguson, 2000; Cohen & Schooler, 1997; Fazio, 2001; Greenwald & Banaji, 1995; Hameroff, Kaszniak, & Scott, 1996; Kihlstrom, 1994; Lambie & Marcel, 2002; Leventhal, 1984; Shallice, 1972; Schneider & Shiffrin, 1977) suggests a number of adjectival pairs, in addition to conscious and unconscious, that are regularly used: explicit versus implicit, controlled versus automatic, effortful versus effortless, and conceptual/

Type of affective state: brief definition (examples)	Intensity	Duration	Synchronization	Event/situation focus	Intrinsic appraisal	Transactional appraisal	Rapidity of change	Behavioral impact	Induction via art/music
Preferences: evaluative judgments of stimuli in the sense of liking or disliking, or preferring or not, over another stimulus (*like, dislike, positive, negative*)	L	M	VL	VH	VH	M	VL	M	H
Utilitarian emotions: relatively brief episodes of synchronized response of all or most organismic subsystems to the evaluation of an external or internal event as being of major significance for personal goals and needs (*angry, sad, joyful, fearful, ashamed, proud, elated, desperate*)	H	L	VH	VH	M	VH	VH	VH	H
Aesthetic emotions: evaluations of auditory or visual stimuli in terms of intrinsic qualities of form or relationship of elements (*moved, awed, surprised, full of wonder, admiration, bliss, ecstasy, fascination, harmony, rapture, solemnity*)	L–M	L	M	H	VH	L	VH	L	VH
Mood: diffuse affect state, most pronounced as change in subjective feeling, of low intensity but relatively long duration, often without apparent cause (*cheerful, gloomy, irritable, listless, depressed, buoyant*)	M	H	L	L	M	L	H	H	M
Interpersonal stances: affective stance taken toward another person in a specific interaction, coloring the interpersonal exchange in that situation (*distant, cold, warm, supportive, contemptuous*)	M	M	L	H	L	L	VH	H	L
Attitudes: relatively enduring, affectively colored beliefs and predispositions toward objects or persons (*loving, hating, valuing, desiring*)	M	H	VL	VL	L	L	L	L	M
Personality traits: emotionally laden, stable personality dispositions and behavior tendencies, typical for a person (*nervous, anxious, reckless, morose, hostile, envious, jealous*)	L	VH	VL	VL	L	VL	VL	L	L

FIGURE 13.1. Design feature definitions for major types of affect. VL, very low; L, low; M, medium; H, high; LH, very high. From Scherer (2004b). Copyright 2004 by the *Journal of New Music Research* (www.tandf.co.uk). Reprinted by permission.

propositional versus schematic. Although individual authors may make sharper distinctions, there is a common tendency to assume a high degree of overlap between unconscious, implicit, automatic, effortless, and schematic, on the one hand, and conscious, explicit, controlled, effortful, and conceptual/propositional, on the other. In addition, there is a tendency to view these pairs as binary, dichotomous alternatives rather than as opposite poles on an underlying dimension. Both of these assumptions seem to require more extensive debate (see also Clore & Ketelaar, 1997).

To what extent are these modalities interrelated? It is likely that there is a high degree of empirical covariation between some of the modalities. But these relationships are probably much too complex to justify treating the terms *unconscious, implicit, automatic*, and *effortless* as synonyms. For example, on the one hand, an automatically triggered reflex may require little effort and could remain opaque to consciousness unless it is externalized as overt behavior, as in the case of the knee jerk. On the other hand, reflexes should, by definition, be explicit. Implicit processes should be effortful because they require a lot of inference to determine the behavioral meaning. If attention is one of the required resources, it is unlikely that the process will be automatic and remain entirely unconscious. The lack of appropriate conceptual distinctions may actually hinder the careful analysis of the precise nature of the processes involved in the emotion mechanism. Thus the modalities or dimensions discussed earlier should be treated as independent, continuous dimensions in a multidimensional space. In consequence, the processes under study in a particular research project should be qualified, at least roughly, with respect to their position on each of these dimensions separately. Although difficult and necessarily speculative, such an approach could produce interesting insights into the nature of the mental processes that underlie emotion. It would certainly force us to be more precise in the conceptualizations and potentially even in the operationalizations used in this research.

THE DETECTION AND EVALUATION OF THE SIGNIFICANCE AND IMPLICATIONS OF A STIMULUS EVENT FOR THE INDIVIDUAL

The presence of an emotion is an indicator that the individual has detected an event that is likely to have significant consequences for his or her needs, goals, and values. The reason that we can be confident of this statement is that the principle of economy underlying much of evolution would not permit an important investment of resources, as constituted by a massive, synchronized response across several organismic systems, unless there were a real need for adaptation. The better we understand the process of significance detection and evaluation, the better we understand emotion. The significance of a stimulus event resides in its meaning, and its meaning, in its behavioral (as compared with semantic) sense, is defined by potential consequences for the individual's needs, goals, and values. There seem to be two major mechanisms for meaning assignment: pattern matching and rule-based inference (see also Smith & Neumann, Chapter 12).

It is generally assumed that, from an individual's past experience, the matched schemas or the inferences from specific features will produce a certain type of behavioral meaning. For example, if one has had negative experiences with doctors, a negative attitude may be activated each time one sees a man in a white coat, independent of the context. However, in many cases, the current context, and particularly the current motivational state of the person, contributes massively to the emergence of the behavioral meaning of an event (and the consequent emotional reaction). In other words, *behavioral meaning* is, in large part, constituted by an individual's assessment of the probable consequences of a particular stimulus event occurring at a particular time, and this assessment is determined by the individual's motivational state, available resources, and the respective socionormative context. This point is so important that it bears restating: *Although some of the behavioral meaning of a schema or an inference is stored in memory in the form of association with other memory and knowledge content as well as past affective reactions, much of the behavioral meaning in a particular situation is determined by an interaction between these stored meaning components and their evaluation in the light of the current motivational state and available resources for outcome control.*

To my knowledge, until recently (see Ekman, 2004), neither basic emotion theorists nor dimensional theorists have been centrally concerned with the nature of the processes that detect pertinent events, evaluate their consequences and meaning for the individual, and thus differentiate the resulting emotions and their behavioral effects (Scherer, 2000b). In contrast, this evaluation is the major focus of interest in componential appraisal theories of emotion (see Ellsworth & Scherer, 2003; Scherer, 1999; Scherer, Schorr, & Johnstone, 2001, for overviews), which attempt to conceptualize the behavioral meaning of an event for the individual (and thus the resulting emotion) on the basis of profiles of evaluation criteria such as novelty, agreeableness, goal conduciveness, coping potential, and norm compatibility (see Scherer, 2001a). For example, appraisal theorists might describe the behavioral meaning of an event, such as being threatened by a mugger, as novel, disagreeable, goal obstructive, difficult to cope with, and immoral. The predicted emotion would be a variant of a fear–anger blend. Importantly, appraisal theorists consider the evaluation and the resulting emotion as a continuous and constantly changing process. The variability is due to situational changes as well as to reappraisals of the consequences. Furthermore, the motivational state of the individual as well as his or her resource supply are likely to change, sometimes rather abruptly. In consequence, behavioral meaning must be an emergent quality, subject to constant and often sudden change.

In consequence, all stimulation impinging on the organism must be constantly monitored for dynamic behavioral meaning. This meaning is emergent, based on an interaction between the nature of the event, its consequences, and the individual's motivational state. Given the complexity and changeability of the factors involved, it is unlikely that behavioral meaning can be constituted simply by matching situational features with schemas stored in long-term memory. The only exception might be powerful stimuli that have an unconditional impact, such as evolutionary threat, or other unconditioned stimuli that represent powerful aversive (pain) or appetitive (food, sex) functions. Yet even these might be mediated by motivational states. Thus it seems that pain sensitivity is mediated by both dispositional and state differences (Coderre, Mogil, & Bushnell, 2003).

In general, the ongoing evaluation of most day-to-day stimulus events will require comparative evaluation of an event with the current motivational and resource state. These operations go far beyond simple feature detection or even schema matching and are thus likely to be effortful. However, they must be largely automatic, given that they operate almost constantly. It would hardly be feasible to imagine a higher-order monitoring system controlling this process in any depth. For the same reason, much of this process is likely to operate outside of consciousness, because the attentional resources mobilized by conscious processing could not be invested in a continuous fashion. Because the significance-evaluation mechanism is *on* all the time, one might expect a shallow filter to operate to screen incoming stimulation for significant consequences, on the basis of a particular tuning or setting of the organism's motivational state. Only stimuli that are not filtered out as inconsequential will elicit deeper processing.

How does this process work? The enormous amount of research on the amygdala that has been stimulated by the pioneering work of LeDoux (2000) and Davis (1998; Davis & Whalen, 2001) suggests some beginning answers. There is much evidence to suggest that direct projections from the sensory thalamus to the amygdala serve to activate rudimentary defense reactions to powerful threats such as evolutionarily prepared stimuli (e.g., snakes, facial anger expression) or conditioned stimuli based on painful unconditioned stimuli (Lunsqvist & Öhman, Chapter 5; de Gelder, Chapter 6; Atkins & Adolphs, Chapter 7; Dolan & Morris, 2000; Vuilleumier, Armony, Driver, & Dolan, 2001; Vuilleumier & Schwartz, 2001; Whalen,

1998; Whalen, Curran, & Rauch, 2001; Whalen, Shin, et al., 2001). From this evidence, there is reason to believe that the amygdala plays an important role in the filtering process referred to earlier. This role is all the more probable because, contrary to popular opinion, the amygdala does not seem to be exclusively focused on the recognition of threat- or fear-relevant stimulation. In a careful review of the literature, Sander, Grafman, and Zalla (2003) have accumulated evidence that suggests that the amygdala is a generalized device for the low-level detection of significance or pertinence in a general sense. In other words, the amygdala seems capable of deciding, on the basis of rather rudimentary information conveyed directly from the sensory thalamus, that a particular stimulus is potentially significant for the needs and the well-being of an organism. The baffling question is, of course, how the amygdala does it. Could it be that a certain number of pertinent schemas, "the most significant of . . . , " are stored in this subcortical structure, and if so, in which form? Or does the amygdala, which is highly connected to most subcortical and cortical regions, rely on schemas stored in a distributed fashion? Is the inventory of the schemas that reflects vital behavioral meaning the same for every individual, that is, genetically determined by evolutionary preparation? Or does the experience and the motivational makeup of the individual influence the target patterns stored in this central gatekeeper structure? Does the information processing that takes place in the amygdala take into account the current motivational and resource state of the organism, implying some kind of comparison, or at least tuning, or is it limited to matching the input features to invariant schemas? The research agenda for affective neuroscientists specializing on the amygdala should keep the discipline busy for some time.

Most important, despite the fascinating demonstration of the existence of a "low road" (direct thalamo–amygdala projections) and a "high road" (via the cortical association areas) of information processing by LeDoux and others, one should not forget that the process is generally integrated. Activation triggered by external stimulation speeds along both roads, and although the more rapid lower road may start producing some generalized autononous nervous system (ANS) efference after 80 milliseconds of stimulus onset, travel on the high road is not far behind, and the first results of cortical processing will arrive at the amygdala 50–100 milliseconds later. Thus it cannot be a question of either/or but rather of how processing along the two routes is integrated and coordinated. One can assume that this integration and coordination can take many different forms, ranging from predominance of the lower road, with only minor involvement of the higher level (as in the case of stimulation to which satisfactory adjustment can be made on the basis of low-level regulation), to almost exclusive involvement of the cortical level (as in the case of logical deductions in a philosophy seminar). In addition, it is not only the level but also the quality of process-ing that is at stake. Is simple schema matching sufficient or are inference and comparison required? Is the process highly routinized and able to unfold automatically or is an active, effortful, and controlled search required? How many tasks have to be dealt with at the same time and how much attention is available for each? As suggested earlier, we can expect that the quality of the respective evaluation process must be described as a trajectory through a multidimensional space formed by the dimensions of effort, automaticity, explicitness, and consciousness. Leventhal and Scherer (1987) have suggested that the type of processing with regard to content (types of appraisal) and level (sensory–motor, schematic, and conceptual) is determined by the need to arrive at a conclusive evaluation result (yielding a promising action tendency). If automatic, effortless, unconscious pro-cesses do not produce a satisfactory result, more controlled, effortful, and possibly conscious mechanisms are brought into play to determine the behavioral meaning of a stimulus event and prepare an adaptive response.

THE PREPARATION OF RESPONSE TENDENCIES

The function of emotion is to prepare adaptive behavioral reactions. In con-sequence, one of the most important processes is the preparation of appro-priate action tendencies. The conceptualization of this essential set of processes varies considerably over the three theoretical traditions. Dimen-sional theorists, in line with their emphasis on valence, mostly discuss the preparation of approach or avoidance tendencies (Carver, 2001). Discrete or basic emotion theorists assume highly integrated response patterns for each of the basic emotions, particularly with regard to motor expression and physiological response specificity (Ekman, 1972; Izard, 1971). In con-trast, many appraisal theorists postulate that response preparation depends directly on the results of the appraisal process (Roseman, 2001; Scherer, 1984, 2001a; Smith & Scott, 1997). I have postulated that each significant result on an appraisal dimension triggers a response in all components of emotion and that these sequential changes are cumulatively integrated. Each result of a particular check in the cognitive component is expected to affect every other component of the emotion process (even though the effect may be slight in many cases). The effects of subsequent checks cumu-latively add to the pattern of change (see Scherer, 2001a, Fig. 2). Given the theoretical prediction of a fixed but recursive, sequence and of detailed response characteristics in different peripheral domains (e.g., motor ex-pression and physiological responding), these claims can be empirically investigated (for a discussion, see Barrett, Chapter 11). This is particularly interesting with regard to the temporal unfolding of these processes, for which there is currently little evidence in the literature. Electroencephalographic work in progress in our lab (Grandjean & Scherer, 2003) provides the first evidence for the assumption that the checks underlying the appraisal process are not simultaneous but occur sequentially, as predicted. For example, the cerebral processes at the cortical level related to the experimental manipulation of novelty, investigated with electroencephalographic methods, seem to occur earlier than the processes related to the relevance appraisal.

THE INTEGRATION OF EVALUATIVE AND PROPRIOCEPTIVE INFORMATION AND THE EMERGENCE OF SUBJECTIVE FEELING STATES

As suggested earlier, an emotion episode essentially consists of synchronized processes of event evaluation and response preparation involving several components. Each of these processes can be expected to have its own projections and proprioceptive feedback loops, allowing for rudimentary, largely automatic regulation. However, if these processes are to be controlled and regulated at a higher level, the information needs to be centrally represented and, at least in part, to emerge into consciousness. The reason is that the complete process of central evaluation and peripheral responses is unlikely to be centrally stored over an extended period of time, both because of capacity limitations and the need for meaning analysis on a macro level that can guide control and regulation efforts. In consequence, we need to model the process that underlies the emergence of integrated representations of central processing and proprioceptive feedback into consciousness.

Figure 13.2 illustrates these notions. A Venn diagram with a set of overlapping circles represents the different aspects of monitoring (see also Kaiser & Scherer, 1997; Scherer, 1994). The first circle (A) represents the raw reflection or representation of changes in all synchronized components in a monitoring structure in the central nervous system, integrating the representation of central processing and somatosensory feedback (Iwamura, 1998). This structure is expected to receive massive projections from both cortical and subcortical central nervous system (CNS) structures (including proprioceptive feedback from the periphery). Even though this representation will only become partly conscious, the information represented here is of central importance for response preparation (and thus behavioral adaptation), learning, and rudimentary coping and regulation. One might call the content of the circle *integrated process representation*.

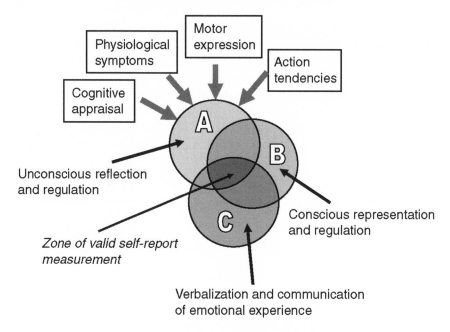

FIGURE 13.2. Three modes of the representation of changes in emotion components: unconsciousness, consciousness, and verbalzation.

The second circle (B), only partially overlapping with the first, represents that part of the integrated process representation that enters awareness (possibly when a high degree of component synchronization requires a high level of controlled regulation and social communication) and thereby becomes conscious. This circle represents the quality and intensity of the conscious feeling state generated by the eliciting event. It would seem that the content of this circle is close to what philosophers and psychologists have referred to as *qualia*.

The third circle in Figure 13.2 represents the individual's ability (which may or may not be realized) to *verbally report* the subjective experience during the emotion episode and thus share it with significant others (including emotion researchers). The fact that this verbalization circle overlaps only partially with the conscious feeling circle is meant to suggest that we can verbalize only a small part of our conscious experience, as a result of (1) the limited availability of appropriate verbal categories (in a particular language and/or to a particular individual), and (2) the individual's intentions to control or hide some of his or her innermost feelings. Most important, the constant flow of consciousness cannot be completely described by a discrete utterance. Thus verbal report must, by necessity, be an approximation that identifies the most salient elements of the experience in the form of a state definition that uses concepts provided by the emotion-related semantic concepts in a language (for a more complete description of the Venn diagram, see Scherer, 2004a; for an alternative view, see Barrett, Chapter 11).

Admittedly, this schema does not do much to advance our understanding of the processes involved, but it may help us ask appropriate research questions concerning (1) the nature of the integration of information from different modalities into a coherent representation, (2) the conditions for emergence of this representation into consciousness, and (3) the encoding of conscious representations into verbal statements.

The central projections from both the cognitive processing and the motor and physiological responding need to be integrated within each domain, across the different domains, and over time. I believe that these extremely complex dynamic integration processes have been severely neglected by past work on emotion. They constitute a major challenge for investigators in this area, because the processes of integration are likely to be largely unconscious but result in a holistic, phenomenal experience or feeling that is at least, in part, conscious. In what follows, I briefly sketch the integration processes that seem to be required: (1) the integration of appraisal results, (2) the integration of peripheral component effects, and (3) integration across components and time.

Integration of Appraisal Results

In trying to predict the emotions resulting from different patterns of appraisal, theorists in this tradition have generally used profile matching or regression analysis (for a review, see Scherer, 1999) without paying too much attention to the problem of the integration of the appraisal results with regard to both the different evaluation criteria or dimensions and the changes over time. In my own model, I have proposed a recursive sequence of stimulus evaluation checks, with an accumulation of the expected efferent effects (see Scherer, 2001a, Figure 2). What remains to be done is to specify the nature of the integration functions that must underlie these cumulative processes. I have suggested attacking this issue by starting from a suggestion made by Anderson (1989), who postulates different types of integration functions based on the current goals of the organism, which transform subjective appraisal results into an implicit response (see Scherer, 2004a). It would be a major breakthrough to be able to model information integration in appraisal and to predict integration rules for combinations of specific appraisal criteria. For example, we found empirically (van Reekum et al., 2004) that the perceived coping potential has a dif-

ferent effect on psychophysiological responses as a function of goal conduciveness. As one might expect, coping ability is of less relevance and has
less of an impact on the ANS when things are going according to plan. In
Anderson's approach, this pattern would be modeled by a *configuration
rule*, which predicts that the importance of one of the criteria depends on
the level of another.

To what extent are these processes available to consciousness? Appraisal theorists are often chided for relying on verbal report in order to
study event evaluation (Parkinson, 1997). The argument is that, given the
rapidity and complexity of the underlying inference processes, individuals
are unlikely to have access to the inner workings of the process. This is
quite likely. However, it does not rule out that the individual is aware of the
outcome of the inference process, for example, the realization of being
faced with a goal obstruction that he or she is powerless to remove. This
issue is related, of course, to the even more complex issue of what the
objects of consciousness are. It is unlikely that the results of evaluations on
individual appraisal dimensions enter awareness directly, in raw form, so to
speak, because it is probably the interaction between different dimensions
that is central rather than the nature of the individual ingredients. Despite
this complexity, we may need to be more specific about these objects if we
want to advance our understanding of the nature of emotion-antecedent
evaluation processes. In order to address these issues in research, we obviously need to rely on self-report (heeding the problems of incomplete overlap of circles B and C in the schema described earlier). However, if we want
to get at the integrated representation of the appraisal results, we may need
to change our instruments and procedures, which, so far, have focused on
individual appraisal dimensions.

Integration of Peripheral Component Effects

Proprioceptive feedback information is available from different response
components such as vocal and facial expression or psychophysiological
symptoms. The question of how different patterns of feedback from the somatic nervous system (SNS) and the ANS are integrated and when they
enter consciousness has not been extensively studied to date. One possibility is that integration is, in part, predetermined by major functional circuits
that underlie peripheral responding. For example, in Gellhorn's (1964) theory of ergotropic and trophotropic systems (or the more general notion of
sympathetic and parasympathetic systems), individual responses are synchronized by the activation of the superordinate systems. One could
assume that feedback integration reassembles those functional interrela-
tionships. Although such a form of autoorganization might be a feasible

mechanism for ANS integration (albeit there is increasing doubt as to the unity of such large-scale systems), such a mechanism is unlikely to be operative in somatic integration, in particular, facial expression and action-related movement. In the case of adaptive behavior, the underlying determinant, and possibly the focus of integration, may be some form of motivational urge, such as an action tendency (Frijda, 1986). In the case of facial expression, there is much debate between theorists who suggest that the face expresses basic emotions (Ekman, 1972; Izard, 1971), a "social message" point of view (Fridlund, 1994; see also Owren, Rendall, & Bachorowski, Chapter 8), and appraisal theorists, who suggest that elements of facial expression might be directly triggered by the results of evaluation on particular combinations of appraisal dimensions (Scherer, 1992; Smith & Scott, 1997). Each of these assumed functions seems to imply a different type of integration process.

How do these processes enter awareness? Although we know that interoception, that is, the *conscious proprioceptive representation* of internal physiological changes, does not accurately reflect the physiological parameters (Barrett, Chapter 11; Vaitl, 1996), there might be more precise nonconscious representations that provide input to the process of integrating the various response domains in the ANS and SNS. In other words, raw proprioceptive feedback from peripheral physiological responses may not project directly to brain structures that underlie the emergence of consciousness but, rather, may contribute to a representation that integrates the changes in several response components. This integrated representation, in turn, may then reach consciousness without allowing the specification of details for individual classes of responses.

One of the problems with studies of interoception (or, for that matter, of emotion-specific physiological response patterns, in general) is that, to the best of my knowledge, not a single study has studied interoception during serious emotional upheavals, such as trying to flee from a terrorist bomb attack, being enraged by an unbearable insult, or experiencing extreme joy in seeing one's baby. Much of the experimental research, to date, has induced mild emotional states, if any, and it is not surprising that people are not good at verbally indexing subtle variations in physiological parameters. Nor is it surprising that it is difficult to find emotion-specific patterns in physiological responding if no specific emotions have been induced. Thus the issue remains open until more representative emotional states with higher specificity and higher intensity have been studied (if this will ever be possible). From the standpoint of evolutionary architecture, it seems functional that humans should not have a detailed conscious representation of minor adjustments of ANS parameters, because minor regulation should be performed automatically without taxing the control center.

In contrast, in the case of a strong emotion with massive, highly synchronized deviations from baseline across several response modalities, one would expect the changes to be represented in consciousness to allow high-level coping and regulation. The question is whether that emergence into consciousness happens in the form of an integrated representation (e.g., becoming aware of high arousal or excitation) or in the form of domain-specific representations (e.g., increased heart rate, short breath, perspiration, etc.). Most likely, both processes operate. People often do report specific symptoms in connection with an emotional experience (and, as suggested earlier, there is little evidence that strong symptoms during intense experiences cannot be accurately reported). At the same time, people also readily evaluate the degree of their arousal or excitation (to name but one possible integrated representation). So far, few studies have been conducted to evaluate the correlation between these impressions and objective indicators. Past research has shown, however, that there does not seem to be a single indicator of arousal. This is as it should be if, as one would expect, arousal or excitation reflects an integrated representation across several modalities.

As this brief overview suggests, an important effort of conceptualization and much basic research are needed to better understand the underlying feedback and integration mechanisms and the specificity of each domain. It is to be hoped that neuropsychological research on the projection and organization of proprioceptive feedback in different domains can provide fresh insight on these complex phenomena.

Integration across Components and Time

Although the issue of integration and the form in which raw or integrated representations reach consciousness are difficult to address, they are even harder to conceptualize and study across domains. If emotional episodes are subjectively experienced as an integrated whole, as one may assume from the way in which people normally talk about their emotions, there must be some kind of overall integration and representation *across the different components and across time*. Although we can focus on micro-momentary changes of feeling and particular cognitive processes or peripheral responses, it seems that we more typically become aware of our feelings in experiential chunks. In other words, there is some phenomenal unity to the feeling in a particular emotion episode, possibly linked to a cause–effect chain as well as to some type of closure. In consequence, there must be a powerful process of integration across components and over time. What is the structure of this integration, its gestalt or organizing principle? Here I again contrast the different suggestions made by dimensional theories, discrete emotion theories, and my own version of componential appraisal theory.

Dimension theorists suggest that subjective experience is integrated along the dimensions of valence and arousal. Recently, Russell and Barrett (Russell, 2003; Russell & Barrett, 1999) have suggested that the representation of feeling in this two-dimensional space, prior to further elaboration, is the primitive *core affect* (see also Barrett, Chapter 11). This idea has a venerable history, having been first articulated by Wundt (1874), who proposed a tension–relaxation dimension in addition to valence and activation. The assumption is that the feeling constituted by these dimensions is a conscious phenomenon and accessible to introspection.

Basic emotion theorists have not felt the need to extensively discuss the issue of feeling and the role of consciousness, because the assumption of homogeneous emotion patterns entails the existence of feeling states that correspond to the patterning provided by the respective basic emotions. These states are accessible to consciousness and labeled by the respective verbal emotion labels. Thus, in this tradition, feeling states are integrated with regard to basic emotion families.

The position of appraisal theorists is less clear and possibly less homogeneous. Therefore, I describe my own position in greater detail (summarized from Scherer, 2004a). I have argued earlier (Scherer, 1984) that there are as many different emotions as there are distinguishable patterns of appraisal results. This explanation translates directly into the issue of integration and feeling. Briefly put, I suggest that multidomain integration is unique to the specific stimulus event and the appraisal results it generates. These results, and the proprioceptive feedback of the response patterns they produce, are integrated across components and over time, in the form of *qualia*—specific emotional experiences that are unitary, indivisible phenomena. I further suggest that it is the very process of synchronization, which I have proposed as the hallmark of emotion as an affective phenomenon, that elicits and organizes this process of integration. It seems safe to assume that this integration occurs outside of awareness. As Anderson (1989, p. 147) suggested earlier: "What does attain consciousness is often, perhaps always, a result integrated across different sense modalities at preconscious stages."

What processes might mediate the emergence into consciousness of preconsciously integrated content? In a chapter urging the use of nonlinear dynamic systems theory for the description of emotion processes (Scherer, 2000a), I suggested that this point might be marked by a qualitative change in a monitor system that reacts to a degree of coupling or synchronization of the subsystems that surpasses the normal baseline fluctuations.

What is the justification for claiming that emotional experience is integrated in the form of qualia, or myriad different representations? Claiming such a mechanism seems to contradict the postulate for efficiency and parsimony I have advocated in several places earlier. However, if feelings represent a monitoring system that serves to regulate, it seems appropriate to assemble as much detailed information as possible in a central representation to fine-tune regulation attempts. Specifically, the integration of proprioceptive information from response components should maintain a maximal amount of detail in unconscious short-term memory (as symbolized by circle A in Figure 13.2). Many low-level regulation processes are likely to operate at this level and can benefit from a comprehensive representation of the behavioral meaning of the eliciting event and the response profile that was produced by the associated appraisal process.

When part of the unconscious representation becomes conscious or is to be stored in long-term memory (e.g., passing from circle A to circle B in Figure 13.2), further integration will be required. One could argue that it is at this point that integration along the lines of dimensions or basic emotion categories occurs. Yet based on the fact that we can obtain self-report on appraisal patterns, or experienced symptoms, or expression patterns in addition to emotion labels, it is likely that even at this level, detailed information is retained in less integrated form. Self-report is certainly biased by social representations concerning emotions, including stereotypes, but it is highly likely that individuals do have conscious access to central representations of their appraisals and response patterns, at least in the sense of *outcome consciousness* (as compared with process consciousness).

Further integration occurs when conscious experience is verbalized (the intersection of circles B and C in Figure 13.2). Although the common path for integration is constituted by the semantic field for emotional phenomena in the respective language, this does not mean that the integration necessarily occurs along the lines of discrete emotion categories, as represented by single words or concepts or by valence and arousal dimensions. Verbal report is not limited to simple naming; it can use complex expressions and even analogies or metaphors (Lakoff & Kövecses, 1987). Clearly, if respondents are forced to respond to a limited number of categories, as identified by labels or dimensions, they will integrate the information retrieved from memory in a form that allows them to decide among the alternatives or determine the overall valence or arousal level. However, this form of report does not constitute evidence that preformed categories or dimensions determine the integration early on in the process. Functionally, it makes sense to keep as much detailed representation as possible and to perform only as much integration as necessary.

The conceptualization of conscious affective feeling suggested here does not contradict the proposals made by dimensional or discrete emotion theorists but, rather, integrates these proposals. Although I would continue to hold that there are as many different emotional states as there are potential appraisal patterns, it is true that some appraisal profiles occur much more frequently than others, producing what I have called *modal emotions* (Scherer, 1994). These emotions correspond to the basic emotion categories that exist in all languages, reflecting the well-known fact that discrete verbal labels reflect objects, events, or concepts for which there is a strong need to communicate. Most likely, conscious feeling states corresponding to frequently encountered appraisal profiles form already coherent qualia even before verbalization (circle B in Figure 13.2). The act of verbal encoding probably serves to focus the feeling further and structure it around social and individual schemas.

With respect to dimensional theories, I suggested many years ago that the Wundtian dimensions of feeling might reflect underlying criteria of emotion processing (Scherer, Abeles, & Fischer, 1975, p. 138). Translated into the more recent notion of stimulus/evaluation checks, this means that (1) the valence dimension reflects appraisal of intrinsic pleasantness and goal conduciveness, (2) activation reflects pertinence and urgency, and (3) power/control reflects coping potential (see also Scherer, 2004a; Scherer, Dan, & Flykt, in press). Here I would disagree with Russell and Barrett's view that the valence and activation dimensions are somehow primary or reflect a primitive "core" of affective feeling. Rather, I see them as derivative or secondary in the sense that the individual is able to synthesize or project more complex feeling states onto those dimensions when required to do so. However, the issue is open to debate and focused empirical investigation.

CONCLUSION

It is common knowledge that the relationship between emotion and consciousness is extremely complex. The current contribution renders the issue even more complex by (1) insisting on multiple dimensions, facets of consciousness, and associated processes, and (2) highlighting the importance of the neglected phenomena of subsystem synchronization and integration as decisive determinants of the emergence of feeling into consciousness. The latter processes, which have rarely been addressed in the literature, are central features of emotion. I do not tire of suggesting that multicomponent synchronization is the essential feature that distinguishes emotional from nonemotional states, and I have speculated that the emergence of conscious feeling may be related to the degree of synchronization, which is related to the need for high-level controlled regulation (Scherer, 1984, 2001a). In discussing neuroscience approaches of relevance to current debates in emotion psychology (Scherer, 1993), I suggested that Damasio's (1990) model of time-locked or synchronized multiregion activation as a potential mechanism for memory recall might be an interesting example of CNS-based synchronization. Over the last 15 years, the notion of neural synchronization as a basis for multimodal temporal binding (Treisman, 1996) has become extremely popular. Partly because of an influential paper by Crick and Koch (1990), there have been several attempts to link neural synchronization to the emergence of awareness and consciousness. In a comprehensive overview of this literature, Engel and Singer (2001) point out that any theory about the neural correlates of consciousness must explain how multiple component processes can be integrated and how large-scale coherence can emerge within distributed neural activity patterns (see Dennett, 1991, for an alternative view). This is exactly what is required to understand emotion as conceptualized by the component process model. Engel and Singer review evidence showing that cross-system coherence and dynamic response selection can be achieved through dynamic binding of distributed information via temporal synchronization of neuronal discharges (with precision in the millisecond range). Concretely, Engel and Singer (p. 23) suggest that synchrony may be ideally suited to promote access of selected contents to working memory ("Synchronized assemblies may stabilize in some reverberatory state, endowing them with competitive advantage over temporarily disorganized activity"), thus becoming conscious. According to Engel and Singer (p. 24), the process of neural synchronization also explains integration: "Temporal binding may establish patterns of large scale coherence, thus enabling specific cross-system relationships that bind subsets of signals in different modalities."

To date, most of the empirical work has been done on perceptual and somatosensory processes in animals, apart from some pioneering work on human perception (Tallon-Baudry, Bertrand, Delpuech, & Pernier, 1996). However, the general framework is extremely pertinent to the issue of emotion emerging into consciousness, as discussed in this chapter. I hope that the effort to disentangle different aspects of consciousness and to start speculating about underlying processes may help, in the long run, to pose more specific questions, amenable to systematic experimental research. It seems obvious to me that progress in understanding the underlying mechanisms critically depends on the development of a truly interdisciplinary domain of affective sciences and effective collaboration with the behavioral neurosciences.

ACKNOWLEDGMENTS

I gratefully acknowledge helpful comments and suggestions by David Sander Didier Grandjean, and Ursula Scherer.

REFERENCES

Anderson, N. H. (1989). Information integration approach to emotions and their measurement. In R. Plutchik & H. Kellerman (Eds.), *Emotion: Theory, research, and experience: Vol. 4. The measurement of emotion* (pp. 133–186). New York: Academic Press.

Bargh, J. A. (1994). The four horsemen of automaticity: Awareness, intention, efficiency, and control in social cognition. In R. S. Wyer, Jr., & T. K. Srull (Eds.), *Handbook of social cognition: Vol. 1. Basic processes* (2nd ed., pp. 1–40). Hillsdale, NJ: Erlbaum.

Bargh, J. A., & Ferguson, M. J. (2000). Beyond behaviorism: On the automaticity of higher mental processes. *Psychological Bulletin, 126*(6), 925–945.

Carver, C. S. (2001). Affect and the functional bases of behavior: On the dimensional structure of affective experience. *Personality and Social Psychology Review, 5*, 345–356.

Clore, G., & Ketelaar, T. (1997). Minding our emotions: On the role of automatic, unconscious affect. In R. S. Wyer, Jr. (Ed.), *The automaticity of everyday life: Advances in social cognition: Vol. 10. Advances in social cognition* (pp. 105–120). Mahwah, NJ: Erlbaum.

Coderre, T. J., Mogil, J. S, & Bushnell, M. C. (2003). The biological psychology of pain. In M. Gallagher & R. J. Nelson (Eds.), *Handbook of psychology: Vol. 10. Biological psychology* (pp. 237–268). New York: Wiley.

Cohen, J. D., & Schooler, J. W. (Eds.). (1997). *Scientific approaches to consciousness.* Hillsdale, NJ: Erlbaum.

Crick, F., & Koch, C. (1990) Towards a neurobiological theory of consciousness. *Seminars in the Neurosciences, 2*, 263–275.

Damasio, A. R. (1990). Synchronous activation in multiple cortical regions: A mechanism for recall. *Seminars in the Neurosciences, 2*, 287–296

Davis, M. (1998). Are different parts of the extended amygdala involved in fear versus anxiety? *Biological Psychiatry, 44*(12), 1239–1247.

Davis, M., & Whalen, P. J. (2001). The amygdala: Vigilance and emotion. *Molecular Psychiatry, 6*(1), 13–34.

Dennett, D. C. (1991). *Consciousness explained.* Boston: Little, Brown.

Dolan, R. J., & Morris, J. S. (2000). The functional anatomy of innate and acquired fear: Perspectives from neuroimaging. In R. D. Lane & L. Nadel (Eds.), *Cognitive neuroscience of emotion* (pp. 225–241). New York: Oxford University Press.

Ekman, P. (1972). Universals and cultural differences in facial expression of emotion. In J. R. Cole (Ed.), *Nebraska symposium on motivation* (pp. 207–283). Lincoln: University of Nebraska Press.

Ekman, P. (2004). What we become emotional about. In A. S. R. Manstead, N. H. Frijda, & A. H. Fischer (Eds.), *Feelings and emotions: The Amsterdam symposium* (pp. 119–135). Cambridge, UK: Cambridge University Press.

Ellsworth, P. C., & Scherer, K. R. (2003). Appraisal processes in emotion. In R. J. Davidson, H. Goldsmith, & K. R. Scherer (Eds.), *Handbook of the affective sciences* (pp. 572–595). New York: Oxford University Press.

Engel, A. K., & Singer, W. (2001). Temporal binding and the neural correlates of sensory awareness. *Trends in Cognitive Sciences, 5*(1), 16–25.

Fazio, R. H. (2001). On the automatic activation of associated evaluations: An overview. *Cognition and Emotion, 15*(2), 115–141.

Fridlund, A. J. (1994). *Human facial expression: An evolutionary view.* San Diego, CA: Academic Press.

Frijda, N. H. (1986). *The emotions.* Cambridge, UK: Cambridge University Press.

Gellhorn, E. (1964). Motion and emotion: The role of proprioception in the physiology and pathology of the emotions. *Psychological Review, 71,* 457–472.

Grandjean, D., & Scherer, K. R. (2003, June). *Appraisal processes in emotion elicitation: A topographic electrophysiological approach.* Poster presented at the Human Brain Mapping conference, New York.

Greenwald, A. G., & Banaji, M. R. (1995). Implicit social cognition: Attitudes, self-esteem, and stereotypes. *Psychological Review, 102*(1), 4–27.

Hameroff, S. R., Kaszniak, A. W., & Scott, A. C. (Eds.). (1996). *Toward a science of consciousness: The first Tucson discussions and debates.* Cambridge, MA: MIT Press.

Iwamura, Y. (1998). Hierarchical somatosensory processing. *Current Opinion in Neurobiology, 8,* 522–528.

Izard, C. E. (1971). *The face of emotion.* New York: Appleton-Century-Crofts.

Kaiser, S., & Scherer, K. R. (1997). Models of "normal" emotions applied to facial and vocal expressions in clinical disorders. In W. F. Flack, Jr., & J. D. Laird (Eds.), *Emotions in psychopathology* (pp. 81–98). New York: Oxford University Press.

Kihlstrom, J. F. (1994). The rediscovery of the unconscious. In H. Morowitz & J. L. Singer (Eds.), *Santa Fe Institute studies in the sciences of complexity: Vol. 22. The mind, the brain, and complex adaptive systems* (pp. 123–143). Reading, MA: Addison Wesley.

Lakoff, G., & Kövecses, Z. (1987). *Women, fire, and dangerous things: What categories reveal about the mind.* Chicago: University of Chicago Press.

Lambie, J. A., & Marcel, A. J. (2002). Consciousness and the varieties of emotion experience: A theoretical framework. *Psychological Review, 109*(2), 219–259.

LeDoux, J. (2000). Cognitive–emotional interactions: Listen to the brain. In R. D. Lane & L. Nadel (Eds.), *Cognitive neuroscience of emotion* (pp. 129–155). New York: Oxford University Press.

Leventhal, H. (1984). A perceptual motor theory of emotion. In K. R. Scherer & P. Ekman (Eds.), *Approaches to emotion* (pp. 271–292). Hillsdale, NJ: Erlbaum.

Leventhal, H., & Scherer, K. R. (1987). The relationship of emotion to cognition: A functional approach to a semantic controversy. *Cognition and Emotion, 1,* 3–28.

Parkinson, B. (1997). Untangling the appraisal–emotion connection. *Personality and Social Psychology Review, 1*(1), 62–79.

Roseman, I. J. (2001). A model of appraisal in the emotion system: Integrating theory, research, and applications. In K. R. Scherer, A. Schorr, & T. Johnstone (Eds.), *Appraisal processes in emotion: Theory, methods, research* (pp. 68–91). Oxford, UK: Oxford University Press.

Russell, J. A. (2003). Core affect and the psychological construction of emotion. *Psychological Review, 110*, 145–172

Russell, J. A., & Barrett, L. F. (1999). Core affect, prototypical emotional episodes, and other things called emotion: Dissecting the elephant. *Journal of Personality and Social Psychology, 76*, 805–819.

Sander, D., Grafman, J., & Zalla, T. (2003). The human amygdala: An evolved system for relevance detection. *Reviews in the Neurosciences, 14*(4), 303–316.

Scherer, K. R. (1984). On the nature and function of emotion: A component process approach. In K. R. Scherer & P. Ekman (Eds.), *Approaches to emotion* (pp. 293–317). Hillsdale, NJ: Erlbaum.

Scherer, K. R. (1992). What does facial expression express? In K. Strongman (Ed.), *International review of studies on emotion* (Vol. 2, pp. 139–165). Chichester, UK: Wiley.

Scherer, K. R. (1993). Neuroscience projections to current debates in emotion psychology. *Cognition and Emotion, 7*, 1–41.

Scherer, K. R. (1994). Toward a concept of "modal emotions." In P. Ekman & R. J. Davidson (Eds.), *The nature of emotion: Fundamental questions* (pp. 25–31). New York: Oxford University Press.

Scherer, K. R. (1999). Appraisal theories. In T. Dalgleish & M. Power (Eds.), *Handbook of cognition and emotion* (pp. 637–663). Chichester, UK: Wiley.

Scherer, K. R. (2000a). Emotions as episodes of subsystem synchronization driven by nonlinear appraisal processes. In M. D. Lewis & I. Granic (Eds.), *Emotion, development, and self-organization: Dynamic systems approaches to emotional development* (pp. 70–99). New York: Cambridge University Press.

Scherer, K. R. (2000b). Psychological models of emotion. In J. Borod (Ed.), *The neuropsychology of emotion* (pp. 137–162). Oxford, UK: Oxford University Press.

Scherer, K. R. (2001a). Appraisal considered as a process of multi-level sequential checking. In K. R. Scherer, A. Schorr, & T. Johnstone (Eds.), *Appraisal processes in emotion: Theory, methods, research* (pp. 92–120). New York: Oxford University Press.

Scherer, K. R. (2001b). The nature and study of appraisal: A review of the issues. In K. R. Scherer, A. Schorr, & T. Johnstone (Eds.). *Appraisal processes in emotion: Theory, methods, research* (pp. 369–391). New York: Oxford University Press.

Scherer, K. R. (2004a). Feelings integrate the central representation of appraisal-driven response organization in emotion. In A. S. R. Manstead, N. H. Frijda, & A. H. Fischer (Eds.), *Feelings and emotions: The Amsterdam symposium* (pp. 136–157). Cambridge, UK: Cambridge University Press.

Scherer, K. R. (2004b). Which emotions can be induced by music? What are the underlying mechanisms? And how can we measure them? *Journal of New Music Research, 33*(3), 239–251.

Scherer, K. R., Abeles, R. P., & Fischer, C. S. (1975). *Human aggression and conflict: Interdisciplinary perspectives*. Englewood Cliffs, NJ: Prentice Hall.

Scherer, K. R., Dan, E., & Flykt, A. (in press). What determines a feeling's position in three-dimensional affect space? *Cognition and Emotion*.

Scherer, K. R., Schorr, A., & Johnstone, T. (Eds.). (2001). *Appraisal processes in emotion: Theory, methods, research*. New York: Oxford University Press.

Schneider, W., & Shiffrin, R. M. (1977). Controlled and automatic human information processing: I. Detection, search, and attention. *Psychological Review, 84*(1), 1–66.

Shallice, T. (1972). Dual functions of consciousness. *Psychological Review, 79*(5), 383–393.

Smith, C. A., & Scott, H. S. (1997). A componential approach to the meaning of facial expressions. In J. A. Russell & J. M. Fernandez-Dols (Eds.), *The psychology of facial expression* (pp. 229–254). New York: Cambridge University Press.

Tallon-Baudry, C., Bertrand, O., Delpuech, C., & Pernier, J. (1996). Stimulus specificity of phase-locked and non-phase-locked 40 Hz visual responses in human. *Journal of Neuroscience, 16*, 4240–4249.

Treisman, A. (1996). The binding problem. *Current Opinion in Neurobiology, 6*, 171–178.

Vaitl, D. (1996). Interoception. *Biological Psychology, 42*(1–2), 1–27.

van Reekum, C., Banse, R., Johnstone, T., Etter, A., Wehrle, T., & Scherer, K. R. (2004). Psychophysiological responses to emotion-antecedent appraisal in a computer game. *Cognition and Emotion, 18*(5), 663–688.

Vuilleumier, P., Armony, J. L., Driver, J., & Dolan, R. J. (2001). Effects of attention and emotion on face processing in the human brain: An event-related fMRI study. *Neuron, 3*, 829–841.

Vuilleumier, P., & Schwartz, S. (2001). Beware and be aware: Capture of spatial attention by fear-related stimuli in neglect. *NeuroReport, 12*(6), 1119–1122.

Whalen, P. J. (1998). Fear, vigilance, and ambiguity: Initial neuroimaging studies of the human amygdala. *Current Directions in Psychological Science, 7*(6), 177–188.

Whalen, P. J., Curran, T., & Rauch, S. L. (2001). Using neuroimaging to study implicit information processing. In D. D. Dougherty & S. L. Rauch (Eds.), *Psychiatric neuroimaging research: Contemporary strategies* (pp. 73–100). Washington, DC: American Psychiatric Association.

Whalen, P. J., Shin, L. M., McInerney, S. C., Fischer, H., Wright, C. I., & Rauch, S. L. (2001). A functional MRI study of human amygdala responses to facial expressions of fear versus anger. *Emotion, 1*(1), 70–83.

Wundt, W. (1911). *Grundzüge der physiologischen Psychologie*, 6th ed. [Principles of physiological psychology]. Leipzig, Germany: Engelmann. (Original work published 1874)

CHAPTER 14

Emotion, Behavior, and Conscious Experience

Once More without Feeling

PIOTR WINKIELMAN

KENT C. BERRIDGE

JULIA L. WILBARGER

This chapter focuses on the relation of unconscious components of emotion to conscious feeling. By *conscious feeling* we mean the experiential, phenomenological, "what-it's-like" aspect of emotion. We ask whether valenced states—affect and emotion—can exist as well as drive the organism's behavior without participation of conscious feeling. The question is controversial because, as we will see shortly, there is a tradition in the human emotion literature to view conscious feeling as central for emotion.

The chapter is structured as follows. First, we summarize the traditional view on emotion and conscious feeling. Second, we argue for the idea of unconscious or unfelt emotion. Third, we address some of the empirical and philosophical challenges of this idea. Fourth, we address the relation between conscious and unconscious components of emotion.

EMOTION WITH FEELING

Definitions

An old line says there are more emotion definitions than emotion researchers. However, if there is one definition on which most researchers agree, it

1. *What is the scope of your proposed model? When you use the term* emotion, *how do you use it? What do you mean by terms such as* fear, anxiety, *or* happiness?

We think of emotion as a state in which several systems of the organism are directed toward a specific valence. As we discuss in the section titled "Definitions," it is typically assumed that emotion is characterized by loosely coordinated changes in several components, including (a) conscious feeling, (b) perception and cognition, (c) action tendency, (d) bodily expression, and (e) physiology. Our chapter examines whether the conscious feeling component is indeed necessary for emotion in human and nonhuman animals. We conclude that it is not.

2. *Define your terms:* conscious, unconscious, awareness. *Or say why you do not use these terms.*

One important aspect of consciousness is the potential of the organism to introspect about a state and to express it verbally or nonverbally. As we argue in the chapter, sometimes an emotion state can be principally unconscious, that is, unavailable to the systems responsible for expression and introspection, even under proper motivational and cognitive conditions.

3. *Does your model deal with what is conscious, what is unconscious, or their relationship? If you do not address this area specifically, can you speculate on the relationship between what is conscious and unconscious? Or if you do not like the conscious–unconscious distinction, or if you do not think this is a good question to ask, can you say why?*

The relation between conscious and unconscious aspects of emotion involves a complex set of psychological and neural factors. Conscious aspects of emotion probably emerge from a hierarchy of unconscious emotional processes, implemented by interactive brain systems that form reciprocal connections across subcortical and cortical networks. Some specific factors are discussed in our section "What Makes Emotion Unconscious or Conscious?"

---

is probably close to this. Emotion is a state characterized by loosely coordinated changes in the following five components: (1) *feeling*—changes in subjective experience; (2) *cognition*—changes in attentional and perceptual biases, low-level appraisals, and high-level beliefs; (3) *action*—changes in the predisposition for specific responses and the general behavioral direction; (4) *expression*—changes in facial, vocal, postural appearance; and (5) *physiology*—changes in the central and peripheral nervous systems. This definition is presented in several classic textbooks on emotions and is used throughout this volume (e.g., Atkinson & Adoplphs, Chapter 7; Scherer, Chapter 13; but for a critical position, see Barrett, Chapter 11).

It is also useful to distinguish between affect and emotion. The term *affect* describes a state that can be identified primarily by its positive–negative valence. The term *emotion* describes a state that can be identified by more than its valence and includes specific types of negative states (e.g., fear, guilt, anger, sadness, disgust) and specific positive states (e.g., happiness, love, pride). Throughout this chapter we primarily use the term *emotion* because we believe that our arguments also apply to specific emotion states, even though the empirical evidence for our position has been obtained primarily in the domain of affect. We return to this issue later.

Theories of Emotion: Feeling as a Central Component

Theorists have long recognized that there are many components of emotion. Typically they have considered feeling as a central or even a necessary component. Consider some of the influential theorists. In "What Is An Emotion?" William James proposes that *conscious feeling*, generated through the perception of bodily changes, is exactly what distinguishes emotion from other mental states. Without it, "we find that we have nothing left behind, no 'mind-stuff' out of which the emotion can be constituted" (James, 1884, p. 193). Similarly, Freud, though often portrayed as the father of the unconscious, specifically excluded emotions from the realm of states that can exist without being experienced. Freud believed that emotions are always conscious, even if their underlying causes sometimes are not: "It is surely of the essence of an emotion that we should feel it, i.e. that it should enter consciousness." (Freud, 1950, pp. 109–110). These assumptions are shared by contemporary theorists. Clore (1994) titled one of his essays "Why Emotions Are Never Unconscious" and declared subjective feeling as a necessary (although not a sufficient) condition for emotion (see also Clore, Storbeck, Robinson, & Centerbar, Chapter 16). In defining affect, Frijda says that the term "primarily refers to hedonic *experience*, the experience of pleasure and pain" (1999, p. 194; emphasis added). In short, past and present theorists of human emotion emphasize the centrality of conscious feeling.[1]

Emotion Research: Feeling as a Central Agenda

The feeling component is emphasized not only in theories but also in research on human emotion. In social-psychological studies, for example, the presence of an emotion is typically determined by self-reports of feelings (e.g., mood questionnaires, affective checklists, interviews). When studies collect multiple measures of emotion, including the cognitive, behavioral, expressive, or physiological components, the self-report is often considered as the "gold standard" for determining whether emotion had occurred (Larsen & Fredrickson, 1999). There is also a lot of substantive interest in the nature of feelings. For example, some of the debates in emotion literature concern the contribution of bodily responses to feelings (Niedenthal, Barsalou, Ric, & Krauth-Gruber, Chapter 2; Prinz, Chapter 15), the dimensional structure of feelings (Russell, 2003), individual differences in the valence versus arousal component of feelings (Barrett, Chapter 11), the role of culture in type and frequency of feelings (Mesquita & Markus, 2004), and the simultaneous coexistence of positive and negative feelings (Cacioppo, Larsen, Smith, & Berntson, 2004).

Most important, conscious feeling is seen as a central causal force in emotional impact on behavior. One example comes from research on judgment. A dominant model, tellingly called "feeling-as-information," proposes that emotions influence judgment via changes in conscious feelings, which people use as a shortcut to judgment, following the "how-do-I-feel-about-it-heuristic" (Clore et al., Chapter 16; Schwarz & Clore, 2003). The feeling-as-information model has received strong empirical support and certainly captures many cases of affective influence on judgment. However, most studies testing this model relied on manipulations designed to produce conscious feeling states, using stimuli such as music, movies, recall of autobiographical memories, etc. Yet the model is silent on the mechanism by which emotional stimuli that do not change feelings could influence judgments and behavior.

EMOTION WITHOUT FEELING

As we have just shown, conscious feeling has a central place in both the theoretical thinking and empirical practice of human emotion research. However, do emotions always require consciousness? Can one meaningfully talk about "unfelt" or "unconscious" emotions? Over the last several years, researchers have increasingly started to consider these possibilities.

Unconscious Elicitation of Emotion

The first challenge to the role of consciousness in emotion came from demonstrations that subliminal stimuli trigger emotional reactions. These demonstrations are now widely accepted in the emotion research community. In fact, in a recent *Emotion Researcher*, newsletter of the International Society for Emotion Research (2004), on the issue of "unconscious emotion," no contributor expressed doubts that emotion can be elicited outside of awareness or attention.

An example of a subliminal elicitation of positive affect comes from research on the mere-exposure effect, or the increase in preference to repeated items (Kunst-Wilson & Zajonc, 1980). In one study, participants were first subliminally exposed to several repeated neutral stimuli consisting of random visual patterns. Later those participants reported being in a better mood than participants who had been subliminally exposed to different nonrepeated neutral stimuli (Monahan, Murphy, & Zajonc, 2000). An example of a subliminal induction of negative affect comes from studies in which subliminal stimuli, such as gory scenes embedded in a movie or pictures of snakes presented to phobic participants, led to an increase in self-reported anxiety (Öhman & Soares, 1994; Robles, Smith, Carver, & Wellens, 1987).

Note, however, that in these studies only the affect-triggering stimulus is unconscious; the affective reaction itself is conscious. Indeed, the very presence of the affective reaction is determined by asking people to self-report. Thus it is useful, instead, to look at other studies that tested the presence of an affective reaction using physiological measures. For example, skin conductance response, an indicator of sympathetic arousal, can be triggered by subliminally presented emotional words (Lazarus & McCleary, 1951) and by pictures of fear-relevant objects (Lundqvist & Öhman, Chapter 5). Similarly, subliminal facial expressions activate the amygdala, a structure involved in assigning affective significance to stimuli (Whalen et al., 1998), and elicit facial reactions detectable with electromyography (Dimberg, Thunberg, & Elmehed, 2000) (for a review, see Lundqvist & Öhman, Chapter 5; de Gelder, Chapter 6; Atkinson & Adolphs, Chapter 7; and Öhman, Flykt, & Lundqvist, 2000). Unfortunately, these studies are not conclusive on the question of unconscious emotion. First, the physiological measures used in these studies cannot distinguish between the arousal and valence components of a response, or may reflect other processes such as facial mimicry. Thus it is not clear if a valenced reaction actually occurred. Second, in these studies self-reports of emotion were either not collected or collected after the physiological measure of affective reactions, so it is not clear if the reaction registered in physiology was itself conscious or not. Third, because these studies did not measure behavioral consequences, it is possible that any emotion reaction was extremely weak and possibly inconsequential. Still, the physiological studies are suggestive and raise the possibility that under right conditions, people could have genuine affective reactions that are not manifested in their conscious experience.

Unconscious Emotion

Over the last several years we have offered theoretical arguments and empirical support for the idea of unconscious emotion (Berridge & Winkielman, 2003; Winkielman & Berridge, 2004). Our views are in agreement with several other authors. For example, Kihlstrom (1999) suggested that the term *implicit emotion* could be used to refer to "changes in experience, thought or action that are attributable to one's emotional state, independent of his or her conscious awareness of that state" (p. 432). Damasio (1999) and LeDoux (1996) described how deep brain structures participate in generating an unconscious stage of fear, anger, happiness, and sadness reactions. Lambie and Marcel (2002) suggested that there are "several kinds of unawareness of genuine concurrent emotion" (p. 220), including "an entirely nonconscious emotion state" (p. 229).[2]

In the next several sections we review the main theoretical and empirical arguments for the idea that emotion may exist independent of conscious experience. First, we present functional and evolutionary considerations. Second, we review evidence from research on the emotional brain. Third, we discuss relevant psychological studies. Fourth, we address theoretical and empirical challenges to the notion of unconscious emotion and address outstanding issues.

Functional and Evolutionary Considerations

Does the capacity for emotional behavior evolutionarily precede, follow, or co-occur with the capacity for conscious feeling? This is a difficult question as it involves making historical assumptions about the conjunction of two complex mental faculties: emotion and consciousness (Heyes & Huber, 2001). It is more manageable to ask whether basic affective reactions require conscious processing. Consider simple positive/negative reactions that animals produce to stimuli such as predators, prey, strangers, conspecifics, food, drink, or mates (Konorski, 1967). The function of these affective reactions is to allow animals to react appropriately to favorable or unfavorable events by adjusting sensory apparatus (e.g., prioritizing certain stimuli), physiology (e.g., cardiovascular and hormonal changes), and action (e.g., priming of motor programs). From a design standpoint, it would be disadvantageous if performing this basic function required the organism to possess a cognitive apparatus capable of consciousness (Cosmides & Tooby, 2000). Though little is known about the exact mechanisms of consciousness, it is unlikely it can be implemented by the computational architecture of simple organisms (Dennett, 1991; Prinz, Chapter 15). Further, even in humans, conscious mechanisms are often too slow and imprecise to coordinate an emotional response (Smith & Neumann, Chapter 12). Most important, consciousness is often unnecessary. After all, many relatively complex coordination functions in organisms are efficiently performed without experiential representation (e.g., coupling between the cardiovascular, respiratory, and digestive systems, Porges, 1997). In short, it is reasonable to assume that at least basic affective reactions can be performed without engaging mechanisms responsible for conscious feelings (LeDoux, 1996).

One standard challenge psychologists sometimes offer to the above arguments is that positive/negative reactions of simple organisms should not be called *affective*. For example, paramecia can approach a variety of stimuli, but it makes little sense to use the term *positive affect* for an organism that does not even have neurons. Further, even in more complex organisms, many reactions to favorable or unfavorable stimuli are more aptly classified as reflexes, than affective behaviors. For example, when a spider jumps to kill a prey, it makes little sense to explain this behavior by proposing an underlying negative affect state. We agree, and along with most authors, require that to count as affective, the behavior should meet several criteria (Scherer, Chapter 13). First, the organism must be able to assess the input in terms of valence. Second, this assessment must lead to a temporary state that involves several synchronized components (i.e., perceptual, hormonal, cardiovascular, muscular). Importantly, these criteria do not require the organism to explicitly represent its goals or explicitly make emotional "judgments"—only to respond in a coherent way to challenges and opportunities in their environment (see Prinz, Chapter 15).

Given these criteria, affect perhaps should *not* be assigned to reflexes or to creatures such as paramecia. However, it should be assigned to organisms that respond in a coherent, multisystemic fashion to challenges and opportunities, even if these organisms have little cognitive capacity for consciousness. For example, under these criteria, reptiles are capable of affect because they show coherent cardiovascular, hormonal, perceptual, and behavioral responses to favorable and unfavorable stimuli (Cabanac, 1999). In fact, there are many structural homologies between the reptilian and the mammalian limbic system (Martinez-Garcia, Martinez-Marcos, & Lanuza, 2002), and there are also remarkable similarities in the affective neurochemistry in reptiles, fish, birds, and mammals (Goodson & Bass, 2001).

In short, the available data suggest that vertebrates are capable of coordinated, multisystemic responses to emotionally relevant stimuli, via homologous neural circuitry that regulates these responses across a diversity of vertebrate groups. Thus, while it seems inarguable that the neural substrates required for conscious experience are quite different across these groups, there is nonetheless remarkable consistency in other components of affective response. It therefore seems reasonable to propose that neural components of emotional processing can function in a way that is largely uncoupled from the neural components of consciousness.

Neuroscientific Considerations

These evolutionary arguments are consistent with research on modern mammalian brains. As we discuss next, both subcortical and cortical structures participate in affective processes. However, as many have suggested, the "old" subcortical structures might be especially important for basic affective reactions, whereas the "new" cortical structures might be especially important for conscious feelings. The locations of the most important structures of the generalized emotional brain are indicated in Figure 14.1. Below we provide a brief overview of what is known about the roles of these structures in generating positive and negative affect. However, we remind the reader that our presentation here is very simplified and does not capture the multiple roles these structures play in both affect and cognition, and their complex neuroanatomy and neurochemistry (see Berridge, 2003).

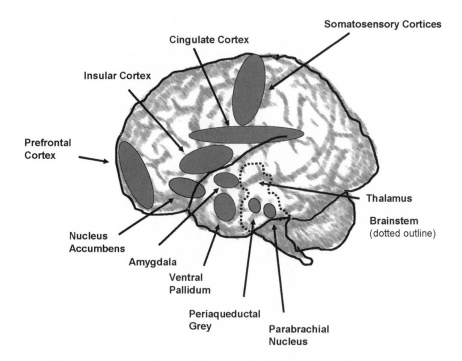

FIGURE 14.1. Approximate location of brain structures important for emotion. The figure does not show the relative depth of any structure and shows only one of each pair of bilateral structures.

Subcortical Networks and Basic Affective Reactions

The subcortical structures involved in causing basic affective reactions range from the "mere" brainstem to the complex network of the "extended amygdala" (Berridge, 2003). Let us illustrate the critical role of these structures in both positive and negative affect with a few examples.

Brainstem. Though some view it as a merely reflexive structure, almost every physical pleasure or pain must climb its way up through the brainstem. Research shows that in both animals and humans basic affective responses are modulated by structures in the brainstem. For example, in the domain of positive affect, research highlights the importance of the parabrachial nucleus (PBN). The PBN receives signals ascending from many sensory modalities, including visceral signals regarding internal bodily functions, and also taste sensations from the tongue.[3] Not surprisingly, PBN plays a role in generating positive responses to tasty foods. For example, when a rat's PBN is tweaked by microinjections that activate its benzodiazepine/gamma-aminobutyric acid (GABA) receptors, the rat produces greater "liking" reactions to sugar, such as tongue protrusions and lip licking (Berridge & Pecina, 1995). In the domain of negative affect, research highlights the importance of the periaqueductal grey (PAG). In animals, the PAG mediates defensive reactions to threatening stimuli (Panksepp, 1998), and in both animals and humans, the PAG mediates responses to pain (Willis & Westlund, 1997). Importantly, the PAG does not simply compile incoming information to relay to the forebrain, but forms reciprocal connections with subcortical forebrain structures, thereby providing an anatomical basis by which sensory stimuli can be processed by the PAG in a context-dependent and coordinated fashion (Panksepp, 1998).

A particularly poignant demonstration of the importance of the brainstem to basic affective reactions is offered by a cruel experiment of nature. As a result of a birth defect, some infants have a congenitally malformed brain, possessing only a brainstem but no cortex and little else of the forebrain (i.e., no amygdala, nucleus accumbens, etc). Yet in these anencephalic infants, the sweet taste of sugar still elicits facial expressions that resemble normal "liking" reactions, such as lip sucking and smiles, whereas bitter tastes elicit facial expressions that resemble "disliking" reactions, such as mouth gapes or nose wrinkling (Steiner, 1973). In this context, it is also interesting that positive facial expressions to sweetness are emitted by chimpanzees, orangutans, gorillas, various monkeys, and even rats (Berridge, 2000; Steiner, Glaser, Hawilo, & Berridge, 2001). The pattern of positive facial expression becomes increasingly less similar to humans as the taxonomic distance increases between a species and us. But all of these species share some reaction components that are homologous to ours, suggesting common evolutionary ancestry and a similar neural mechanism that might be anchored in the brainstem.

Extended Amygdala. The term *extended amygdala* designates a configuration that includes the amygdala, nucleus accumbens, ventral pallidum, bed nucleus of the stria terminalis, and other structures. Recent years have witnessed an explosion of research highlighting the role of the extended amygdala in basic affective reactions.

Amygdala. The amygdala consists of a pair of almond-shaped structures located in the medial temporal lobe, just anterior to the hippocampus. The amygdala is reciprocally connected to a variety of areas, including the visual thalamus and visual cortex, allowing for affective modification of perception; the dorsolateral prefrontal cortex, allowing for upstream and downstream regulation of affect state; and subcortical structures, allowing for affective influence on sympathetic and parasympathetic regulation of cardiovascular activity, respiration, hormone levels, and basic muscular reactions. The role of the amygdala in perceptual and learning aspects of emotion has been confirmed in animal research as well as human neuroimaging and lesion studies (Phelps, Chapter 3; Atkinson & Adolphs, Chapter 7). Thus patients with congenital or acquired amygdala damage show impairments in conditioned fear responses, fear-potentiated startle responses, and arousal-enhanced perception and memory. Remarkably, patients with damage to the amygdala show little, if any, impairment in their subjective experience of emotion, at least as measured by the magnitude and frequency of self-reported positive and negative affect assessed by the positive and negative affect schedule (PANAS) (Anderson & Phelps, 2002). This finding suggests a relative independence of the amygdala from the mechanisms underlying the generation of feelings.

There is also evidence that the amygdala can modulate emotional responses independent of any conscious evaluation of the stimulus. Some of this evidence comes from observations that the amygdala can be activated with facial expressions that are not consciously perceived, presumably via a direct pathway from the visual thalamus (see Atkinson & Adolphs, Chapter 7). Thus amygdala activation has been observed with expressions of fear and anger presented subliminally (Morris, Öhman, & Dolan, 1999; Whalen et al., 1998), under condition of binocular suppression (Williams, Morris, McGlone, Abbott, & Mattingley, 2004), or to a patient's blind visual field (de Gelder, Chapter 6).

Additional evidence for the independence of basic affective reactions and conscious stimulus evaluation comes from autism—a neurodevelopmental disorder characterized by deficits in communicative and social skills, restricted interests, repetitive behaviors, and impairments in emotional abilities (Hobson, 1993; Kasari, Sigman, Yirmiya, & Mundy, 1993). There are several reports of amygdala abnormalities in people with autism (Baron-Cohen et al., 2000). Thus one can expect individuals with autism to be impaired in their basic affective responses, which are dependent on the amygdala, and relatively unimpaired on affective responses that rely on more deliberate, conscious strategies. We have recently obtained such evidence in studies of affective startle modulation (Wilbarger, McIntosh, & Winkielman, 2004) which refers to a phenomenon that when individuals are startled by a loud noise, their defensive reflexes, such as the eyeblink, are larger in the context of negative than positive stimuli. This penomenon presumably reflects the modulation of an aversive versus approach response system (Lang, 1995). The amygdala is critical for such modulation, as suggested by the finding that electrical stimulation of the amygdala enhances startle amplitude, whereas lesions diminish it (Davis, 1997; Funayama, Grillon, Davis, & Phelps, 2001; Phelps, Chapter 3). In our studies the individuals without autism replicated the classic startle modulation pattern: potentiation of an eyeblink response to a loud noise after negative pictures and reduction of the eyeblink after positive pictures. In contrast, the individuals with autism spectrum disorder (ASD) showed startle potentiation after both negative *and* positive stimuli. Importantly, the ASD individuals did not differ from typical individuals on conscious, explicit evaluation of the stimuli, as reflected in self-reports of valence and arousal (Wilbarger et al., 2004). In sum, these data again suggest that the impact of affective stimuli on basic behavioral responses can be dissociated from conscious responses to the same stimuli.

Ventral Pallidum. The ventral pallidum borders on the lateral hypothalamus at its front and lateral sides and is a part of the extended amygdala. In rats, this structure is involved in producing positive reactions to tasty foods, as suggested by the facts that (1) ventral pallidal neurons fire to tasty rewards, (2) behavioral "liking" reactions to sweetness are increased by opioid drug microinjections in the ventral pallidum, and (3) excitotoxin lesions of the ventral pallidum abolish hedonic reactions and cause aversive reactions (e.g., gaping and headshakes) to be elicited even by normally palatable foods (Cromwell & Berridge, 1993; Tindell, Berridge, & Aldridge, 2004). The ventral pallidum may also be crucial to sexual and social pair bonding in rodents (Insel & Fernald, 2004). Less is known regarding the role of the ventral pallidum in affect mediation for humans, because the structure is too small to study via brain imaging. However, there are a few intriguing observations. For example, electrical stimulation of the adjacent structure, the globus pallidus, has been reported to sometimes induce bouts of affective mania that can last for days (Miyawaki, Perlmutter, Troster, Videen, & Koller, 2000). In addition, the induction of a state of sexual or competitive arousal in normal men was found to be accompanied by increased blood flow in the ventral globus pallidus (Rauch et al., 1999).

Nucleus Accumbens. The nucleus accumbens, which lies at the front of the subcortical forebrain and is rich in dopamine and opioid neurotransmitter systems, is as famous for positive affective states as the amygdala is for fearful ones. The accumbens systems are often portrayed as reward and pleasure systems. In fact, activation of dopamine projections to the accumbens and related targets has been viewed by many neuroscientists as a neural "common currency" for reward. There is actually evidence that the accumbens reflects not "pleasure" or "liking" of the stimulus, but rather an incentive salience, or "wanting," of the stimulus (Berridge & Robinson, 1998). However, for the purpose of our argument here it is only important to highlight the role of the accumbens in positive affective reactions. For example, in rats, brain microinjections of drug droplets that activate opioid receptors in the nucleus accumbens cause increased "liking" for sweetness (Pecina & Berridge, 2000). In humans, the accumbens activates to drug cues and to other desired stimuli, including foods, drinks, and even money (Knutson, Adams, Fong, & Hommer, 2001).

Cortical Networks and Subjective Experience

We cannot talk about the emotional brain of mammals without discussing the cortex. In fact, when human subjects spontaneously recall emotional events, a host of cortical structures activate, including the prefrontal cortex, the insular cortex, the somatosensory cortices, and the cingulate cortex (Damasio et al., 2000). The approximate location of these structures is shown in Figure 14.1. Several chapters in this volume address the role of cortical structures in more detail (Niedenthal et al., Chapter 2; Phelps, Chapter 3; Gray, Schaefer, Braver, & Most, Chapter 4; Atkinson & Adolphs, Chapter 7; Prinz, Chapter 15; other chapters suggest it: Barrett, Chapter 11; Clore et al., Chapter 16). Here we only mention research most relevant to the proposition that the cortex mediates conscious experience by hierarchically monitoring and rerepresenting subcortical processes.

Prefrontal Cortex. The prefrontal cortex lies, not surprisingly, at the very front of the brain. The ventral or bottom one-third of the prefrontal cortex is called the orbitofrontal cortex and is the most elaborately developed in humans and other primates. There is some evidence that subcortical projections to the prefrontal cortex contribute to conscious affective experience. For example, the intense feeling of pleasure experienced by heroin users appears to involve accumbens-to-cortex signals that are relayed to cortical regions via the ventral pallidum and thalamus (Wise, 1996). In another example, self-reports of excitement in typical participants are related to the degree of activation in the nucleus accumbens and prefrontal cortex (Knutson et al., 2004). The prefrontal cortex is important not only for conscious feelings; it also participates in affective reactions by modulating lower brain structures via descending projections (Damasio, 1999; Phan, Wagner, Taylor, & Liberzon, 2002). For example, the orbitofrontal cortex projects back to the accumbens (Davidson, Jackson, & Kalin, 2000), and the dorsolateral prefrontal cortex projects back to the amygdala (Ochsner & Gross, 2004).

Somatosensory Cortex and Insula. The primary (S1) and secondary (S2) somatosensory cortices are located behind the central sulcus and are responsible for monitoring the state of the body, including sensations (e.g., touch) and proprioception (i.e., state of muscles and joints), and for creating the internal "image" of the body (Ramachandran & Blakeslee, 1998). The insula is located near the bottom of the somatosensory cortices, almost at the intersection of the frontal, parietal, and temporal lobes, and receives inputs from limbic structures, such as the amygdala, and cortical structures, such as the prefrontal and posterior parietal cortices and the anterior cingulate. It appears to be particularly important for introception: monitoring the state of internal organs (Craig, 2003; Critchley, Wiens, Rothstein, Öhman, & Dolan, 2004).

There is evidence that the somatosensory cortices and the insula might jointly contribute to emotional experience by generating a model of the current body state. The neuropsychological evidence for this mechanism is extensively discussed by Atkinson and Adolphs (Chapter 7), and psychological evidence is reviewed by Niedenthal et al. (Chapter 2). For example, neuroimaging studies show that recall of emotional memories is associated with extensive activation of the somatosensory cortices (Damasio et al., 2000). In another example, lesions to the right somatosensory cortex are associated with both impaired perception of facial expressions and impaired touch perception (Adolphs, Domasio, Tranel, Cooper, & Domasio, 2000). Finally, human studies show involvement of the insula in pain (Peyron, Laurent, & Garcia-Larrea, 2000), disgust (Wicker, Keyers, Plailly,

Royet, Gallese, & Rizzolatti, 2003), and appreciation of sweet tastes and related rewards (O'Doherty, Deichmann, Critchley, & Dolan, 2002).

Cingulate Cortex. The cingulate cortex consists of a longitudinal strip running front to back along the midline of each brain hemisphere. It is a richly interconnected structure thought to interface between the limbic system and the prefrontal cortex. The cingulate cortex has been implicated in human clinical conditions such as pain, depression, anxiety, and other distressing states (Davidson, Abercrombie, Nitschke, & Putnam, 1999; Peyron et al., 2000). Interestingly, some research suggests that a conscious experience of emotion, per se (e.g., "I'm angry"), is associated with the dorsal anterior region of the cingulate cortex, whereas more reflective parts of the emotional awareness (e.g., "I know I'm angry"), are associated with the rostral anterior region (Lane, 2000).

Interactions of Cortical and Subcortical Networks

As our brief review indicates, both subcortical and cortical systems participate in emotion as a complex network connected in multiple loops. Within those loops, however, the subcortical systems seem essential for triggering basic affective reactions, whereas the cortical systems seem essential for supporting conscious affective experience. Specifically, the conscious experience appears to emerge from the interaction between the cortical and subcortical loops, as the cortex hierarchically rerepresents and feeds back on the causally active subcortical processes. Importantly, we are not diminishing the causal role of the cortex in emotion; as obviously, for humans, many events trigger an emotional response after extensive cortical processing. We are simply suggesting that in order to have a conscious emotional experience, the cortical networks may need to receive and reprocess input from subcortical networks.

Is it possible that conscious feelings exist subcortically, perhaps in structures as deep as the brainstem's periaqueductal grey (PAG)? For example, Panksepp argued that "the most basic form of conscious activity . . . arises from the intrinsic neurodynamics of the PAG" (1998, p. 314) and suggested that "it is the PAG that allows creatures to first cry out in distress and pleasure" (p. 314). We agree that it is logically possible that brainstem circuits generate a rudimentary but real consciousness. This possibility can never be conclusively disproved. For now, it seems more likely that these subcortical circuits simply instantiate unconscious affective process. Those processes do not give rise to conscious feelings by themselves. They are not even directly accessible to conscious introspection in a normal brain, as evidenced by people's inability to report subliminally induced affect (discussed shortly). Accordingly, we propose that the isolated brainstem is capable of unconscious "likes" and "dislikes," which it reflects behaviorally, but not of conscious feelings of pleasure or displeasure.

Finally, it is worth highlighting that our point really is not about anatomical separation—a neat division of labor in which subcortical networks instantiate unconscious processes, whereas cortical networks instantiate conscious processes. Our point is that the *mechanisms* of consciousness are computationally demanding and require ability to rerepresent the input, integrate across multiple sources of input, and probably create some rudimentary representation of the self (Dennett, 1991). On that view, different mechanisms could be mixed together in the same brain divisions, or the same brain divisions could have both conscious and unconscious modes.

In sum, the multiplicity of loops and levels within brain networks raises the possibility for functional decoupling, possibly producing emotional reactions without conscious feelings, as well as conscious feelings without emotional reactions reflected in physiology or behavior. In fact, some research reviewed earlier could be interpreted as showing a double dissociation (A occurs without B, and B occurs without A). For example, "liking" responses in anacephalic babies represent the preservation of basic affective reactions after damage to mechanisms supporting consciousness (Steiner, 1973), whereas intact conscious feelings in patients without the amygdala (Anderson & Phelps, 2002) represent preservation of conscious experience after damage to subcortical mechanisms supporting basic affective reactions. This possibility is consistent with research in experimental psychology, as we review next.

Experimental Psychology

All statements about whether emotion can or cannot be divided into conscious versus unconscious are mere speculations. Without actual evidence of unconscious emotion, even positing its existence is a matter of taste. Neuroscientific evidence by itself is suggestive, but not enough—it could be consistent with either possibility. Further, much of neuroscientific evidence comes from animal studies and studies of brain-damaged patients. What is needed is an unambiguous demonstration of unconscious emotion—if it indeed exists—in typical individuals who are not brain damaged, not drug addicted, not under hypnosis, not under extreme circumstance, and not lacking in verbal or intellectual skills. If evidence could actually be obtained, then the discussion would shift from *whether* unconscious emotion is possible to *how* it is possible and *what it means* for psychology and neuroscience. So—is there any clear evidence?

Uncorrected and Unremembered Affective Reactions to Facial Expression

An initial approach to the question of whether participants can be unaware of their affective responses was made in a study that asked participants to rate novel and neutral stimuli, such as Chinese ideographs (Winkielman, Zajonc, & Schwarz, 1997). Unbeknownst to the participants, some ideographs were preceded by subliminally presented happy or angry faces. As mentioned earlier, neuroimaging studies suggest that subliminal angry and fearful faces activate the amygdala and related limbic structures, and are particularly likely to trigger unconscious affective reactions. As participants were making judgments of the ideographs, some were asked to monitor changes in their conscious feelings and told not to use their feelings as a source of their preference ratings. Those participants were also given instructions containing plausible alternative explanations for why their feelings might change, such as music playing in the background, or, closer to the truth, participants were told about invisible subliminal stimuli that might influence their mood. In effect, these instructions encouraged corrective attributions that typically eliminate the contaminating influence of conscious feelings on evaluative judgments (Clore, 1994). However, even for participants who knew to disregard their "contaminated" feelings, the subliminal happy faces increased, and the subliminal angry faces decreased, preference ratings. Most relevant to the question of unconscious emotion, participants did not remember experiencing any changes in their mood when asked after the experiment about their emotions. Still, these studies are subject to criticism. Affective memory is not infallible. A skeptic could well argue that participants had a conscious emotional experience when exposed to subliminal affective faces, but simply failed to remember it later. Further, misattributional manipulations can fail for a variety of cognitive and motivational reasons.

Unconscious Affective Reactions Strong Enough to Change Behavior

We agree that stronger evidence is needed. Such evidence would show that cognitively able and motivated participants are *unable to report a conscious feeling* at the same time that their behavior reveals the *presence of an affective reaction*. Ideally, the affective reaction should be strong enough to change even behavior that has real consequences for the individual. To obtain such evidence, we assessed consumption behavior, requiring ingestion of a novel substance, after exposing participants to several subliminal emotional facial expressions (either happy, neutral, or angry). Each of the subliminal expressions was masked by a clearly visible neutral face on which participants performed a simple gender detection task (Winkielman, Berridge, & Wilbarger, 2005). Immediately after the subliminal affect induction, some participants rated their feelings (mood and arousal) and then consumed a fruit beverage. Other participants performed consumption behavior and feeling ratings in opposite order. In Study 1, the consumption behavior involved pouring themselves a cup of a novel drink from a pitcher and then drinking it. In Study 2, participants were asked to take a small sip of the drink and rate it on different dimensions (e.g., monetary value). In both studies, there was no evidence of any change in conscious mood or arousal, regardless of whether participants rated their feelings on a simple scale from positive to negative or on a multi-item scale asking about specific emotions. That is, participants did not feel more positive after viewing subliminal happy expressions, nor did they feel more negative after angry expressions. Yet participants' consumption behavior and drink ratings were influenced by those subliminal affective stimuli, especially when participants were thirsty. Specifically, thirsty participants exposed to subliminal happy faces poured significantly more drink from the pitcher and drank more from their cup than those exposed to subliminal angry faces (Study 1). Thirsty participants were also willing to pay about twice as much more for the drink after exposure to happy, rather than angry, expressions (Study 2). That is, subliminal emotional faces evoked affective reactions that altered participants' consumption behavior and evaluation of the beverage, but produced no mediating change in their conscious feelings at the moment the affective reactions were caused. Since participants rated their feelings of mood immediately after the subliminal affect induction, these results cannot be explained by the failure of affective memory. Thus we propose that these results demonstrate unconscious affect in the strong sense—an affective process strong enough to alter behavior, but of which people are simply not aware, even when attending to their feelings.

CHALLENGES TO UNCONSCIOUS EMOTION

Findings such as the one just described constitute some evidence for the independence of affect and conscious experience. But there are several challenges to be met.

How Does Unconscious Affect Work?

One challenge involves specifying the mechanisms by which affect can influence behavior toward an object without eliciting conscious feelings.

One possibility is that unconscious affect directly modulates the object's ability to trigger affective and motivational responses via a "front-end" or perceptual–attentional mechanism (Phelps, Chapter 3). That is, instead of triggering feelings, the affect could modify the position of relevant target objects on the organism's "incentive landscape." For example, in our beverage studies, the exposure to subliminal happy or angry expressions could transiently multiply up or down the incentive value of the drink, leading to differential behavior and ratings. To give a neuroscientific account of a possible mechanism, we speculate that subliminal facial expressions might activate the amygdala, which then might activate the adjacent accumbens and related structures responsible for processing natural incentives (Berridge, 2003; Rolls, 1999; Whalen et al., 1998). Altered neuronal activity in the nucleus accumbens (constituting unconscious "liking") could then change the human affective reaction to the sight and taste of a drink, leading to differential behavior and ratings, all without eliciting conscious feelings. In other words, we propose a mechanism that is not unlike what happens when a morphine microinjection into a rat's shell of accumbens enhances the rat's affective reaction to sweetness and leads to behavioral reaction of greater "liking." This proposal awaits empirical testing.

Affect or Emotion?

Some skeptics accept *unconscious affect* but deny *unconscious emotion* (e.g., Barrett, Chapter 11). They point out that much of the evidence concerns basic unconscious positive–negative or liking–disliking reactions, and not the categorically different states associated with emotion (e.g., fear, anger, disgust, sadness, joy, love, pride). However, note that subcortical circuitry is capable of at least some qualitative differentiation. For example, animals, even reptiles, show some categorical reactions to situations demanding different emotional response (Panksepp, 1998). In another example, human neuroimaging studies reveal different patterns of amygdala activation to consciously presented facial expressions of fear, anger, sadness, and disgust (Phan et al., 2002; Whalen, 1998). If future research shows that masked expressions of fear, anger, disgust, or sadness can create different physiological reactions with different behavioral consequences, all without eliciting conscious feelings, then there might indeed be processes fully deserving the label "unconscious emotion." Studies that measure psychophysiological, behavioral, and self-report manifestations of emotion within a single design could be particularly useful to address such issues (Winkielman, Berntson, & Cacioppo, 2001).

Affect or Cognition?

A critic may challenge the idea of unconscious affect by explaining the relevant empirical phenomena using a cognitive framework (e.g., Clore et al., Chapter 16). For example, the critic could argue that in our beverage studies, facial expressions influenced behavior via cognitive reinterpretation of the consumption situation. In general, note that such an explanation is divorced from the larger animal and human literature suggesting involvement of subcortical mechanisms in the processing of facial expressions and consumption stimuli. More specifically, note that the cognitive account cannot explain several findings from the beverage studies. First, the cognitive account predicts that all evaluations should be influenced by subliminal facial expressions. However, subliminal expressions influenced only ratings related to the incentive value of the drink, as predicted by our account, but not ratings of mood or ratings of the drink that were irrelevant to its incentive value (e.g., sweetness), as would be predicted by the cognitive account. Second, a cognitive account cannot easily explain why the influence of facial expressions was selectively amplified by a motivational state (thirst), whereas that prediction naturally follows from our incentive value account. In short, our proposed explanation in terms of unconscious affect changing the drink's incentive value is more consistent with the literature as well as the obtained data.

Unnoticed, Unverbalized, or Unconscious Affect?

Yet another challenge comes from the difficulty of conclusively establishing the absence of feelings. For one, there is the pesky problem of "proving the absence." This problem can be addressed, however, through converging replications, such that the presence of conscious feelings is established as unlikely (just as Santa Claus cannot be proven nonexistent, but can be proven unlikely to exist). A more substantive problem involves the very nature of reporting on phenomenal states. Several writers point out the difference between primary "experiencing" or "raw" consciousness and secondary "reflecting" or "meta" consciousness (Charland, Chapter 10; Lambie & Marcel, 2002; Schooler, 2002). This distinction suggests that people can "feel" without being "aware that they feel." Thus, perhaps in our drinking experiments, angry facial expression did indeed elicit "raw" anger, but our participants never reached a conscious, reportable belief that they "feel angry." Or perhaps participants' feelings were too subtle to be reflectively appraised. Or perhaps participants' attempts to reflect destroyed their fleeting feelings. These are all interesting possibilities.

However, we find them unlikely. First, the impact of the unconscious affect was sufficiently strong to change our participants' behavior, so it should have been sufficiently strong to change their reports of experience. Second, our participants were able to self-report on other aspects of their mood and sensations, as reflected in individual differences in reports of their baseline mood states and in their precise reports of drink experience (see Winkielman et al., 2005). Still, future research should examine to what extent the absence of self-reported feelings in human studies represents a genuine absence of phenomenology or an inability to reflect on that phenomenology. Several writers have suggested that these questions could be addressed by providing participants with training in (1) introspection, (2) use of beepers, ratings scales, or momentary affect dials, and (3) alternative, nonverbal ways of expressing emotion (Bartoshuk, 2000; Lambie & Marcel, 2002; Nielsen & Kaszniak, in press; Schooler & Schreiber, 2004). Finally, neuroscience may be of help. If it is possible in the future to reliably identify a neural correlate of subjective experience, the presence of conscious feelings could be suggested by changes in relevant neural activation.

CONSCIOUS AND UNCONSCIOUS EMOTION

In the preceding section we have presented a variety of arguments for the existence of "unfelt" affect and emotion. So are feelings just "icing on the cake"—nice, but not necessary? Are they the "red herring" of emotion research? We do not believe so. In the following section we offer speculation on the role of conscious feelings in emotion and the relation between conscious and unconscious components in emotion.

What Good Is Conscious Feeling?

Just like it makes functional sense that emotion can be "unfelt," there are good reasons why at least some creatures are capable of conscious feelings. In general, there are several benefits for a mental state, whether emotional or cognitive, to be conscious (see Gray et al., Chapter 4; Smith & Neumann, Chapter 12; Prinz, Chapter 15). Consciousness allows flexibility and depth. The organism can go beyond simple, habitual reactions and design novel, complex, context-sensitive forms of responding (Dennett, 1991; Rolls, 1999). Consciousness also allows control. The organism can stop undesirable responses and promote the desirable ones, deciding how and when to respond (Ochsner & Gross, 2004). On top of these standard perks of consciousness, the capacity for conscious feelings may give emotion a specific communicative and motivational function. Conscious feelings give internal feedback about how well the organism is doing with the current pursuits, telling it to maintain or change its path (Clore et al., Chapter 16). Feelings also come with psychological immediacy and urgency, making the organism "care" about its fate in a way that may not available to any other mechanism (Searle, 1997). This immediacy and urgency applies to simple hedonic states, such as pain and pleasure, and to complex emotions. Thus, pangs of guilt propel us to make amends, whereas green eyes of jealousy make us watch for trespasses of our mates (Frank, 1988).

What Makes Emotion Unconscious or Conscious?

Given the many benefits of consciousness, why then are humans sometimes unaware of their emotion? We suppose that a variety of neuroscientific and psychological factors play a role. Most of these factors probably apply regardless of whether the process is emotional or cognitive. Earlier we speculated that under some circumstances, relevant neural processes could simply bypass the circuitry for subjective experience and feed directly into behavioral circuitry. That is, sometimes emotion can be unconscious for the same reason why vision can be unconscious. As documented in research on "vision for perception vs. vision for action" (Goodale & Milner, 2004) and in research on "blindsight" (de Gelder, Chapter 6; Weiskranz, 1996), the relevant information can feed into the action system without ever reaching brain areas responsible for subjective experience. Further, sometimes rudimentary affective processes may be like other neural processes, such as thermoregulation or fluid regulation which can run unconsciously and elicit conscious experience (e.g., feeling cold, or feeling thirsty) only when there is a need for conscious intervention. Another important factor might be the brain's inability to construct a coherent percept, as when alternative sources of activation compete for interpretation (Crick & Koch, 2003).

Still other factors preventing the emergence of conscious representation are more psychological. The input might be too weak or too brief, as amply demonstrated in the work on backward masking (Enns & DiLollo, 2000). Or the input may be strong but inconsistent with the perceivers' expectations and thus escape attentional processing, as demonstrated in research on change blindness (Simons & Chabris, 1999). Or the input may not make sense in the context of the current situation (Dennett, 1991). Yet, in all these cases, the input may be sufficient to influence behavior.

Unfortunately, there is little empirical work on factors that determine the emergence of conscious emotional feelings. Future work could make some progress by, for example, systematically examining what determines whether subliminal stimuli elicit conscious mood. As we discussed earlier, in our research, exposure to subliminal facial expressions did not elicit feeling (Winkielman et al., 2005). However, other studies observed feeling changes after subliminal bloody pictures (Robles et al., 1987) or mere-exposed ideographs (Monahan et al., 2000). These findings suggest that perhaps simple or highly practiced stimuli, such as happy and angry faces used in our studies, are less likely to elicit feelings than more complex or novel stimuli, such as visual scenes or ideographs. The impact on feelings could also depend on the individual's sensitivity to a particular emotion inducer. For example, subliminally presented snakes increased conscious anxiety in phobic but not typical participants (Öhman & Soares, 1994). Similarly, introspectively sensitive participants are better at detecting the impact of subliminal stimuli and use their own reactions in behavior (Katkin, Wiens, & Öhman, 2001). Another interesting factor is the salience of the self representation. That is, when the self is salient, a change in an affective state might be channelled to a conscious feeling, rather than a representation of an external object (Clore et al., Chapter 16; Lambie & Marcel, 2002). Finally, motivational factors could also channel the affect to the representation of the external object or to the conscious feeling. For example, in our drinking studies, the only hint of change in subjective experience as a result of subliminal expression was observed among nonthirsty participants (for discussion, see Berridge & Winkielman, 2003). In sum, the emergence of conscious feelings may be determined by a host of stimulus, personal, and motivational factors. Though little is known at this point, it seems clear that the question of when and how emotion becomes conscious can be fruitfully investigated in an empirical manner, especially given all the new experimental and neuroscientific techniques now available.

CONCLUSION

In this chapter we argued for the existence of verifiable but unconscious emotional reactions. These reactions may be grounded in the oldest part of the emotional brain and may be similar in humans and animals. Nevertheless, they can be powerful enough to guide even human behavior and judgments. Thus emotion researchers should not limit themselves to subjective experiences when theorizing about emotion and conducting relevant empirical research. However, we also believe that conscious feelings are critical for understanding the mechanisms of emotion and its impact on behavior. Thus self-reports of feelings and other techniques that tap subjective experience have a major place in emotion theory and research. In fact, we see some of the most exciting topics in emotion research as understanding how and when emotion becomes conscious. Investigations of implicit emotional processes, techniques from human and animal affective neuroscience, and refinements in self-report methodology all can help us better understand the relation between conscious and unconscious emotions.

ACKNOWLEDGMENTS

We thank Jerry Clore, Lisa Feldman Barrett, Jim Goodson, Brian Knutson, and Paula Niedenthal for helpful discussions. Preparation of this chapter was supported by National Science Foundation Grant No. BCS-0350687 to Piotr Winkielman.

NOTES

1. Emotion theorists grounded in animal research typically do not consider subjective experience as a central or necessary component of emotion (e.g., Bouton, Chapter 9).
2. Lambie and Marcel's (2002) endorsement of nonconscious emotion is qualified by their statement that "to be in an emotion state is almost always to be in a phenomenal state" (p. 229).
3. Some have suggested that in humans the PBN participates in generating the "protoself," an unconscious but coherent representation of the momentary state of the body (Damasio, 1999).

REFERENCES

Adolphs, R., Damasio, H., Tranel, D., Cooper, G., & Damasio, A. R. (2000). A role for somatosensory cortices in the visual recognition of emotion as revealed by 3-D lesion mapping. *Journal of Neuroscience, 20,* 2683–2690.

Anderson, A.K., & Phelps, E. A. (2002). Is the human amygdala critical for the subjective experience of emotion? Evidence of intact dispositional affect in patients with lesions of the amygdala. *Journal of Cognitive Neuroscience, 14,* 709–720.

Baron-Cohen, S., Ring, H. A., Bullmore, E. T., Wheelwright, S., Ashwin, C., & Williams, S. C. R. (2000). The amygdala theory of autism. *Neuroscience and Biobehavioral Reviews, 24,* 355–364.

Bartoshuk, L.M. (2000). Psychophysical advances aid the study of genetic variation in taste. *Appetite, 34,* 105.

Berridge, K. C. (2000). Measuring hedonic impact in animals and infants: Microstructure of affective taste reactivity patterns. *Neuroscience and Biobehavioral Reviews, 24,* 173–198.

Berridge, K. C. (2003). Comparing the emotional brain of humans and other animals. In R. J. Davidson, H. H. Goldsmith, & K. Scherer (Eds.), *Handbook of affective sciences* (pp. 25–51). New York: Oxford University Press.

Berridge, K. C., & Pecina, S. (1995). Benzodiazepines, appetite, and taste palatability. *Neuroscience and Biobehavioral Reviews, 19,* 121–131.

Berridge, K. C., & Robinson, T. E. (1998). What is the role of dopamine in reward: Hedonic impact, reward learning, or incentive salience? *Brain Research—Brain Research Reviews, 28,* 309–369.

Berridge, K. C., & Winkielman, P. (2003). What is an unconscious emotion?: The case for unconscious "liking." *Cognition and Emotion, 17,* 181–211.

Cabanac, M. (1999). Emotion and phylogeny. *Journal of Consciousness Studies, 6,* 176–190.

Cacioppo, J. T., Larsen, J. T., Smith, N. K., & Berntson, G. G. (2004). The affect system: What lurks below the surface of feelings? In A. S. R. Manstead, N. H. Frijda, & A. H. Fischer (Eds.), *Feelings and emotions: The Amsterdam symposium.* Cambridge, UK: Cambridge University Press.

Clore, G. L. (1994). Why emotions are never unconscious. In P. Ekman & R. J. Davidson (Eds.), *The nature of emotion: Fundamental questions* (pp. 285–290). New York: Oxford University Press.

Cosmides, L., & Tooby, J. (2000). Evolutionary psychology and the emotions. In M. Lewis & J. Haviland-Jones (Eds.), *Handbook of emotions* (2nd ed., pp. 91–115). New York: Guilford Press.

Craig, A. D. (2003). Interoception: The sense of the physiological condition of the body. *Current Opinion in Neurobiology, 13,* 500–505.

Crick, F., & Koch, C. (2003). A framework for consciousness. *Nature Neuroscience, 6,* 119–126.

Critchley, H. D., Wiens, S., Rothstein, P., Öhman, A., & Dolan, R. J. (2004). Neural systems supporting interoceptive awareness. *Nature Neuroscience, 2,* 189–195.

Cromwell, H. C., & Berridge, K. C. (1993). Where does damage lead to enhanced food aversion: The ventral pallidum/substantia innominata or lateral hypothalamus? *Brain Research, 624*(1–2), 1–10.

Damasio, A. R. (1999). *The feeling of what happens: Body and emotion in the making of consciousness.* New York: Harcourt Brace.

Damasio, A. R., Grabowski, T. J., Bechara, A., Damasio, H., Ponto, L. L., Parvizi, J., & Hichwa, R. D. (2000). Subcortical and cortical brain activity during the feeling of self-generated emotions. *Nature Neuroscience, 3,* 1049–1056.

Davidson, R. J., Abercrombie, H. C., Nitschke, J., & Putnam, K. (1999). Regional brain function, emotion and disorders of emotion. *Current Opinion in Neurobiology, 9,* 228–234.

Davidson, R. J., Jackson, D. C., & Kalin, N. H. (2000). Emotion, plasticity, context, and regulation: Perspectives from affective neuroscience. *Psychological Bulletin, 126,* 890–909.

Davis, M. (1997). The neurophysiological basis of acoustic startle modulation: Research on fear motivation and sensory gating. In P. Lang, R. Simons, & M. Balaban (Eds.), *Attention and orienting: Sensory and motivational processes* (pp. 69–98). Mahwah, NJ: Erlbaum.

Dennett, D. (1991). *Consciousness explained.* Boston: Little, Brown.

Dimberg, U., Thunberg, M., & Elmehed, K. (2000). Unconscious facial reactions to emotional facial expressions. *Psychological Science, 11*, 86–89.

Emotion Researcher: Official Newsletter of the International Society for Research on Emotions. (2004). Special issue on unconscious emotion, *19*, 1.

Enns, J. T., & DiLollo, V. (2000). What's new in visual masking? *Trends in Cognitive Sciences, 4*, 345–352.

Frank, R. (1988). *Passions within reason: The strategic role of the emotions.* New York: Norton.

Freud, S. (1950). *Collected papers* (Vol. 4) (J. Riviere, Trans.). London: Hogarth Press and The Institute of Psychoanalysis.

Frijda, N. H. (1999). Emotions and hedonic experience. In D. Kahneman, E. Diener & N. Schwarz (Eds.), *Well-being: The foundations of hedonic psychology* (pp. 190–210). New York: Russell Sage Foundation.

Funayama, E. S., Grillon, C. G., Davis, M., & Phelps, E. A. (2001). A double dissociation in the affective modulation of startle in humans: Effects of unilateral temporal lobectomy. *Journal of Cognitive Neuroscience, 13*, 721–729.

Goodson, J. L., & Bass, A. H. (2001). Social behavior functions and related anatomical characteristics of vasotocin/vasopressin systems in vertebrates. *Brain Research Reviews, 35*, 246–265.

Goodale, M. A., & Milner, M. A. (2004). *Sight unseen: An exploration of conscious and unconscious vision.* Oxford, UK: Oxford University Press.

Heyes, C. M., & Huber, L. (Eds.). (2001). *Evolution of cognition.* Cambridge, MA: MIT Press.

Hobson, P. (1993). Understanding persons: The role of affect. In S. Baron-Cohen, H. Tager-Flusberg, & D. J. Cohen (Eds.), *Understanding other minds: Perspective from autism* (pp. 204–227). New York: Oxford University Press.

Insel, T. R., & Fernald, R. D. (2004). How the brain processes social information: Searching for the social brain. *Annual Reviews: Neuroscience, 27*, 697–722.

James, W. (1884). What is an emotion? *Mind, 9*, 188–205.

Kasari, C., Sigman, M., Yirmiya, N., & Mundy, P. (1993). Affective development and communication in children with autism. In A. P. Kaiser & D. B. Gray (Eds.), *Enhancing children's communication: Research foundation for early language interventions* (pp. 201–222). Baltimore: Brookes.

Katkin, E.S., Wiens, S., & Öhman, A. (2001). Nonconscious fear conditioning, visceral perception, and the development of gut feelings. *Psychological Science, 12*, 366–370.

Kihlstrom, J. F. (1999). The psychological unconscious. In L. A. Pervin & O. P. John (Eds.), *Handbook of personality: Theory and research* (2nd ed., pp. 424–442). New York: Guilford Press.

Knutson, B., Adams, C.M., Fong, G.W., & Hommer, D. (2001). Anticipation of increasing monetary reward selectively recruits nucleus accumbens. *Journal of Neuroscience, 21*, 1–5.

Knutson, B., Bjork, J. M., Fong, G. W., Hommer, D. W., Mattay, V. S., & Weinberger, D. R. (2004). Amphetamine modulates human incentive processing. *Neuron, 43*, 261–269.

Konorski, J. (1967). *Integrative activity of the brain: An interdisciplinary approach.* Chicago: University of Chicago Press.

Kunst-Wilson, W. R., & Zajonc, R. B. (1980). Affective discrimination of stimuli that cannot be recognized. *Science, 207,* 557–558.

Lambie, J. A., & Marcel, A. J. (2002). Consciousness and the varieties of emotion experience: A theoretical framework. *Psychological Review, 109,* 219–259.

Lane, R. D. (2000). Neural correlates of conscious emotional experience. In R. D. Lane & L. Nadel (Eds.), *Cognitive neuroscience of emotion* (pp. 345–370). New York: Oxford University Press.

Lang, P.J. (1995). The emotion probe: Studies of motivation and attention. *American Psychologist, 50,* 372–385.

Larsen, R. J., & Fredrickson, B. L. (1999). Measurement issues in emotion research. In D. Kahneman, E. Diener, & N. Schwarz (Eds.), *Well-being: Foundations of hedonic psychology* (pp. 40–60). New York: Russell Sage Foundation.

Lazarus, R. S., & McCleary, R. A. (1951). Autonomic discrimination without awareness: A study of subception. *Psychological Review, 58,* 113–122.

LeDoux, J. (1996). *The emotional brain: The mysterious underpinnings of emotional life.* New York: Simon & Schuster.

Martinez-Garcia, F., Martinez-Marcos, A., & Lanuza, E. (2002). The pallial amygdala of amniote vertebrates: Evolution of the concept, evolution of the structure. *Brain Research Bulletin, 57,* 463–469.

Mesquita, B., & Markus, H. R. (2004). Culture and emotion: Models of agency as sources of cultural variation in emotion. In N. H. Frijda, A. S. R. Manstead, & A. Fisher (Eds.), *Feelings and emotions: The Amsterdam symposium* (pp. 341–358). Cambridge, MA: Cambridge University Press.

Miyawaki, E., Perlmutter, J. S., Troster, A. I., Videen, T. O., & Koller, W. C. (2000). The behavioral complications of pallidal stimulation: A case report. *Brain and Cognition, 42,* 417–434.

Monahan, J. L., Murphy, S. T., & Zajonc, R. B. (2000). Subliminal mere exposure: Specific, general and diffuse effects. *Psychological Science, 11,* 462–466.

Morris, J. S., Öhman, A., & Dolan, R. J. (1999). A subcortical pathway to the right amygdala mediating "unseen" fear. *Proceedings of the National Academy of Sciences, 96,* 1680–1685.

Nielsen, L., & Kaszniak, A.W. (in press). Conceptual, theoretical, and methodological issues in inferring subjective emotion experience: Recommendations for researchers. In J. A. Coan & J. J. B. Allen (Eds.), *The handbook of emotion elicitation and assessment.* New York: Oxford University Press.

Ochsner, K. N., & Gross, J. J. (2004). Thinking makes it so: A social cognitive neuroscience approach to emotion regulation. In R. F. Baumeister & K. D. Vohs (Eds.), *Handbook of self-regulation: Research, theory, and applications* (pp. 229–255). New York: Guilford Press.

O'Doherty, J., Deichmann, R., Critchley, H. D., & Dolan, R. J. (2002). Neural responses during anticipation of a primary taste reward. *Neuron, 33,* 815–826.

Öhman, A., Flykt, A., & Lundqvist, D. (2000). Unconscious emotion: Evolutionary perspectives, psychophysiological data and neuropsychological mechanisms.

In R. D. Lane, L. Nadel, & G. Ahern (Eds.), *Cognitive neuroscience of emotion* (pp. 296–327). New York: Oxford University Press.

Öhman, A., & Soares, J. J. F. (1994). "Unconscious anxiety": Phobic responses to masked stimuli. *Journal of Abnormal Psychology, 103,* 231–240.

Panksepp, J. (1998). *Affective neuroscience: The foundations of human and animal emotions.* Oxford, UK: Oxford University Press.

Pecina, S., & Berridge, K. C. (2000). Opioid eating site in accumbens shell mediates food intake and hedonic "liking": Map based on microinjection Fos plumes. *Brain Research, 863,* 71–86.

Peyron, R., Laurent, B., & Garcia-Larrea, L. (2000). Functional imaging of brain responses to pain: A review and meta-analysis. *Clinical Neurophysiology, 30,* 263–288.

Phan, K. L., Wagner, T., Taylor, S. F., & Liberzon, I. (2002). Functional neuro-anatomy of emotion: A meta-analysis of emotion activation studies in PET and fMRI. *Neuroimage, 16,* 331–348.

Porges, S. W. (1997). Emotion: An evolutionary by-product of the neural regulation of the autonomic nervous system. In C. S. Carter, B. Kirkpatrick, & I. I. Lederhendler (Eds.), The integrative neurobiology of affiliation. *Annals of the New York Academy of Sciences, 807,* 62–77.

Ramachandran, V. S., & Blakeslee, S. (1998). *Phantoms in the brain.* New York: William Morrow.

Rauch, S. L., Shin, L. M., Dougherty, D. D., Alpert, N. M., Orr, S. P., Lasko, M., Macklin, M. L., Fischman, A. J., & Pitman, R. K. (1999). Neural activation during sexual and competitive arousal in healthy men. *Psychiatry Research, 91,* 1–10.

Robles, R., Smith, R., Carver, C. S., & Wellens, A. R. (1987). Influence of subliminal images on the experience of anxiety. *Personality and Social Psychology Bulletin, 13,* 399–410.

Rolls, E. T. (1999). *The brain and emotion.* Oxford, UK: Oxford University Press.

Russell, J. A. (2003). Core affect and the psychological construction of emotion. *Psychological Review, 110,* 145–172.

Schooler, J. W. (2002). Re-representing consciousness: Dissociations between experience and meta-consciousness. *Trends in Cognitive Sciences, 6,* 339–344.

Schooler, J. W., & Schreiber, C. A. (2004). Consciousness, meta-consciousness, and the paradox of introspection. *Journal of Consciousness Studies, 11,* 17–29.

Schwarz, N., & Clore, G. L. (2003). Mood as information: 20 years later. *Psychological Inquiry, 14,* 296–303.

Searle, J. (1997). *The mystery of consciousness.* New York: New York Review Press.

Simons, D. J., & Chabris, C. F. (1999). Gorillas in our midst: Sustained inattentional blindness for dynamic events. *Perception, 28,* 1059–1074.

Steiner, J. E. (1973). The gustofacial response: Observation on normal and anencephalic newborn infants. *Symposium on Oral Sensation and Perception, 4,* 254–278.

Steiner, J. E., Glaser, D., Hawilo, M. E., & Berridge, K. C. (2001). Comparative expression of hedonic impact: Affective reactions to taste by human infants and other primates. *Neuroscience and Biobehavioral Reviews, 25,* 53–74.

Tindell, A. J., Berridge, K. C., & Aldridge, J. W. (2004). Ventral pallidal representation of Pavlovian cues and reward: Population and rate codes. *Journal of Neuroscience, 24,* 1058–1069.

Watson, D., & Tellegen, A. (1985). Toward a consensual structure of mood. *Psychological Bulletin, 98,* 219–235.

Weiskrantz, L. (1996). Blindsight revisited. *Current Opinion in Neurobiology, 6,* 215–220.

Whalen, P. J. (1998). Fear, vigilance and ambiguity: Initial neuroimaging studies of the human amygdala. *Current Directions in Psychological Science, 7,* 177–188.

Whalen, P. J., Rauch, S. L., Etcoff, N. L., McInerney, S. C., Lee, M. B., & Jenike, M. A. (1998). Masked presentations of emotional facial expressions modulate amygdala activity without explicit knowledge. *Journal of Neuroscience, 18,* 411–418.

Wicker, B., Keyers, C., Plailly, J., Royet, J.-P., Gallese, V., & Rizzolatti, G. (2003). Both of us disgusted in my insula: The common neural basis of seeing and feeling disgust. *Neuron, 40,* 655–664.

Wilbarger, J. L., McIntosh, D. N., & Winkielman, P. (2004). Affective startle modification in autism. Manuscript submitted for publication.

Williams, M.A., Morris, A.P., McGlone, F., Abbott, D.F., & Mattingley, J.B. (2004). Amygdala responses to fearful and happy facial expressions under conditions of binocular suppression. *Journal of Neuroscience, 24,* 2898–2904.

Willis, W. D., & Westlund, K. N. (1997). Neuroanatomy of the pain system and of the pathways that modulate pain. *Journal of Clinical Neurophysiology, 14,* 2–31.

Winkielman, P., Berntson G. G., & Cacioppo J. T. (2001). The psychophysiological perspective on the social mind. In A. Tesser & N. Schwarz (Eds.), *Blackwell handbook of social psychology: Intraindividual processes* (pp. 89–108). Oxford, UK: Blackwell.

Winkielman, P., & Berridge, K. C. (2004). Unconscious emotion. *Current Directions in Psychological Science, 13,* 120–123.

Winkielman, P., Berridge, K. C., & Wilbarger, J. (2005). Unconscious affective reactions to masked happy versus angry faces influence consumption behavior and judgments of value. *Personality and Social Psychology Bulletin, 1,* 121–135.

Winkielman, P., Zajonc, R. B., & Schwarz, N. (1997). Subliminal affective priming resists attributional interventions. *Cognition and Emotion, 11,* 433–465.

Wise, R. A. (1996). Addictive drugs and brain stimulation reward. *Annual Review of Neuroscience, 19,* 319–340.

CHAPTER 15

Emotions, Embodiment, and Awareness

JESSE J. PRINZ

In ordinary talk, we sometimes refer to emotions as feelings. Feelings are conscious mental episodes. Therefore, it is tempting to presume that emotions cannot be unconscious. Freud (1915/1984, p. 191) tells us, "It is surely of the essence of an emotion that we should be aware of it, i.e., that it should become known to consciousness." In recent years, some researchers have argued that there can be unconscious emotions (see Damasio, 1994; Berridge & Winkielman, 2003; Winkielman, Berridge, & Wilbarger, Chapter 14). I think these authors are right (but for an alternative view, see Clore, Chapter 16). Following Williams James (1883), I believe that emotions are perceptions of bodily changes. In this chapter I defend that thesis and use it to explain various ways in which emotions can be both conscious and unconscious. Along the way, I propose parallels between emotion and vision: Both are forms of perception, both are hierarchically organized, both can occur unconsciously, and, I speculate, both give rise to consciousness via similar mechanisms (see Prinz, 2004).

WHAT ARE EMOTIONS?

Two Pathways

James argued that emotions are perceptions of patterned, instrumental changes in our visceral organs, muscles, and other bodily systems. Fear, for example, is a perception of changes that prepare us for flight. Call this the

1. *What is the scope of your proposed model? When you use the term* emotion, *how do you use it? What do you mean by terms such as* fear, anxiety, *or* happiness?

The theory that I am proposing is intended to encompass all emotions. I think all emotions are structurally and functionally alike. Every emotion is an embodied appraisal; an inner state that registers a patterned bodily change and carries information about an organism/environment relation that bears on well-being. Fear, for example, carries the information that one is in danger, and it does so by registering a bodily pattern that reliably occurs in dangerous situations (e.g., a racing heart, constricted blood vessels, wide-open eyes, and strained respiration).

2. *Define your terms:* conscious, unconscious, awareness. *Or say why you do not use these terms.*

A mental state or episode is conscious if it feels like something to the organism. In philosophers' jargon, conscious states have phenomenological character. Unconscious states do not feel like anything. Most of our mental states are unconscious. Awareness occurs when mental states become available to central cognitive processes and executive control. Awareness and consciousness are intimately linked, because mental states become conscious when they become available in this way. In addition to becoming aware *of* a mental state, we can become aware *that* the state is occurring. This happens when we categorize or label our own mental states ("This is fear that I am feeling").

3. *Does your model deal with what is conscious, what is unconscious, or their relationship? If you do not address this area specifically, can you speculate on the relationship between what is conscious and unconscious? Or if you do not like the conscious–unconscious distinction, or if you do not think this is a good question to ask, can you say why?*

I am interested in how emotions become conscious. Because emotions register bodily changes, they are perceptions. I think the mechanisms underlying emotion consciousness are therefore exactly parallel to the mechanisms underlying perceptual consciousness more generally. Also, like all perceptions, emotions can be unconscious. Unconscious emotions are unavailable to central processes. In addition, we can experience conscious emotions without awareness of which emotion we are having. We can experience an emotion without categorizing it.

---

embodiment thesis. To defend this thesis, James asked his readers to imagine being in an emotional state and then to mentally subtract each bodily component. Imagine anger without tensed muscles, a pounding heart, and a scowl. When all bodily changes are gone, there doesn't seem to be anything left that we would call an emotion. This imaginative exercise is suggestive but not demonstrative. Stronger evidence comes from several new lines of research (see Damasio, 1994; Niedenthal, Barsalow, Ric, & Krauth-Gruber, Chapter 2; Niedenthal et al., in press; Prinz, 2004).

First, some researchers have found that the six basic emotions (fear, anger, joy, sadness, surprise, and disgust) can be distinguished by a pattern of autonomic response (Levenson, Ekman, & Friesen, 1990). That is not to say that each emotion has just one physiological manifestation; in fact, each emotion may correspond to several patterns (see Cacioppo, Berntson, Larsen, Poehlmann, & Ito, 2000; Zajonc & McIntosh, 1992; Barrett, Chapter 11).

Second, providing subjects with false feedback about some their autonomic states can influence emotions. False bodily feedback, for example, has been shown to increase judgments of attractiveness (Valins, 1966); bodily changes caused by drugs can make subjects feel as if they were in emotional states (Marañon, 1924); and people are more likely to be angered by an insult if their bodies have just been aroused by physical exercise (Zillmann, 1978). Real body feedback can also influence emotion. Changes in facial expression can cause changes in experienced affect and in evaluative judgments (Levenson et al., 1990; Zajonc, Murphy, & Inglehart, 1989).

Third, there is evidence from neuroimaging. Again and again, neuroimaging studies of emotion show activation in brain structures that have been independently associated with bodily response. For example, Damasio et al. (2000) performed a functional magnetic resonance imaging (fMRI) study in which subjects recalled emotional events. They found different overlapping patterns of activation for different emotions, but it is premature to conclude that each emotion corresponds to the same identifiable pattern on every occasion. Different studies have obtained different results (Barrett, Chapter 11; Murphy, Nimmo-Smith, & Lawrence, 2003; Phan, Wager, Taylor, & Liberzon, 2002). The crucial point is that emotions always seem to involve activity in neural structures that play a role in body perception. These include the anterior cingulate cortex, the insula, and the somatosensory cortices (see Atkinson & Adolphs, Chapter 7; Winkielman, Berridge, & Wilbarger, Chapter 14). All of these structures have been found to play a role in the perception of bodily states (e.g., Aziz et al., 2000).

Fourth, consider how disorders in body perception affect emotional experience. There is a degenerative disorder known as pure autonomic failure, whose victims cannot modulate activity in their autonomic nervous systems. Critchley, Mathias, and Dolan (2001) examined a group of patients with this condition and found that their emotions were significantly reduced (although the effect sizes were small). In a self-report study, they were more likely to more strongly endorse statements such as "I can no longer feel sad."

This evidence indicates a close relationship between bodily responses and emotions. Some researchers are unconvinced, however. They concede that emotions are typically correlated with perceptions of bodily changes, but they deny that they are identical to such changes. There are two strategies for trying to refute the embodiment thesis. One can argue that perceptions of the body are not *necessary* to be in an emotional state, or one can argue that perceptions of the body are not *sufficient*.

First consider the allegation that perceived bodily changes are unnecessary for emotions. Introspectively, some emotions do not seem to involve bodily perturbations. Harré (1986) cites loneliness as an example, and Frank (1988) notes that guilt lacks the expressive behavior associated with embodied emotions. I think introspection is misleading in these cases. Evidence shows that loneliness does have a somatic grounding. Caccioppo et al. (2002) found that lonely people have lower cardiac contractility, heart rate, and cardiac output than people who are not lonely. Loneliness may also incorporate sadness, which has known bodily analogues (Levenson et al. 1990). Guilt gives us bodily pangs; neuroimaging studies of guilt show activation in the insular and anterior cingulate cortices, which are associated with bodily response (Shin et al., 2000).

Another argument against the necessity of bodily states comes from Chwalisz, Diener, and Gallagher (1988), who found that individuals with spinal cord injuries have emotions despite the fact that their body perception is severely compromised. Damasio (1999) offers a decisive response. First, he points out that spinal patients can perceive bodily states through the bloodstream and the vagus nerve, and they can perceive facial changes through the head and neck. Second, Damasio points out that the brain can generate imagery of bodily changes when no such changes have taken place. Spinal patients can have brain states that are just like normal bodily perceptions, regardless of their injuries.

Now consider the objection that perceptions of bodily changes are *insufficient* for emotional states. According to this line, William James may have been right to insist on an embodied component, but emotions have a cognitive component as well. Every emotion, the objection goes, is bound to an appraisal judgment. This is a widespread view in psychology (e.g., Lazarus, 1991; Roseman, Spindel, & Jose, 1990; Scherer, 1993, Chapter 13). The structure and content of emotional appraisals vary a bit from theory to theory, but the gist is usually the same. Sadness occurs when there is an appraisal of loss; anger occurs when there is an appraisal concerning insult; fear occurs when there is an appraisal of danger; and so on. Appraisal theorists claim that a perception of a bodily perturbation without an accompanying appraisal would not be an emotion.

Appraisal theories are usually defended in one of two ways. Experimenters purport to show that emotions can be influenced (i.e., elicited or altered) by manipulating appraisals, or they show that subjects systematically associate appraisal meanings with their emotions (e.g., Lazarus, 1991; Roseman et al., 1990; Scherer, 1993). Neither form of evidence is decisive. The fact that appraisals can induce emotions shows that appraisals are sufficient for emotions, not necessary. If appraisals are merely sufficient, they may not be components of emotions. A roller-coaster ride is sufficient for inducing fear, but the ride is not a component of the fear. The fact that people associate appraisal meanings with their emotions does not establish appraisal theories either. It shows that emotions are responses to specific kinds of external *events*, not that they contain internal *judgments*. Consider, by analogy, the case of pain. If asked, subjects would report that pain occurs when they are wounded. An experience of pain does not entail an inner judgment, "I have been wounded." Pain can occur without any judgment. Likewise, emotions can be caused by perceptions of external events without any intermediating appraisal. For example, fear can be directly triggered by seeing a bug or hearing a loud noise. Sometimes fear follows a judgment, but it need not. Appraisal theorists sometimes conjecture that appraisals take place unconsciously in these cases, but that is ad hoc. It seems more plausible that we move directly from a perception of a stimulus to a patterned bodily response, rather than imposing an unnecessary appraisal in between the two.

LeDoux (1996) has provided evidence in support of this conjecture. He has shown that fear can be triggered subcortically by a pathway that extends from the sensory thalamus into the amygdala (see also Morris et al., 1999; Phelps, Chapter 3). At the psychological level, this pathway is consistent with certain dual-processing models (Smith & Neumann, Chapter 12). The amygdala sends afferents to structures that regulate different kinds of bodily responses. Seeing a bug can trigger a cascade of bodily changes before the visual stimulus has even been processed in the neocortex. The perception of those changes is experienced as fear. Some authors describe the amygdala itself as an appraisal center. This is implausible. The cells in the amygdala can directly link perceptual images to structures that control bodily response. The amygdala has no intervening cells representing the fact that, for example, a snake is a threat to me.

I think we must distinguish between two kinds of information-processing pathways that are involved in emotional response. First, there are pathways implicated in emotion elicitation. Emotions can be elicited either by judgments or perceptions of emotionally significant stimuli. Therefore, emotion elicitation pathways in the brain include structures involved in high-level cognition as well as structures involved in low-level perception. We can think of the large, heterogeneous class of inner states that can trigger a given emotion as comprising an elicitation file. The file for fear includes visual images of crawling insects, proprioceptive images of falling, auditory images of loud, sudden noises, and cognitive judgments about danger. These representations are distributed across the brain, united only by the fact that they reliably trigger the same physiological responses. They trigger those responses through what might be termed *somatic association areas*. These are areas that record and coordinate associations between thoughts or images and patterned bodily response. The amygdala is a somatic association area; presumably, there are others.

When a thought or image causes excitation in a somatic association area, signals are sent to structures that modulate bodily states. Those structures affect changes in our visceral organs, muscles, hormones, and so on. These changes are then perceived. The move from bodily change to perceptions thereof takes place in what can be called the response pathway. The brain structures that perceive bodily states lie in this pathway, and, if James is right, they contain the neural correlates of emotion. Emotions do not reside in the elicitation pathways. Emotion research that focuses on elicitation without addressing bodily perception is incomplete. It is like studying the history of warfare by investigating precipitating events and never examining the wars themselves. If we want to study emotions themselves, we must look at the events that occur after the amygdala and its attendant body regulators have done their work—which is the topic to which I turn next.

Levels of Emotional Processing

Once bodily responses have been initiated, they can be perceived. Information about parts of the body outside of the central nervous system comes in through the brainstem via structures such as the nucleus of the solitary tract. Bodily perception has been less thoroughly investigated than visual perception, but we know enough to make informed speculations. For example, changes in different aspects of the body are likely to be perceived independently at first (e.g., see Saper, 2002; Critchley, Wiens, Rothstein, Öhman, & Dolan, 2004). Structures that register changes in heart rate may differ from structures that register respiratory changes, muscle tension, goose bumps, or intestinal twinges. We know that different brain areas are involved in kinesthesia, interoception, and cutaneous touch.

Local changes in the body are separately perceived, but the brain presumably registers co-occurrence as well. A racing heart could indicate elation or terror; its significance depends on accompanying bodily states. In elation, there may be increased blood flow to the head, whereas in terror blood flows to the extremities and vessels in the head may become constricted (the pallor of fear). To keep track of this sequence of bodily events, the brain must register *patterns* of bodily response—not unlike the level in visual processing in which edges are bound together into shapes and contours.

We can also postulate a higher level of processing. Recall that the same emotion can correspond to different patterns of physical response. In fear, we freeze, flee, or fight, depending on the nature of the threat (see Bouton, Chapter 9; Gray & McNaughton, 2000). If you are home alone at night and hear a glass shatter in the next room, you may freeze momentarily. If you are strolling outside and see a tornado cloud on the nearby horizon, you may run with fear. If an assailant physically aggresses against you, you may be forced to fight. All of these behaviors are different and, hence, differently represented within the brain. However, we identify all of these as fear responses. Thus the brain must be able to recognize that distinct bodily patterns correspond to the same emotion. We must, in other words, recognize patterns of patterns. I speculate that there is a categorical level of emotion processing (see also, Barrett, Chapter 11).

The categorical level of emotion processing may be quite useful. It allows us to classify our current emotional states, and that, in turn, helps in the selection of appropriate responses. If you know that you are afraid, you can try to pick an appropriate coping strategy. If you believe that the fear is justified, you may try to pursue behaviors that increase the distance between you and the object of your fear. If you think the fear is unjustified, you may try to find ways of reducing it rather than escaping its object. Categorical emotion recognition may also be an entry point for culturally informed emotional scripts (see Tomkins, 1979; D'Andrade, 1992). If your culture imparts values about what frightened people should do, categorical recognition of fear may be an essential precondition for complying with those values. The categorical level may also be used to self-ascribe emotions when physiological responses are absent. Indeed, it may be crucial for those individuals who are deficient in bodily awareness (see p. 377), and it may help us appreciate the emotional significance of a situation even when lower-level processes have not been engaged (in this sense, it may be comparable to the "propositional" emotion system postulated by Philippot & Schaefer, 2001).

If the preceding considerations are correct, then the emotion response pathways must be hierarchically organized (for related ideas, see Critchely et al., 2001; Damasio, 1999; Leventhal & Scherer, 1987; Panksepp, 1998). After a pattern of bodily changes has been triggered, it is perceived. Perception begins locally, as each component of the bodily pattern is registered separately. Thereafter, the local changes are integrated, and the global pattern is perceived. And, finally, any given pattern may be recognized as an instance of a range of patterns that arise in related circumstances. The stages of perception can be termed *low*, *intermediate*, and *high*, or, more descriptively, *local*, *integrative*, and *categorical*.

It is not easy to pinpoint the exact location of these stages in the brain. We do not yet know the neural correlates of discrete emotions, and there has not been a concerted effort to look for hierarchical organization in the response pathways. Still, it is worth offering some provisional speculations. I suggest that low-level processes within the emotion hierarchy are largely located in the brainstem, the thalamus, and the primary somatosensory cortex. These structures may themselves be hierarchically organized, both internally and with respect to each other. I locate low-level processing here because I suspect that these structures contain representations of local bodily changes rather than integrated patterns of change. The intermediate level, where patterns are perceived, must be distributed across structures that get inputs from earlier sites of processing. Of particular interest in this regard are the secondary somatosensory cortex, the insular cortex, and portions of the anterior cingulate cortex, including Brodmann areas 23 and 24. All these structures seem well situated to represent patterns of bodily response. That leaves us with the high-level processing. Earlier I said that high-level emotion recognition may involve representations that relate emotion categories to cultural knowledge and scripts. Such knowledge is presumably distributed across the frontal lobe and association cortices. However, there may be more localized representations of emotion categories that monitor patterned bodily changes and fire categorically when related patterns occur. Regions involved in this process must receive inputs from intermediate-level emotion processing areas. I think especially good candidates include the more rostral portion of the anterior cingulate cortex (area 32) and neighboring areas of the medial and orbitofrontal cortices. In a positron emission tomography (PET) study, Lane, Fink, Chau, and Dolan (1997) presented subjects with emotionally evocative pictures and asked them to make either a neutral location judgment (indoor or outdoor) or an emotional judgment (positive or negative). The latter requires categorical recognition of one's emotional states. Subjects in the emotional judgment condition showed greater activation in the rostral anterior cingulate and medial frontal areas as compared to the location condition. These areas, then, are likely to be involved in high-level emotion processing.

Above I claimed that emotions reside within the response pathways. Given the hierarchical organization that I have been describing, the question about where emotions reside can be made more precise. We can ask whether emotions reside at a single level of processing or at multiple levels, and, if they reside at a single level, we can ask which one. I think that emotions reside at the intermediate or integrative level. The low level represents bodily changes that occur independently. No somatic component of an emotional state corresponds to an emotion on its own. Integration is necessary. There is a different problem with locating emotions at the high level. These representations seem too abstract. As I envisage the high level, it is the place where we recognize that we are in emotional states, not the locus of those states. To recognize that you are afraid, you must have experienced a prior state that constitutes the fear (for an opposing view, see Barrett, Chapter 11). If you were to form the judgment that you are afraid without perceiving a patterned bodily response, there would be grounds for thinking you were mistaken. You cannot be afraid without perceiving some specific pattern of bodily response. Such perceptions arise at the intermediate level. Here, I submit, is where emotions reside. This analysis will help focus the discussion of emotional consciousness, to which I turn now.

CONSCIOUS AND UNCONSCIOUS EMOTIONS

Awareness of Elicitors

Any discussion of emotion awareness should distinguish between processes in the two kinds of pathways that we have been considering. When an emotion occurs, we can be aware of the elicitor, and we can be aware of the elicited response. I have said that the emotion itself resides at the intermediate level in the response pathway. Before turning to the emotion itself, however, I want to consider awareness of elicitors.

Let me begin with a distinction. We can be aware of an elicitor, and we can be aware that the elicitor is, in fact, responsible for our emotional state. Suppose someone cuts you off while driving, causing you to get angry. You are aware of the offending event, and you are aware that the event is responsible for your anger. To be aware of the offending event in this case is to have a conscious visual experience of the car cutting in front of you. To be aware that this event is responsible for your anger involves awareness of the offending event, awareness of the anger (which I address in the next section), and awareness of the link between these two. There has been little research on how we become aware of such links. One possibility is suggested by the research on the "binding problem" in sensory perception. In perception we bind colors, shapes, sounds, and other separately processed features of experience into coherent representations of objects. There are various theories about how such bindings are achieved. A popular suggestion is that the cells responding to a visual stimulus fire synchronously with the cells responding to the corresponding auditory stimulus (Gray & Singer, 1989). Perhaps emotions get bound to elicitors using the same kind of mechanism.

Another possibility is that we have no direct awareness of the links between emotions and their elicitors. If this is right, then we would form beliefs about those links by inference ("I wonder what's making me mad . . . "). That would help to explain why we seem to be at risk for misidentifying the sources of our emotions (compare Bargh, 1992). In the car example, there is little room for error. The perception of the car is close in time to the resulting anger and appropriate in content. In other cases, the cause of an emotion is harder to discern. Consider a case in which anger lingers after being cut off in traffic, and then gets vented elsewhere. We sometimes unleash our aggravations inappropriately and mistake hapless victims for rightful causes. We may do so because the link between emotion and object cannot be a direct object of awareness.

Misidentification of emotion elicitors can also arise in cases in which those elicitors are themselves unconscious (see Winkielman, Berridge, & Wilbarger, Chapter 14). Consider, for example, Zajonc's work on mere-exposure effects. In a representative study, monolingual English-speaking subjects were asked to speculate about the meaning of Chinese characters (reviewed in Zajonc, 2000). Unbeknownst to the subjects, some of those characters had been previously viewed during a training phase of the experiment. Subjects were significantly more likely to judge that the familiar characters expressed positive meanings than unfamiliar characters, despite the fact that they had no recollection of which characters they had seen. Familiarity caused positive feeling, and these feelings were misattributed to the imagined meanings of the characters, because the factor that elicited those positive feelings (familiarity) was not itself an object of awareness.

In other experiments emotions are induced by presenting eliciting stimuli below the threshold of awareness. In a PET study Morris, Öhman, and Dolan (1999) briefly presented subjects with angry faces, followed by expressionless faces. The expressionless faces masked the angry faces for all the subjects. Compared to a neutral control condition, there was amygdala activation associated with the unconscious presentations of the angry faces. Given the amygdala's role in emotion induction, this activation suggests that we can have an emotional response to a stimulus that we have not experienced consciously (see also Esteves, Dimberg, & Öhman, 1994; Lundquist & Öhman, Chapter 5; de Gelder, Chapter 6; Atkinson & Adolphs, Chapter 7; Winkielman et al., Chapter 14; but for a critical view, see Clore et al., Chapter 16).

In sum, there is reason to think that the elicitor of an emotion and the link between emotion and elicitor can both be unconscious. In many circumstances, of course, we are aware of emotion elicitors, but it is currently unknown whether we are ever directly aware of the link between elicitor and emotion. So far, I have said nothing about awareness of emotions themselves, the topic which I take up next.

Awareness of Emotions

In the Jamesian view outlined above, emotions are perceptions of patterned changes in the body. These perceptions occur in emotion response pathways. We can now ask where in those pathways awareness takes place.

To approach this question, I want to consider an analogy with visual perception. Elsewhere I have defended a theory of visual consciousness (Prinz, 2000) and argued that it can be extended to other sensory modalities (Prinz, in press). That theory begins with a hypothesis expounded by Jackendoff (1987) that states that consciousness always arises at an intermediate level in hierarchically organized perceptual systems. In visual object recognition, there is presumed to be a hierarchy that begins with detection of simple edges, extends to representations of viewpoint-specific contours and depth, and culminates with object representations that are invariant across a rage of vantage points (Marr, 1982; Zeki, 1993). This process parallels the hierarchical organization that I postulated in the case of emotions, which extends from local to integrative and finally to categorical representations. Jackendoff argued that we are conscious only of the integrative level in vision. We experience objects from a particular vantage point, rather than invariant representations of disconnected edges. I think the same holds true in the case of emotion (Prinz, 2003, 2004). In emotional processing, we are aware of integrated bodily patterns rather than local bodily changes or categorical representations of discrete emotions. At present, the best evidence for this conjecture is introspective. When we experience emotions, they seem to be based in the body, but they do not seem to be collections of wholly independent bodily states. Nor do conscious emotions seem to fully categorical. A freezing response feels different from a fleeing response, for example.

Above I argued that the intermediate level within emotion response pathways is the level at which emotions reside. If that is right, then the conscious experiences that issue from emotion response pathways are experiences of emotions themselves, rather than merely causes and effects of emotions. This proposition accords with the presumption that emotions can be felt. But can emotions also occur without conscious feelings?

To answer this question, it is helpful to return to the case of vision. It is widely believed that there can be unconscious visual perception (Dixon, 1981). We need an account of how this type of perception occurs. Jackendoff's intermediate-level theory implies that visual consciousness arises whenever there is activity in intermediate-level visual processing systems. This view is probably incorrect. Neuroimaging studies have shown that activity can arise in intermediate-level visual areas without awareness (Rees, 2001; Vuilleumier et al., 2001)—which is presumably what happens in some cases of unconscious perception. Information is processed all the way through the visual system, but it does not enter consciousness.

What ingredient distinguishes conscious and unconscious processing in vision? The answer that I defend elsewhere is attention (Prinz, in press). There is evidence that visual awareness wanes with attention (Mack & Rock, 1998; Simons & Chabris, 1999), and that brain areas associated with attention are active in those conditions when visual stimuli are consciously perceived (Rees, 2001). These findings are consistent with everyday experience. We often fail to notice one thing when we are attending to another. For these reasons, I believe that consciousness arises whenever an intermediate-level perceptual representation is modulated by attention. Conscious states are attended intermediate-level representations (AIRs).

These observations lead to the prediction that emotional consciousness (i.e., the feeling of an emotion) will arise only when attention is allocated to the patterned changes in the body. This claim is supported by the finding that individuals who are less skilled at attending to changes in their bodies experience emotions less intensely (Wiens, Mezzacappa, & Katkin, 2000; Critchley et al., 2004). However, I do not mean to imply that conscious emotional experience requires an *effortful* or *intentional* deployment of attention. Attention can be captured bottom-up. Indeed, emotional processing generally captures our attention. This makes sense, because emotions arise under conditions of concern. If emotions do generally engage attention, then they are generally conscious. But there may be conditions under which emotions fail to capture or sustain attention. When that happens, I would predict that emotions would be unconscious. Let me consider two kinds of cases.

First, consider cases in which the bodily response triggered by an emotionally evocative stimulus is too weak to capture attention. Emotions can vary in intensity. There is a difference between the joy of a decent meal and the joy of a great meal, and there is a difference between being slightly concerned and stricken with anxiety. If the Jamesian approach is right, these differences in intensity may correspond to different degrees of bodily response. Minor concern may increase the heart rate slightly, whereas anxiety causes the heart to pound. Minor perturbations may be less likely to engage attention. This hypothesis is borne out by recent experiments. For example, Strahan, Spencer, and Zanna (2002) found that subjects who had been subliminally presented with sad faces were more likely to choose to listen to uplifting music than controls. The subliminal presentations had no effect, however, on the subjects' self-reported moods. It is possible that the subliminal emotion induction did not cause a response that was strong enough to engage attention. Unconscious emotions may have also been induced in the Morris et al. study mentioned above, and in Zajonc's mere-exposure effects. The experimenters do not systematically report their subjects' subjective feelings in these studies, but it is possible that the induced changes in affective states were too subtle to be detected consciously.

Another way to elicit emotions unconsciously is to give subjects a demanding or distracting task alongside an emotion induction task. If subjects are distracted by a concurrent task, perturbations in their bodies may fail to capture their attention. Indeed, distraction is a familiar coping strategy. Suppose a person with a flight phobia is aboard an airplane and experiencing fear. She might try to distract herself by reading an in-flight magazine. Distracting herself with the magazine's articles may alleviate the conscious experience of fear, but her body may continue to exhibit signs of that emotion. She may clutch the magazine, perspire, and so forth. I am not aware of studies that directly investigate this phenomenon in the lab, but related findings may be available. Consider an experiment by Winkielman, Berridge, and Wilbarger (2005), who had subjects pour and consume a fruit-flavored drink after subliminally presenting happy, neutral, and angry faces. The thirsty subjects in the experiment reported no change in their emotions, but their drinking behavior was affected by the subliminal presentations. They poured and drank more juice after subliminally perceiving happy faces than after seeing neutral faces, and less juice after seeing angry faces. We might explain this result by saying that subliminally induced emotions are too weak to engage attention, as I suggested for the Strahan et al. study. But this interpretation *may* be mistaken. In the Winkielman et al. study, subjects who were not thirsty before the experiment reported a change in emotional state after the subliminal induction. The effect is small but intriguing. Perhaps the thirsty subjects failed to experience that minute change because their thirst was drawing attention away from this subtle emotional state. The thirst, then, may have functional as a distraction. Winkielman (personal communication) suggests that an emotion elicitor stronger than pictures of faces might have resulted in a conscious emotion experience for all participants in this study. Future research should try to identify conditions under which subliminally induced emotions go unfelt. Weakness of the response and the demands of concurrent tasks may both play a role in muting subjective experience.

The findings of Strahan, Winkielman, Berridge, and Wilbarger are compelling in that they suggest that we can have emotions in the absence of awareness. The perceptual theory of emotion predicts this possibility. After all, unconscious perception is possible in other modalities. The AIR theory predicts that consciousness will wane with attention, and that prediction is consistent with available results. However, the claim that emotions can be unconscious is not universally accepted (e.g., see Clore et al., Chapter 16).

To some critics, the concept of an unconscious emotion is simply incoherent. Such critics might concede that the AIR theory of consciousness is correct while denying that we ever have unconscious emotions. These individuals would say that perceptions of patterned bodily changes qualify as emotions only when they are conscious. This move is simply verbal, and I see no reason to take it seriously. Unconscious perceptions of bodily changes can play a role comparable to their conscious analogues: They can (1) affect semantic evaluations (Zajonc), (2) lead to conditioned aversions (Morris et al.), (3) increase and reduce beverage consumption (Winkielman et al.), and (4) promote coping behavior, such as listening to pleasant music (Strahan et al.). Denying that these are emotions is like denying that unconscious states in the visual system are perceptions. Neither move is motivated.

Similar considerations undermine an argument against unconscious emotions that has been advanced by Clore (1994, although compare Clore & Ortony, 2000). He argues that emotions cannot be unconscious, because unconscious emotions would fail to serve a role that is essential to emotional states. Emotions stand out like red flags to draw our attention to matters of concern. Unconscious emotions, Clore says, would not do this. Therefore, unconscious emotions are not possible. I find the argument doubly problematic. First, I see no reason why an unconscious state could not draw our attention to something. A subliminally presented anger face could, in principle, make an accompanying tone highly salient even if the face and the resulting anger were not. Second, I have already pointed out that unconscious perceptions of the body can play roles that are similar to roles played by conscious emotions. Emotions do not merely serve as red flags; they alter our preferences, influence learning, and help us cope. I see no reason, therefore, to deny that unconscious emotions exist.

If conscious and unconscious emotions play similar roles, one might wonder why emotions ever become conscious. Can't we get by with unconscious emotions? I think not. In general, the difference between conscious and unconscious perceptions is that conscious perceptions allow us to engage in behaviors that require control practices. Unconscious perceptions can trigger innate, stereotypical responses, or highly rehearsed responses. Responses that are novel, plastic, or deliberative require consciousness. Our capacity for controlled responses helps to explain the link between consciousness and attention. There is reason to think that attention is a process of changing the way information flows in the brain (Olshausen, Anderson, & van Essen, 1994). In particular, attention may open up information flow between perceptual systems and systems associated with working memory (Prinz, in press). Working memory areas are implicated in controlled responses. If this view is right, then the process that makes perception conscious, in the case of vision and emotion alike, is identical to the process that makes perceptual states available for control.

Awareness of Emotion Categories

In discussing the hierarchical organization of the emotion response pathway, I suggested that categorical recognition is achieved at the high level. Representations at this level are not components of emotions themselves but, rather, ways we identify the emotions to ourselves. We might say that these representations are concepts of emotions, because they are used to classify particular emotional states as belonging to discrete emotion categories. To be aware of an emotion category is to be aware *that* one is experiencing a particular emotion, in contrast with being aware *of* the emotion, which occurs at the intermediate level. In other words, high-level awareness is metacognitive. In this section, I discuss how high-level awareness is possible.

To recognize that we are having an emotion, we must deploy emotion concepts. Emotion concepts may involve both schematized representations of the body and knowledge of emotional significance (see also Fehr & Russell, 1984; Niedenthal et al., Chapter 2; Barrett, Chapter 11). Sometimes people deploy emotion concepts without awareness of the underlying bodily states, particularly those individuals who are bad at perceiving changes in their bodies (Katlin, 1985; Duclos & Laird, 2001). Such individuals can infer from context that they are afraid without feeling their racing hearts. They may infer: "I am facing a serious danger, so I must be afraid."

High-level emotion categorization can increase awareness of lower-level emotion processes and increase our awareness of our bodily states. If someone points out that you are angry when you begin raising your voice in a heated debate, you might introspect and discover a feeling of anger. Before the high-level judgment, you might have been consciously feeling your anger, but you were not *aware* of it. Such awareness can be helpful in emotion regulation (Barrett, Gross, Conner, & Benvenuto, 2001).

We can also become aware of high-level emotion representations themselves. When we categorize a state as fear, typically we are aware of the fear (the bodily state) and of the fact that we are afraid (the emotion category). A hypothesis of this kind of high-level awareness faces an immediate problem regarding the theory of emotion consciousness that I have been defending. I suggested that high-level representations in the emotion response pathway are never conscious. This conjecture parallels Jackendoff's claims about conscious vision. Categorical representations that are highly invariant across sensory inputs are not objects of direct experience. A person in a state of fear may experience self-reports, such as

"I am afraid" or "That's scary," but these representations in our language centers are merely our attempts to label the categorical representations used by our emotion systems, which are not available to consciousness.

Above I said that there are individual differences in sensitivity to body change. People who are inept at body perception can deploy an emotion category in the absence of experiences of bodily changes. The converse is also true: We can experience bodily changes without deploying emotion categories. There are significant individual differences in the categorical awareness of emotions. Some people are highly skilled at identifying their emotional states, whereas others are not (Barrett, 2004; Feldman, 1995; Lane, 2000). Alexithymia is characterized as an inability to verbalize what emotion one is experiencing (Sifneos, 1973). The condition may involve an impairment or lack of development in categorical emotion recognition. Indeed, in functional imaging studies, people with alexithymia show lower than normal response in the anterior cingulate and adjacent medial frontal areas when viewing emotional stimuli (Berthoz et al., 2002; see also Lane, Ahern, Schwartz, & Kaszniak, 1997). Without a well-functioning high level in the emotion response pathways, we may experience emotions without being able to identify them; we might not even recognize an emotion as such, mistaking it for some other kind of state. This confusion is one reason why alexithymia is associated with somatization disorders, in which emotions are mistaken for mere bodily discomforts (Parker, Bagby, & Taylor, 1989). Honing one's capacity to identify emotional states is a core component of emotional intelligence (Salovey & Mayer, 1990).

Before closing this section, I want to note that there may be a clinical syndrome that is the direct inverse of alexithymia. People with alexithymia have emotions, but they fail to identify them as such. I suspect things can also work the other way around. People with deficient emotions can falsely believe that they have emotions—a kind of emotional anosagnosia. Anecdotal evidence for this can be found in Phelps (Chapter 3), who describes a patient with a profound fear deficit due to bilateral amygdala damage. The patient does not seem to have perfect insight into her deficit. If her high-level emotion representations are intact, then it should be possible for her to believe she is afraid when she really is not. That possibility has not, to my knowledge, been tested.

CONCLUSIONS

I conclude by summarizing the three different forms of emotional awareness that I have been discussing.

First, and most basically, we can be aware *of* our emotions themselves. Emotions are perceptions of bodily changes, and to be aware of an emotion is to experience a patterned bodily change in consciousness. In this respect, emotional awareness is just like perceptual consciousness, and I have argued that a unified theory of perceptual consciousness is available and applicable to emotion.

Second, we can be aware *why* we are having a particular emotion. We can know the thought or perception that triggered an emotional response; however, the thoughts and perceptions that trigger emotions are not components of emotions but belong to vastly distributed elicitation pathways. Awareness of activity in these pathways allows us to discern the objects of our emotions. Much of the literature on so-called unconscious emotion is actually investigating unconscious elicitation. These are cases in which the emotion may be conscious, but the person is not conscious of the reason for the emotion; the person does not know *why* the emotion is occurring.

The third kind of awareness is awareness *that* we are having a particular emotion. It is one thing to experience an emotion consciously and quite another to recognize it as such (compare Schooler, 2002, on "meta-consciousness" and Lambie & Marcel, 2002, on "awareness"). Many of our emotions go unlabeled in the course of day-to-day life. High-level emotion processing allows us to know what we are feeling, which can be very useful in electing coping strategies and describing our states to others. Awareness *that* we are in a particular emotional state is not awareness *of* the state, and indeed the two can come apart. We can learn that we are angry without feeling angry, as occurs in psychotherapy and consciousness raising. Ordinarily, however, we learn what emotions we are experiencing by paying attention to what we are feeling.

These three kinds of emotional awareness—awareness-of, awareness-why, and awareness-that—all have corresponding levels of unawareness. We can fail to know that we are having an emotion or why we are having an emotion, and, most strikingly, we can lack awareness of the emotion itself. Presumably, there are functional differences between conditions under which we have awareness and those under which we lack awareness. I have reason to think that unconscious emotions can play a role in priming, conditioning, and preference formation. Conscious emotions may be needed for forms of learning and decision making that require effort or deliberation. But the functions of emotional awareness have not been fully investigated. My goal here has been to help clear the path toward that end.

REFERENCES

Aziz, Q., Thompson, D. G., Ng, V. W. K., Hamdy, S., Sarkar, S., Brammer, M. J., et al. (2000). Cortical processing of human somatic and visceral sensation. *Journal of Neuroscience, 20,* 2657–2663

Bargh, J. A. (1992). Why subliminality does not matter to social psychology: Awareness of the stimulus versus awareness of its influence. In R. F. Bornstein & T. S. Pittman (Eds.), *Perception without awareness: Cognitive, clinical, and social perspectives* (pp. 236–255). New York: Guilford Press.

Barrett, L. F. (2004). Feelings or words?: Understanding the content in self-report ratings of experienced emotion. *Journal of Personality and Social Psychology, 87,* 266–281.

Barrett, L. F., Gross, J., Conner, T., & Benvenuto, M. (2001). Emotion differentiation and regulation. *Cognition and Emotion, 15,* 713–724.

Berridge, K. C., & Winkielman, P. (2003). What is an unconscious emotion?: The case for unconscious "liking." *Cognition and Emotion, 17,* 181–211.

Berthoz, S., Artiges, E., Van De Moortele, P. F., Poline, J. B., Rouquette, S., Consoli, S. M., et al. (2002). Effect of impaired recognition and expression of emotions on frontocingulate cortices: An fMRI study of men with alexithymia. *American Journal of Psychiatry, 159,* 961–967.

Cacioppo, J. T., Berntson, G. G., Larsen, J. T., Poehlmann, K. M., & Ito, T. A. (2000). The psychophysiology of emotion. In R. Lewis & J. M. Haviland-Jones (Eds.), *Handbook of emotions* (2nd ed., pp. 173–191). New York: Guilford Press.

Cacioppo, J. T., Hawkley, L. C., Crawford, L. E., Ernst, J. M., Burleson, M. H., Kowalewski, R. B., et al. (2002). Loneliness and health: Potential mechanisms. *Psychosomatic Medicine, 64,* 407–417.

Chwalisz, K., Diener, E., & Gallagher, D. (1988). Autonomic arousal feedback and emotional experience: Evidence from the spinal cord injured. *Journal of Personality and Social Psychology, 54,* 820–828.

Clore, G. (1994). Why emotions are never unconscious. In P. Ekman & R. J. Davidson (Eds.), *The nature of emotion: Fundamental questions* (pp. 285–290). New York: Oxford University Press.

Clore, G. L., & Ortony, A. (2000). Cognition in emotion: Always, sometimes, or never? In L. Nadel, R. Lane, & G. L. Ahern (Eds.), *The cognitive neuroscience of emotion.* New York: Oxford University Press

Critchley, H. D., Mathias, C. J., & Dolan, R. J. (2001). Neural correlates of first and second-order representation of bodily states. *Nature Neuroscience 4,* 207–212.

Critchley, H. D., Wiens, S., Rotshtein, P., Öhman, A., & Dolan, R. J. (2004). Neural systems supporting interoceptive awareness. *Nature Neuroscience, 7,* 189–195.

Damasio, A. R. (1994). *Descartes' error: Emotion, reason and the human brain.* New York: Gossett/Putnam.

Damasio, A. R. (1999). *The feeling of what happens: Body and emotion in the making of consciousness.* New York: Harcourt Brace.

Damasio, A. R., Grabowski, T. J., Bechara, A., Damasio, H., Ponto, L. L. B., Parvizi, J., et al. (2000). Subcortical and cortical brain activity during the feeling of self-generated emotions. *Nature Neuroscience, 3,* 1049–1056.

D'Andrade, R. G. (1992). Schemas and motivation. In R. G. D'Andrade & C. Strauss (Eds.), *Human motives and cultural models* (pp. 23–44). Cambridge, UK: Cambridge University Press.

Dixon, N. F. (1981). *Preconscious processing.* Chichester, UK: Wiley.

Duclos, S. A., & Laird, J. D. (2001). The deliberate control of emotional experience through control of expressions. *Cognition and Emotion, 20,* 27–56.

Esteves, F., Dimberg, U., & Öhman, A. (1994). Automatically elicited fear: Conditioned skin conductance responses to masked facial expressions. *Cognition and Emotion, 8,* 393–413.

Fehr, B., & Russell, J. A. (1984). Concept of emotion viewed from a prototype perspective. *Journal of Experimental Psychology: General, 113,* 464–486.

Feldman, L. A. (1995). Valence focus and arousal focus: Individual differences in the structure of affective experience. *Journal of Personality and Social Psychology, 69,* 153–166.

Frank, R. H. (1988). *Passions within reason: The strategic role of the emotions.* New York: Norton.

Freud, S. (1984).The unconscious. In A. Richards (Ed.), *The Pelican Freud library: Vol. 11. On metapsychology: The theory of psychoanalysis* (pp. 159–222). London: Penguin. (Original work published 1915)

Gray, C. M., & Singer, W. (1989). Stimulus specific neuronal oscillations in orientation columns of cat visual cortex. *Proceedings of the National Academy of Sciences, 86,* 1698–1702.

Gray, J. A., & McNaughton, N. (2000). *The neuropsychology of anxiety: An enquiry into the functions of the septo-hippocampal system* (2nd ed.). Oxford, UK: Oxford University Press.

Harré, R. (1986). The social constructivist viewpoint. In R. Harré (Ed.), *The social construction of emotions* (pp. 2–14). Oxford, UK: Blackwell.

Jackendoff, R. (1987). *Consciousness and the computational mind.* Cambridge, MA: MIT Press.

James, W. (1884). What is an emotion? *Mind, 9,* 188–205.

Katkin, E. S. (1985). Blood, sweat, and tears: Individual differences in autonomic self-perception. *Psychophysiology, 22,* 125–137.

Lambie, J. A., & Marcel, A. J. (2002). Consciousness and the varieties of emotion experience: A theoretical framework. *Psychological Review, 109,* 219–259.

Lane, R. D. (2000). Neural correlates of conscious emotional experience. In R. D. Lane & L. Nadel (Eds.), *Cognitive neuroscience of emotion* (pp. 345–370). New York: Oxford University Press.

Lane, R. D., Ahern, G. L., Schwartz, G. E., & Kaszniak, A. W. (1997). Is alexithymia the emotional equivalent of blindsight? *Biological Psychiatry, 42,* 834–844.

Lane, R. D., Fink, G. R., Chau, P. M. L., & Dolan, R. J. (1997). Neural activation during selective attention to subjective emotional responses. *NeuroReport, 8,* 3969–3972.

Lazarus, R. S. (1991). *Emotion and adaptation.* New York: Oxford University Press.

LeDoux, J. E. (1996). *The emotional brain.* New York: Simon & Schuster.

Levenson, R. W., Ekman, P., & Friesen, W. V. (1990). Voluntary facial action generates emotion-specific autonomic nervous system activity. *Psychophysiology, 27,* 363–384.

Leventhal, H., & Scherer, K. R. (1987). The relationship of emotion and cognition:

A functional approach to a semantic controversy. *Cognition and Emotion, 1,* 3–28.

Mack, A., & Rock, I. (1998). *Inattentional blindness.* Cambridge, MA: MIT Press.

Marañon, G. (1924). Contribution à l'étude de l'action émotive de l'adrenaline. *Revue Française d'Endocrinologie, 2,* 301–325.

Marr, D. (1982). *Vision: A computational investigation into the human representation and processing of visual information.* New York: Freeman.

Morris, J. S., Öhman, A., & Dolan, R. J. (1999). A subcortical pathway to the right amygdala mediating "unseen" fear. *Proceedings of the National Academy of Science, 96,* 1680–1685.

Murphy, F. C., Nimmo-Smith, I., & Lawrence, A. D. (2003). Functional neuro-anatomy of emotions: A meta-analysis. *Cognitive, Affective, and Behavioral Neuroscience, 3,* 207–233.

Niedenthal, P. M., Barsalou, L., Winkielman, P., Krauth-Gruber, S., & Ric, F. (in press). Embodiment in attitudes, social perception, and emotion. *Personality and Social Psychology Review.*

Olshausen, B. A., Anderson, C. H., & van Essen, D. C. (1994). A neurobiological model of visual attention and invariant pattern recognition based task. *Journal of Neuroscience, 14,* 6171–6186.

Panksepp, J. (1998). *Affective neuroscience.* New York: Oxford University Press.

Parker, J. D. A., Bagby, R. M., & Taylor, G. J. (1989). Toronto Alexithymia Scale, EPQ and self-report measures of somatic complaints. *Personality and Individual Differences, 10,* 599–604.

Phan, K. L., Wager, T., Taylor, S. F., & Liberzon, I. (2002). Functional neuroanatomy of emotion: A meta-analysis of emotion activation studies in PET and fMRI. *Neuroimage, 16,* 331–348.

Philippot, P., & Schaefer, A. (2001). Emotion and memory. In T. J. Mayne & G. A. Bonanno (Eds.), *Emotions: Current issues and future directions* (pp. 82–122). New York: Guilford Press.

Prinz, J. J. (2000). A neurofunctional theory of visual consciousness. *Consciousness and Cognition, 9,* 243–259.

Prinz, J. J. (2003). Consciousness, computation, and emotion. In S. C. Moore & M. Oaksford (Eds.), *Emotional cognition: From brain to behaviour.* Amsterdam: Benjamins.

Prinz, J. J. (2004). *Gut reactions: A perceptual theory of emotion.* Oxford, UK: Oxford University Press.

Prinz, J. J. (in press). A neurofunctional theory of consciousness. In A. Brooks & K. Akins (Eds.), *Philosophy and neuroscience.* Cambridge, UK: Cambridge University Press.

Rees, G. (2001). Neuroimaging of visual awareness in patients and normal subjects. *Current Opinion in Neurobiology, 11,* 150–156.

Roseman, I. J., Spindel, M. S., & Jose, P. E. (1990). Appraisals of emotion-eliciting events: Testing a theory of discrete emotions. *Journal of Personality and Social Psychology, 59,* 899–915.

Salovey, P., & Mayer, J. D. (1990). Emotional intelligence. *Imagination, Cognition, and Personality, 9,* 185–211.

Saper, C. B. (2002). The central autonomic nervous system: Conscious visceral perception and autonomic pattern generation. *Annual Review of Neuroscience, 25*, 433–469.

Scherer, K. (1993). Studying the emotion-antecedent appraisal process: An expert system approach. *Cognition and Emotion, 7*, 325–356.

Schooler, J. W. (2002). Re-representing consciousness: Dissociations between experience and meta-consciousness. *Trends in Cognitive Sciences, 6*, 339–344.

Shin, L. M., Dougherty, D. D., Orr, S. P., Pitman, R. K., Lasko, M., Macklin, M. L., Alpert, N. M., Fischman, A. J., & Rauch, S. L. (2000). Activation of anterior paralimbic structures during guilt-related script-driven imagery. *Biological Psychiatry, 48*, 43–50.

Sifneos, P. E. (1973). The prevalence of alexithymic characteristics in psychosomatic patients. *Psychotherapy and Psychosomatics, 22*, 255–262.

Simons, D. J., & Chabris, C. F. (1999). Gorillas in our midst: Sustained inattentional blindness for dynamic events. *Perception, 28*, 1059–1074.

Strahan, E., Spencer, S. J., & Zanna, M. P. (2002). Subliminal priming and persuasion: Striking while the iron is hot. *Journal of Experimental Social Psychology, 38*, 556–568.

Tomkins, S. S. (1979). Script theory: Differential magnification of affects. In H. E. Howe, Jr., & R. A. Dienstbier (Eds.), *Nebraska symposium on motivation 1978 (Vol. 26, pp. 201–236)*. Lincoln: University of Nebraska Press.

Valins, S. (1966). Cognitive effects of false heart-rate feedback. *Journal of Personality and Social Psychology, 4*, 400–408.

Vuilleumier, P., Sagiv, N., Hazeltine, E., Poldrack, R. A., Swick, D., Rafal, R. D., & Gabrieli, J. D. (2001). Neural fate of seen and unseen faces in visuospatial neglect: A combined event-related functional MRI and event-related potential study. *Proceedings of the National Academy of Sciences, 98*, 3495–3500.

Wiens, S., Mezzacappa, E. S., & Katkin, E. S. (2000). Heartbeat detection and the experience of emotions. *Cognition and Emotion, 14*, 417–427.

Winkielman, P., Berridge, K. C., & Wilbarger, J. (2005). Unconscious affecrive reactions to masked happy vs. angry faces influence consumption behavior and judgments of value. *Personality and Social Psychology Bulletin, 1*, 121–135.

Zajonc, R. B. (2000). Feeling and thinking: Closing the debate over the independence of affect. In J. P. Forgas (Ed.), *Feeling and thinking: The role of affect in social cognition* (pp. 31–58). Cambridge, UK: Cambridge University Press.

Zajonc, R. B., & McIntosh, D. N. (1992). Emotions research: Some promising questions, some questionable promises. *Psychological Science, 3*, 70–74.

Zajonc, R. B., Murphy, S. T., & Inglehart, M. (1989). Feeling and facial efference: Implications of the vascular theory of emotion. *Psychological Review, 96*, 395–416.

Zeki, S. (1993). *A vision of the brain*. Oxford, UK: Blackwell.

Zillmann, D. (1978). Attribution and misattribution of excitatory reactions. In J. H. Harvey, W. Ickes, & R. F. Kidd (Eds.), *New directions in attribution research* (Vol. 2, pp. 335–368). Hillsdale, NJ: Erlbaum.

CHAPTER 16

Seven Sins in the Study of Unconscious Affect

GERALD L. CLORE

JUSTIN STORBECK

MICHAEL D. ROBINSON

DAVID B. CENTERBAR

The subjective experience of emotion plays a primary role in why lovers pine for one another, jealous spouses monitor each other's phone calls, poets write hymns to the moon, depressives go to therapists, and why emotion researchers care to study emotion.[1] Consider the role of subjective experience in the plight of Othello, the jealous protagonist of Shakespeare's play. If Othello had not been aware of the misleading evidence that his wife, Desdemona, had been unfaithful, would he still have been jealous? Similarly, if he had not felt the urgency of his jealousy, would he have been motivated to seek confirmation of his suspicions? Would he have been spurred to the tragic action that he took? On the other hand, the process of his going from perception to emotion was surely not conscious, nor was the process that actually triggered his vengeful actions conscious. But was the emotion of jealousy itself conscious? Would the drama have played out differently (or have transpired at all) if Othello had felt nothing?

This volume provided a welcome opportunity to think about such issues. Our comments about them are framed as critiques of seven assumptions common in the literature. The goal was to be provocative in the faith

1. *What is the scope of your proposed model? When you use the term* emotion, *how do you use it? What do you mean by terms such as* fear, anxiety, *or* happiness?

If cognition concerns categorization, emotion concerns evaluation. We define emotions simply as affective states, where *affective* means that the state is about the goodness or badness of something, and *state* means that multiple systems are dedicated to the same thing at the same time. Thus an emotion exists when the same evaluation is represented at the same time in multiple systems (e.g., thought, physiology, feeling, motivation, expression). If the multiple systems did not include experience, unconscious emotions could exist, in principle. In practice, they are unlikely, because the coactivation of multiple systems is precisely what produces consciousness.

In the affect-as-information approach, *affect* tends to refer to embodied evaluations (e.g., feelings, expressions, affectively significant action). Controversies often arise when one uses *affect* as a noun. By contrast, the adjective *affective* clearly conveys a focus on evaluation, as in *affective thoughts, affective feelings,* and *affective expressions.*

2. *Define your terms:* conscious, unconscious, awareness. *Or say why you do not use these terms.*

In this chapter we employ conventional uses of the terms *conscious* and "awareness" and do not distinguish them. More generally, clarity can be enhanced by using James's distinction between the "I" and the "me." Thus dogs are conscious of objects in the world through vision, audition, and smell, but they are not conscious of themselves having such experiences. The latter "state of consciousness" or "presence" should emerge when multiple representations show sufficient redundancy to make separate registrations computationally intractable, but sufficient disparity to prevent their assimilation into a single registration.

3. *Does your model deal with what is conscious, what is unconscious, or their relationship? If you do not address this area specifically, can you speculate on the relationship between what is conscious and unconscious? Or if you do not like the conscious–unconscious distinction, or if you do not think this is a good question to ask, can you say why?*

It is no longer a claim worth making to say that something is unconscious, because most bodily, cognitive, and psychological processes occur unconsciously. Affective processes too are largely unavailable to consciousness. Indeed, for this reason we say that affective feelings provide information. Affective feelings are conscious, embodied representations of unconscious appraisals. We may have affective feelings that do not reflect appraisals of events, as in endogenous depression, hormonal imbalances, etc. But the system appears designed to handle the canonical case in which conscious feelings signal that something, in particular, is good or bad in some way. As a result, affective feelings tend to require objects or exhibit "aboutness."

that stirring things up is often useful. With more humility than our presumptuous title suggests, we hope that a critical stance toward some assumptions of our own and others may be helpful as we collectively stumble toward a coherent understanding of emotion. In this spirit, our candidates for the seven sins of studying unconscious affect include the following beliefs:

1. There are unconscious emotions.
2. Unconsciousness emotional stimuli are stronger than conscious ones.
3. Conscious feelings cause liking.
4. Preferences precede inferences.
5. Expressive actions have fixed effects.
6. "Low-route" stimulation causes human emotion.
7. Emotions occur too quickly to require appraisals.

SIN 1: THERE ARE UNCONSCIOUS EMOTIONS

In this section, we ask whether the phenomena referred to by the label unconscious emotion *form a coherent category.*

As part of a general rediscovery of unconscious processes (e.g., Wilson, 2002), psychologists now study implicit personality (Robinson, 2004), implicit attitudes (Greenwald, McGhee, & Schwartz, 1998), and implicit memory (Graf & Schachter, 1985). The current volume similarly promotes the study of implicit emotion (but see Barrett, Chapter 11, for an alternative view). Before signing on wholeheartedly to such a quest, however, it might be prudent to ask whether the idea of "unconscious emotion" really defines a coherent category for study.

Cognitive psychologists who have been examining implicit memory for the last 20 years suggest a surprising answer. The implicit–explicit distinction entered the study of memory when Graf and Schachter (1985) wrote a paper referring to "implicit and explicit" measures of memory. They focused on dissociations between these two kinds of measures. But the terms *implicit–explicit* were soon hijacked to refer not only to kinds of *measures*, but also to kinds of *memory*. Some of the phenomena that show dissociations between implicit and explicit measures include blindsight (in which individuals can accurately locate flashes of light despite having no visual experience), prosopagnosia (in which patients show skin conductance responses to faces they have seen many times but cannot recognize), and Alzheimer's disease (in which patients can remember, e.g., how to play golf, but not how many strokes they had taken in a particular game).

These examples make it clear that there is more to memory than what is available to consciousness. But of what does this "more" consist? What do the various implicit measures of memory *measure*? The surprising answer from those who have studied the question is that implicit memory does not exist (Willingham & Preuss, 1995). The point that Willingham and Preuss make is not that there are no implicit memory phenomena, however; on the contrary, there are so many kinds of non-conscious memory phenomena that nothing holds them together. They share neither a common neurology nor a common function, two of the characteristics that might justify a unified category of implicit memory. People continue to talk about *implicit* as a single state or condition, but it is becoming clear that there is no basis for doing so (Willingham & Preuss, 1995). Squire and Zola-Morgan (1991) argue that implicit versus explicit is not a real distinction about memory but simply a way of separating different aspects of *research* on memory. The labels simply correct the misunderstanding we all used to share that memory is necessarily conscious.

Should we conclude that, like implicit memory, unconscious emotion also does not exist? If most emotional processes are unconscious, then the label *unconscious* may not be informative (for an alternative view, see Winkielman, Berridge, & Wilbarger, Chapter 14). *Unconscious emotion* may simply be a catchall term to connote processes united only by *not* being conscious. However, one benefit of thinking about the unconscious aspects of emotion is that we are led to ask about the role of consciousness in emotion (e.g., Edelman, 1989). We turn to this task now.

SIN 2: UNCONSCIOUS EMOTIONAL STIMULI ARE STRONGER THAN CONSCIOUS ONES

In this section we make two points: (1) Neural activation by conscious stimulation is many times stronger than activation from nonconscious stimulation, and (2) rather than being stronger, unconscious affect is less constrained in its object and hence more easily misattributed.

Consciousness Involves Strong Activation

Most of what the brain does is unconscious, but attention both amplifies and prolongs activation, which allows processing at one site to affect processing at other sites, forming a network of activation that can reverberate and give rise to the experience of consciousness (Dehaene & Naccache, 2001; Dehaene et al., 2001). Brain areas involved in emotion can then interact with other areas. The broad recruitment of neural circuits, which occurs when stimuli are strong in duration and intensity, makes emotional stimuli powerful and ensures their consideration by the brain as a whole (Roser & Gazzaniga, 2004).

Of course, briefer, less intense stimulation can be registered without conscious awareness. However, such stimulation probably does not take a different route (contrary to suggestions by several contributors to this volume), but merely produces transitory and weak sensory signals, which are incapable of recruiting frontal areas of the brain (Storbeck, Robinson, & McCourt, in press; but for an alternative view, see Phelps, Chapter 3; Gray, Schaefer, Braver, & Most, Chapter 4). Stimuli that elicit stronger, longer, and broader activation of neural circuits should typically be more consequential than unconscious stimuli. Pavlov too (1927/1960) noted that of several stimuli occurring together as a conditioned stimulus, the strongest and most salient stimulus would control responding, almost totally, following conditioning.

The importance of activation strength can also be seen in processes such as reading. As our eyes fall on each succeeding word in a sentence, multiple meanings of each word are activated. However, we usually remain unaware of any but the most relevant of these candidate meanings. The one meaning that best fits the gist of a sentence and is most compatible with the larger sense of a paragraph usually wins the race (Conrad, 1974). "Winning the race" means influencing meaning, comprehension, insight, and so on. Losers of the race are eliminated and become inconsequential once the race has been won.

What is true of reading meaningful text is presumably no less true of "reading" the emotional meanings of events. Although subliminal frowning or smiling faces can alter judgments under carefully designed circumstances, it is not clear what analogues exist to such primes in the real world of visual objects (for a review, see Lundqvist & Öhman, Chapter 5; de Gelder, Chapter 6; Atkinson & Adolphs, Chapter 7). Since four-millisecond exposures with pattern masks do not occur regularly in the environment, the explanatory power of such demonstrations is unclear. In contrast, optimal visual stimulation gives rise to a wide pattern of activation, recruiting frontal circuits relevant to consciousness and self-regulation (Storbeck et al., in press). Many visual stimuli compete for our attention, but very few have an influence. The window of opportunity for each is brief, and when gone, it never returns. Stimuli that do exercise influence often do so because their activation is amplified by more frontal neural circuits. Unconscious stimuli do have *some* influence on judgment and behavior, but that such effects are stronger than those involving conscious recognition processes seems doubtful.

Consciousness and Constraint

Despite the self-evident nature of the foregoing assertions, social psychologists tend to believe that unconscious emotional stimuli are somehow stronger than conscious stimuli. It is true that priming and mood effects both occur only when people remain unaware of the true cause of the resulting thoughts and feelings (e.g., Murphy & Zajonc, 1993; Schwarz & Clore, 1983). When priming and mood-induction procedures are made salient, respondents may no longer experience their thoughts and feelings as reactions to target stimuli. Priming and mood effects then tend to disappear. However, what consciousness does in these situations is not to weaken affect but to channel its influence. Awareness makes primes less powerful only in the sense that unconstrained affective meaning does not have unlimited potential to color interpretations of other objects (Clore & Colcombe, 2003).

Mere Exposure

One source of the belief that affect is stronger when it is unconscious are studies of the mere-exposure phenomenon. Zajonc (1980) made much of the fact that mere-exposure effects appear greater when exposures are nonconscious than when they are conscious. He relied heavily on this observation as evidence for "the primacy of affect" over cognition. However, those effects succumb to the same analysis given above. In our view, the reason mere-exposure effects are weaker for long exposures is that when stimuli are consciously recognized, the fluency responsible for exposure effects is then correctly experienced merely as familiarity, rather than as liking. Thus increases in mere-exposure effects with unconscious stimulation (for a review, see Bornstein, 1989) probably tell us nothing about "affective primacy." Rather they tell us about the role of consciousness in constraining meaning by making possible proper attributions for affect (Schwarz & Clore, 1983).

More generally, affective processing proceeds from novelty detection to stimulus categorization and identification. In this process, general, diffuse activation gets transformed into specific and localized activation. There is a curious tendency for investigators to think of the early, diffuse activation as the real emotion, and the categorization and localization processes as secondary, regulatory processes (see also Barrett, Chapter 11). In this regard, investigators have tended to reify amygdala activation as emotion, but the amygdala reacts to novelty and stimulus uncertainty as well as possible danger (Whalen, 1998). Hence, the refinement of such signals in the cortex would seem important in defining as well as regulating emotion (Storbeck et al., in press).

In this section we have argued that unconscious primes and other stimuli are weaker, not stronger, than conscious ones. We suggested that the apparent dampening effects of consciousness on affect are due to the constraints on possible meanings of the affect when a specific source is made salient. More generally, we suggested that it may be useful to view the refinement of affect from cortical involvement as part of emotion, rather than as postemotional, regulatory processing. This section focused primarily on unconscious *sources* of affect. We turn next to unconscious *processes* of affect.

SIN 3: CONSCIOUS FEELINGS CAUSE LIKING

In this section we offer an account of the affect-as-information approach that distinguishes possible roles for conscious and unconscious affect in judgment, decision making, attention, and memory. The first part distinguishes between implicit and explicit judgments and decisions. The second focuses on the role of conscious feelings in explicit judgments and decisions. The third part discusses conscious and unconscious consequences of arousal.

Unconscious Causes of Liking

In his book *The Illusion of Conscious Will*, Wegner (2002) has written persuasively about the unconscious wellsprings of action. He notes that by the time we entertain choice options consciously, an implicit choice has often already been made. He suggests that we are often truly authors of our own actions, but the cause of such actions may not lie in the thoughts about acting that we consciously entertain. Instead, we may simply become aware of whatever option has risen to the top. In other words, both willed actions and consciously preferred behavioral options are the products of unconscious processes that precede these occurrences.

Consciously we may entertain an elaborate narrative of choice, but it is likely to be a post hoc construction of left hemisphere processes. Such narratives are designed to make sense and may even be accurate, such that they represent as good reasons for action some of the actual causes for action. But these conscious accounts may be simply a dramatization of the choosing rather than a glimpse of the actual choice process. The implicit choice, at least, is presumably a function of connections between neural representations and neurochemical reactions, neither of which is consciously available.

Extending Wegner's logic suggests a similar account of how affect may influence judgments and decisions. Let us assume that the mind arranges for the conscious feelings of affect and for the conscious representations of potential attitude objects. When associated in time, we may experience our feelings as causing our liking. The experience may lead us to conclude accurately that affect causes liking, but our feelings may not be doing the work. Instead the critical processes may occur at the implicit level (see also Winkielman et al., Chapter 14). Implicit liking might arise when implicit affect (e.g., involving the release of dopamine or other relevant neurochemicals) becomes linked to an implicit neural representation of an attitude object. The affective feelings that occur when we are consciously thinking about the attitude object then provide information for explicit judgments, as discussed below.

Affect as Information

Conscious feelings reflect unconscious affective processes and provide information for making explicit judgments and decisions, as specified by the affect-as-information approach (Clore et al., 2001; Schwarz & Clore, 1983).

Unconscious affective reactions, registered as conscious affective feelings, provide information for explicit judgments and decisions. Because the information is internal, spontaneous, and experiential, it tends to be credible and compelling. Thus we may be informed by our feelings that we have fallen in love, that we hate, or that we do not care. Such conscious feeling may often be the direct basis for explicit evaluative judgments. An elaboration of this view of the affect-as-information account of liking might be something like the following:

> Implicit liking may be caused by implicit affect (e.g., dopamine and perhaps other neurochemicals) toward implicit neural representations of attitude objects. We may become aware of the liking if we experience feelings in response to thoughts of attitude objects. We construct explicit judgments of the liking or disliking of attitude objects by using such conscious thoughts and feelings as information about our implicit evaluations and attitudes.

Conscious consideration of decision alternatives allows the relevance and importance of alternatives to be subjectively registered, which may often be helpful in decision making. Explicit decisions may be made when subjective experiences are sufficient for us to realize that we have decided. As in being asked "Are you feeling feverish?" or "Are you still mad?" often the only way to know if a decision has been made is to consult one's feelings.

For big decisions, such as buying a car or a house, choosing a college or a job, or deciding whether to marry someone, we often expect to be visited by an affective indication of the right decision. Individuals sometimes make comments such as "We knew that was the house for us as soon as we saw it," or "I fell in love with the university during my first visit." And couples may recall intense romantic moments to reinforce their commitment. People also use their affect as information when making small decisions. An acquaintance who went shoe shopping but returned empty-handed commented that although many shoes seemed fine, nothing moved her to make a purchase. One implication of this analysis is that important decisions not associated with strong conscious feelings pose problems for the individual. We may have a hard time deciding, and if forced by time to decide without the subjective experience that says "This is it," we may vacillate and experience postdecisional worry. For example, a young man recently reported feeling depressed after choosing a college to attend, because he never experienced a rush of feelings telling him that he had made the correct decision.

In summary, we have argued that conscious feelings might be correlated with, but not causal in the formation of, implicit liking or implicit decisions. If so, then the functions served by the consciousness of attitude objects and associated feelings may be primarily informational, ensuring explicit judgments and choices that are consistent with already formed implicit judgments and choices. These considerations focus on the valence dimension, wherein positive and negative feelings provide information about goodness and badness. But what about the arousal dimension?

Affect as Importance

Feelings of arousal convey information about urgency and importance. We propose that conscious feelings of arousal play a role in attention, and that unconscious components of arousal play a role in memory.

An enduring observation about conscious emotional experiences is that they have both valence and arousal components (Wundt, 1897), often shown as independent, bipolar dimensions (Barrett, Chapter 11; Russell, 2003). If the valence component provides embodied evaluation information, the arousal component can be thought of as providing importance information (Barrett, Chapter 11; Frijda, Ortony, Sonnemons, & Clore, 1992).

Two things happen when events are marked with arousal as being urgent or important: They commandeer attention (Simon, 1967), and they become memorable (Cahill & McGaugh, 1998). These are fascinating processes, but for current purposes the question is, "Are they are mediated by conscious experience?" Our tentative answer is "yes" in the case of attention and "no" in the case of memory.

Feelings Trigger Attention

Attention appears to be sense driven in humans and other animals. Thus bright lights and loud noises readily capture our attention. It seems plausible that the same principles govern the effect of emotional cues on attention. Our attention is commandeered by subjective experiences that are intense and have a fast rise time. Surprising someone by firing a gun or clapping one's hand loudly behind the person's head completely disrupts what he or she was doing. In a similar manner the experience of fright, anxiety, disgust, embarrassment, or joy is likely to rivet attention on the object of the emotion. Both external sensory stimuli and internal emotional stimuli have this capacity. As with external stimulation, the greater the intensity of these internal feelings, the more completely they should command attention and redirect limited attentional resources (Simon, 1967). We assume that only strong stimuli exercise such control and hence are unlikely to remain unconscious. The parallel ways in which attention is guided by both external sensory and internal emotional stimuli lead to the speculation that the quasi-sensory processes of the emotional system evolved to make use of sensory operating principles. In any case, one function of conscious emotional feelings appears to be to commandeer attention and reset the cognitive processing agenda, as outlined by Simon (1967).

It should be mentioned that some investigators (e.g., Gray et al., Chapter 4; Lundqvist & Öhman, Chapter 5) present compelling data that the affective guidance of attention occurs unconsciously. On the other hand, after reviewing literature on attentional capture, Pashler, Johnston, and Ruthruff (2001) concluded that "a variety of proposals for 'wired-in' attention capture by particular stimulus attributes have been effectively challenged; attention, it turns out, is subject to a far greater degree of top-down control than was suspected 10 years ago" (p. 648).

In addition to guiding attention, the arousal component of affect also has dramatic effects on how memorable experiences are. However, despite the fact that arousal is experienced, the active agent in memory consolidation may not be the experience of arousal but the neurochemistry underlying those feelings, as discussed next.

Epinephrine Release Triggers Memory Consolidation

McGaugh and colleagues (e.g., Cahill & McGaugh, 1998) have shown that the release of epinephrine after learning is associated with enhanced memory after a period of time. For example, Cahill and colleagues (Cahill et al., 1996) showed emotionally evocative film clips depicting themes of animal mutilation or violent crime. Later, these were much better recalled than neutral clips from the same films. The emotional clips were arousing, whereas the neutral clips were similar in style but not arousing. As participants watched the films, the glucose utilization in the brain was measured by positron emission tomography (PET). Three weeks later they were telephoned and asked to recall the films. One set of results concerned the relationship between amygdala activity and recall: Amygdala activity during the emotional scene was related to later recall of emotional, but not of nonemotional, scenes. Thus, although neutral experiences can be remembered without involving stress hormones or the amygdala, for emotional experiences, stress hormones stimulate the amygdala to influence storage in memory.

The enhancement of memory by arousal occurs even when the arousal is irrelevant and comes after learning. For example, after a list of words had already been studied, a bloody film about pulling teeth produced 10% better memory 24 hours later than a control film about dental care (Nielson, 2003; Pearson, 2002). Arousal in response to experiences presumably gives them greater weight than other information during storage so that the most important experiences yield the strongest memories (Christianson & Loftus, 1991). When an event triggers the release of the stress hormone adrenaline, the adrenaline activates the amygdala, which tags that experience for storage.

With respect to questions of consciousness, it is notable that animal data also show memory enhancement when adrenalin is administered after aversive training. The effect occurs when administered at about the time adrenalin would have been released by aversive stimulation under normal conditions. Although there may be conscious concomitants of adrenaline injections, even in rats, the processes that result in memory consolidation presumably occur at a neurochemical, rather than an experiential, level. However, it is possible that behavioral components contribute to memorability. Experienced arousal tends to attract attention to relevant stimuli, and such increased attention has essentially the same effect on memory as practice does.

In summary, the research of the McGaugh group suggests that affective arousal may be more important in memory than previously realized. Since it would be disadvantageous to remember everything, a primary task of the organism is to appraise what is critical to retain and what is not. Part of that process appears to involve the adrenaline of affective arousal.

The goal of the larger section was to think broadly about the relative roles of conscious and unconscious affect in judgment, decision making, attention, and memory. The importance of affective processes in these cognitive processes raises larger questions about how we should think about the relation between affect and cognition. We turn next to this topic, which has dominated much of the past 25 years of affect research.

SIN 4: PREFERENCES PRECEDE INFERENCES

In this section we review recent evidence suggesting that popular ideas about the primacy of affect have been overstated. Some evidence suggests that preferences do need inferences and that the "automatic evaluation effect" may often be an "automatic categorization effect."

A new age of affect in psychology was announced by two important papers published in the early 1980s. Zajonc's (1980) "Preferences Need No Inferences" paper marked his receipt of the American Psychological Association's Distinguished Scientist Award, and the very next year, Bower (1981) marked his receipt of the same award with his paper "Mood and Memory." Both were important in the development of current affective science, but in a sense they made opposite points. Whereas Bower argued that we could use what we know about cognitive processing to understand emotional phenomena, Zajonc argued that affect and cognition are processed independently. He argued that things are evaluated affectively before they are categorized cognitively.

Affective priming is a phenomenon that seemed consistent with that independence hypothesis. Evaluative priming words can be shown to speed up the processing of similarly valenced target words even though they have no descriptive meaning in common (e.g., Bargh, 1997). This phenomenon was found even for stimuli that were only slightly positive or negative in value, including nonsense syllables, and even on nonevaluative tasks. Such data were interpreted as evidence of the primacy of affect.

The initial demonstration of automatic evaluation was an affective priming study by Fazio, Sanbonmatsu, Powell, and Kardes (1986). Participants were asked to evaluate target words after other evaluative words were shown about 300 milliseconds earlier. After positive prime words (e.g., *friend*), people were faster to evaluate other positive words (e.g., *birthday*) than negative words (e.g., *pain*). At the relatively short intervals used, the evaluative influences were assumed to be automatic. Bargh (1997) reviewed similar results, which he refers to as the "automatic evaluation effect." However, neurological and new behavioral considerations suggest otherwise. For example, Rolls (1999) argued cogently that objects must first be categorized descriptively before they are analyzed affectively. In addition, new data (Storbeck & Robinson, 2004) also cast a very different light on the issue.

The fact that evaluative priming occurs in the absence of any descriptive relationship among primes and targets turns out to be a limitation rather than a strength of evaluative priming studies. If people categorize whatever they see, experimental designs that expose them to words with nothing in common but evaluation may force evaluative priming.

As a test of this hypothesis, Storbeck and Robinson (2004) repeated standard priming studies but varied the categorical as well as the evaluative similarity between primes and targets. Thus, their words included positive and negative animal words (e.g., *puppy*, *spider*) as well as positive and negative texture words (e.g., *silky, rough*) or religious words (e.g., *angel, Hell*). In three different priming paradigms—evaluative, descriptive, and lexical decision tasks—they found robust descriptive priming but no evaluative priming. Evaluative priming was found only when they used traditional stimulus word sets that prevented respondents from engaging in descriptive categorization (see De Houwer & Randell, 2004, for similar findings with pronunciation tasks).

A large body of memory research also suggests that declarative memory is organized descriptively, not evaluatively (e.g., McRae & Boisvert, 1998). Indeed, it seems implausible that nature would have saddled us with a memory system in which any slightly positive or negative stimulus would activate all other positive or negative concepts without regard to their descriptive relevance. To the extent that they speak to issues of cognition and emotion generally, Storbeck and Robinson's (2004) results are more compatible with cognitive appraisal theory than with affective primacy theory. That is, evaluative responding may not routinely occur before semantic categorization. Indeed, the data suggest an "automatic categorization effect" rather than an "automatic evaluation effect." If the stimulus conditions allow for a categorical distinction among primes (e.g., animals vs. texture-related words), such a categorical distinction will be used, rather than evaluation. Good versus bad can also be useful categories, of course, but they do not appear to have a special status.

In this section we reviewed results that cast a new light on the meaning of affective priming. A growing number of psychologists, economists, and marketing and politically oriented investigators cite affective priming as evidence of the primacy of affect within their domains. For example, political scientists working on the cutting edge (e.g., Lodge & Taber, in press)[2] have used the names of political figures and policies as priming stimuli with semantically unrelated target words. For the subset of respondents sufficiently sophisticated to have relevant opinions, the researchers found the usual speed advantage following evaluatively congruent primes when respondents evaluated targets. The investigators rightly conclude that such effects show that political figures are attitude objects, that is, that people react to them evaluatively. However, following standard psychological interpretation, these and other authors see wider implications in their findings. For example, since the nonpolitical target words were dissimilar in content to the political primes, they interpret their results as evidence for the "primacy of affect (Zajonc, 1980; Murphy & Zajonc, 1993)" and suggest that "cognitive and affective systems follow separate . . . pathways in the brain, with feelings following a quick and dirty route (Le Doux, 1996)." They see their results as a strong test because their method breaks "any reasonable cognitive connection between the attitudinal prime and the target concepts." This often repeated reasoning fails to recognize that semantic priming is more robust than affective priming. In the end, affective priming appears to be simply a subvariety of general semantic priming and is not evidence of "affective primacy" in any shape or form (Storbeck & Robinson, 2004; Storbeck et al., in press).

SIN 5: EXPRESSIVE ACTIONS HAVE FIXED EFFECTS

This section suggests that there probably are no direct and unmediated effects of expressive and motor actions on affect, and that appearances to the contrary may depend on meaning supplied by the context of the muscle movements.

Both Darwin and James are often cited in studies concerned with expressive action and emotion. However, it is not clear that either believed that actions cause emotions. James (1890/1955) did say that "we are afraid because we run," but his point was that running is part of fear, rather than that motor actions cause emotions. Similarly, Darwin (1872/1965) believed that expressions amplify emotions, but he did not generally hold that expressions *cause* emotions. Nevertheless, there is a general belief that emotional expressions, gestures, and actions such as smiles, nods, and arm flexion might elicit affect directly without cognitive mediation.

Some studies of self-produced facial actions do suggest that smiling elicits positive affect (Laird, 1974) and that head nods leads to persuasion (Wells & Petty, 1980) (for a general discussion, see Niedenthal, Barsalou, Ric, & Krauth-Gruber, Chapter 2). For example, individuals in a well-known study by Strack, Martin, and Stepper (1988) were asked to hold a pencil in their mouths while viewing cartoons. The pencil-in-the-mouth method unobtrusively got people to flex the muscles involved in smiling, which increased their enjoyment of cartoons. This clever experiment clearly showed that expressions such as smiling can intensify relevant affect. However, it did not necessarily show the kind of direct relationship between action and affect that is often assumed. The problem is that muscle contraction within a single context, such as rating cartoons, leaves us uncertain about whether smiles elicit enjoyment generally or whether they elicit enjoyment in the context of viewing cartoons.

To examine this issue, Tamir and colleagues (Tamir, Robinson, Clore, Martin, & Whitaker, 2004) varied the context of expressions and gestures. In multiple experiments that examined actions such as head shaking and brow furrowing, they found no support for a direct link (i.e., main effect) from motor action to affect. Although affective influences were readily observed, they varied depending on the cognitive context provided. For example, the effect of head shaking on affect was examined as participants watched one of two films. One showed an ex-convict who had murdered a young girl in a psychotic delusion. He is shown arguing that he is perfectly fine and should be free to live wherever he wants, without scrutiny from his new neighbors. The other clip showed a pregnant young heroin addict who explains her wretched situation. Head shaking, manipulated in an irrelevant manner, did influence feelings toward the protagonists, but in opposite ways with reference to the two targets. Those shaking their heads while watching the murder clip judged the character more responsible for his actions and were angrier. In contrast, head shaking during the addict clip functioned as commiseration regarding her sad plight and resulted in greater sympathy rather than greater anger. Another of these studies examined the effects of subliminally presented smiles. Again, the results varied by context. In a competitive game, the smiles appeared either as the participant's performance was being scored or while his or her competitor was being scored. In the former group, unconscious smiles increased participants' estimates of how well they had done. By contrast, in the latter group, unconscious smiles decreased participants' estimates of how well they had done. A third study examined the effects of brow tension on decisional confidence. Again, the effects reversed, depending on the contextual variable that was manipulated.

These contextual effects are useful to contrast with standard social cognition theorizing concerning the influence of expressive movements on affect, judgment, and memory. In their essay "Of Men and Mackerels," Dijksterhuis, Bargh, and Miedema (2000) argue that expressive effects have automatic and invariable effects on affect, judgment, and behavior. They contend that the influence of expressive cues is fixed and that people can minimize them only by exercising conscious control. The data of Tamir et al. (2004) suggest that such an account is incorrect, that people have surprising capacities to contextualize unconscious expressive cues. Thus the link between expressive cues and affective reactions appears to be flexible rather than fixed. To predict how automatic affective cues will influence affect, judgment, or behavior, it is important to know something about the context in which such automatic affective cues are manipulated.

Other experiments have examined the idea that arm flexion and extension influence attitudes toward novel stimuli. In a well-known series of experiments Cacioppo, Priester, and Berntson (1993) examined the effects of arm flexion and extension on attitudes toward novel stimuli. Arm flexion (as in approach) consisted of pressing gently down on a table top or exercise bar, and arm extension (as in avoidance) consisted of pressing up from the bottom of the table or exercise bar. They found that evaluations of novel Chinese ideographs were more positive when associated with approach-related behaviors (flexion) than with avoidance-related behaviors (extension). Do such effects implicate invariant affective programs triggered by expressive cues?

A recent series of studies by Centerbar and Clore (2004) examined the "fixed" consequences of such expressive cues, while simultaneously manipulating contextual variables. They found that the effect of arm contraction on attitudes was not direct but, rather, depended on the valence of the attitude object. Chinese ideographs were preselected based on differences in how positive or negative other participants had rated them. They found that flexion (approach) behaviors led to *higher* liking judgments for the positive stimuli but *lower* liking judgments for the negative stimuli. Conversely, extension (avoidance) led to *lower* ratings of positive stimuli but *higher* ratings of negative stimuli. That is, when people's approach–avoidance motor actions matched their motivational orientation toward positive and negative stimuli, their attitudes toward the stimuli were more positive. There were no direct effects of arm contraction on attitudes. Related reversals have been obtained by using primed positive or negative concepts as the mental context (Centerbar, 2003). In those studies, the direction of effects of approach–avoidance motor action again depended completely on the cognitive context at the time.

In summary, muscle contractions relevant to approach–avoidance (Centerbar & Clore, 2004) point to the same conclusions as prior studies related to expression and gesture (Tamir et al., 2004): *Affect is elicited not by the muscles but by the mind.* In both sets of studies, the same actions were shown to have opposite affective consequences simply by changing the mental context. Even when affective cues are unconscious, these results suggest that they nevertheless gain power primarily through interpretive (i.e., cognitive) processes (Clore & Colcombe, 2003). Indeed, investigators of implicit attitudes (e.g., Glaser & Banaji, 1999; Lowery, Hardin, & Sinclair, 2001) seem to have arrived at a similar conclusion. Affective reactions, even those that are presumed to be automatic and to reflect unconscious content, are contingent on the cognitive context active at the time of measurement. The results suggest that humans are remarkably inferential creatures, and that affective consequences depend on sophisticated unconscious inferential processes.

SIN 6: LOW-ROUTE STIMULATION CAUSES HUMAN EMOTION

In this section we review literature suggesting that the "low route" to emotion is largely irrelevant to human emotion.

The one universal citation in discussions of unconscious emotion is to LeDoux's (1996) concept of the low route to emotion (e.g., see Lundqvist & Öhman, Chapter 5; de Gelder, Chapter 6; and Winkielman et al., Chapter 14). That important research established aversive conditioning in rats without participation of the visual cortex by pairing changes in illumination with electric shock (LeDoux, Romanski, & Xagoraris, 1989). The researchers proposed that emotional responses could be elicited via a subcortical path going directly from the sensory thalamus to the amygdala without first going to the cerebral cortex. That is, fear-relevant responses could be triggered before one could feel fear or identify the conditioned stimulus. Emotional responses could thus fire without one knowing either that one was afraid or of what one was afraid.

This work is routinely cited, not only by psychologists but also by scholars in marketing, economics, law, and political science. Despite the absence of appropriate research related to human emotion, it has become accepted wisdom that human emotions are often triggered via this low route. Storbeck et al. (in press) have recently reviewed relevant literature to assess such conclusions and suggest that the low route probably has limited relevance for human emotion. Some of their points include the following: (1) Only very simple stimuli, such as light versus dark, can be detected without involvement of the visual cortex. Hence the low route cannot, in principle, explain the kinds of effects seen in social-psychological studies of emotion that use such complex stimuli as facial expressions, emotional pictures, words, or the stimuli used in studies of mere exposure; (2) the low-route pathway studied by LeDoux among rats may not exist or be active among primates and humans (Dolan, 2000; Kudo, Glendenning, Frost, & Masterson, 1986); (3) despite demonstrating that emotional conditioning is possible via a subcortical route among rats, LeDoux (1996) himself views the cortical route as more important in most emotional situations, even among rats; and (4) research from a variety of perspectives converges on the conclusion that cortical involvement via output from area IT (inferior temporal area) in the visual cortex is critical for the amygdala to respond to affectively significant stimuli (Fukuda, Ono, & Nakamura, 1987; Rolls, 1999). Conversely, there seems to be no evidence that the amygdala is important for the categorization, identification, or recognition of stimuli. These facts favor the view that with visual stimuli, semantic processing is necessary for affect retrieval.

It is not possible to reproduce the detailed review of relevant literature presented by Storbeck et al. (in press), and interested readers are referred to that paper for a more detailed analysis. There is no reason to suppose, of course, that the semantic processing alluded to is conscious. However, they make clear that the weight of research indicates that the low route could the low route could not be the unconscious evaluator proposed by Bargh (1997) and Zajonc (2000).

SIN 7: EMOTIONS OCCUR TOO QUICKLY TO REQUIRE APPRAISALS

In this section we suggest that appraisal theories concern the psychological structure of emotion differentiation. They are not process models, as critics seem to assume. Thus the fact that emotion elicitation involves heuristic or associative processes has no bearing on the validity of appraisal theory.

Questions about appraisal theory inevitably creep into discussions of emotion. For example, Prinz (Chapter 15) suggests that appraisals are no more necessary for emotion than for pain (but for the opposite view, see Scherer, Chapter 13). Prinz suggests that since we do not appraise our wounds before feeling pain, we need not assume that we appraise emotional events before feeling happy or sad. In fact, pain receptors under the skin do offer a kind of "appraisal" of the extent of tissue damage. However, the main reason the analogy fails is that we have no comparable receptors for detecting psychological injury, so that some sort of psychological appraisal is required.

More importantly, critics often misunderstand the assertions of appraisal theory in a fundamental way—a misunderstanding which appraisal theorists themselves have unwittingly promoted (Frijda, personal communication, July 7, 2004). As a rule, appraisal theories are not models of the processes involved in emotion elicitation, as the critics often assume. Scherer (1984) does have an interesting process account, but most appraisal theories focus on the rules that differentiate one emotion from another. They ask what kinds of situations elicit sadness rather than shame. When does pride arise rather than hope? They do not assume that we need explicit knowledge of the rules in order to feel sad or proud any more than we need explicit knowledge of the rules of syntax in order to communicate. Indeed, the analogy between the rules of appraisal and the rules of syntax is a powerful one.

What are the implications of the fact that people speak correctly and effortlessly regardless of whether they know the rules of grammar? Would anyone argue that language use does not depend on syntactical rules, just because people do not think about such rules before they speak? Similarly, what are the implications of the fact that people who no know nothing about the law can spot an injustice just as fast as a doctor of jurisprudence? We hold people accountable to the law, despite our knowledge that they do not routinely consult laws before acting. Further, despite the fact that many concepts and categories have necessary and sufficient conditions for their correct application, people may use them correctly without consulting such conditions. For example, the category *grandmother* applies if and only if a person is a mother of a parent. But when looking for a grandmother, we might simply point to the nearest, older woman with white hair wearing an apron and carrying a plate of cookies. What's going on here?

We suggest that there is confusion between assertions about the underlying structure of domains and assertions about how we negotiate them. Failure to make such distinctions would lead one to conclude that only linguists can speak, only lawyers know the difference between right and wrong, and only appraisal theorists can feel emotions. But the rules of syntax, the rules of law, and the rules of appraisal theory are assertions about the structure of utterances, of justice, and of emotion, respectively. They are not process models of speaking, judging, or feeling, even though they are basic for understanding those processes.

As particular kinds of embodied evaluations, emotions necessarily involve some sort of appraisal, but the term carries no implications about how such evaluations are made. Sloman (1996) has proposed two kinds of reasoning: rule-based and associative reasoning; Clore and Ortony (2000; see also Smith & Neumann, Chapter 12) use this distinction to resolve misunderstandings about appraisal theory. They note that there are two routes to emotional appraisal ("reinstatement" and "computation"). Although we can compute bottom-up evaluations of events in real time, we generally rely instead on associations between present and past. Thus prior types of emotion are reinstated when current situations remind us of past situations—that is, when they elicit appraisals (and hence emotions) typical of an earlier situation. In these cases, as LeDoux (1996) notes succinctly, "emotion *is* memory."

This duality characterizes cognitive processes generally. In addition to two forms of reasoning and two kinds of emotional appraisal, there are two modes of categorization: prototype-based and theory-based categorization, as seen in the grandmother example above (Clore & Ortony, 1991). Prototype-, case-, or exemplar-based categorization is different from theory-based categorization, in which features might be implicitly mapped onto the defining features of particular categories. The point is that cognitive processes—whether in emotion, categorization, or reasoning—come in two flavors. Top-down, heuristic, and associational processes that are fast but error prone, and bottom-up, computational processes that are slower but more reliable.

Why two different kinds of processes? Clore and Ortony (2000) suggest that the two routes to emotional appraisal and categorization serve different behavioral functions: preparedness and flexibility. Preparedness requires speed of processing; categorizing current situations on the basis of the similarity of their surface features to those of prototypic emotional situations allows preparation of a reaction before the identity of a stimulus has been fully established. But flexibility of response is also part of what emotion offers (Scherer, 1984). Flexibility is better achieved through rule-based processing. When preparation is accompanied by subjective experience, emotions offer an alternative to reflexive action, a mind–body way station that allows additional environmental and memorial information to modify action.

In summary, appraisal theories specify the psychological situations that give rise to anger, fear, shame, pride, and so on. But such theories do not address whether a person's appraisal of an event arises instantaneously on the basis of clang associations or is the product of years of psychotherapy. Humans negotiate the world using simple rules of thumb or heuristics because formal cost–benefit calculations, even when possible, are generally infeasible. But understanding emotions requires more than simply mapping those rules of thumb. Theorists also ask about the underlying cognitive structure of emotions with respect to which such heuristics have evolved. The mental health of individuals and the survival of the species ultimately depend on how well the distinctions afforded by those rules of thumb map differences among important psychological situations in relation to which the various emotions evolved. Appraisal theories are attempts to characterize those important differences in the cognitive structure of emotions and emotional situations.

CONCLUSIONS

We have reviewed research by ourselves and others on seven commonly encountered assumptions relevant to the study of unconscious affect. We termed such assumptions *sins* because we wish to state, somewhat strongly, that the presumed evidence for (or in some cases, the logic of) such assumptions is weak or ambiguous. Our goal is to encourage a critical perspective toward explicit assumptions about the independence of affect from cognition and toward implicit assumptions that the evolution of emotional processes came to a halt very early in our phylogenic history. In concluding, it is worth revisiting our suggestions, albeit briefly.

- *Sin 1: There are unconscious emotions.* We agree with Freud (1915/ 1959), James (1890/1955), and LeDoux (1996) that although most emotional *processes* are unconscious, properly speaking, there are not unconscious emotions, per se. We cautioned that the work of cognitive psychologists studying memory implies that unconscious emotion (like implicit memory) may not be a coherent category.

- *Sin 2: Unconscious emotional stimuli are stronger than conscious ones.* Investigators sometimes assume that differences in conscious and unconscious priming mean that affect is most potent when unconscious. We argued that such results concern not strength but the spread of effects when the source of affective stimulation is not salient. Indeed, there is every reason to believe that conscious affect is more potent than unconscious affect.

- *Sin 3: Conscious feelings cause liking.* We offer an account of the affect-as-information approach that suggests that unconscious affective and neural connections, rather than conscious feelings and thoughts, may be responsible for implicit judgments and decisions. Affective feelings then provide information about implicit processes for making explicit judgments and decisions. If the valence component of feelings signifies value, the arousal component signifies importance. We suggested that conscious arousal may guide attention, whereas unconscious arousal creates memorability.

- *Sin 4: Preferences precede inferences.* We described research indicating that semantic priming may be more robust than affective priming, and that evaluative aspects of encoding typically follow, rather than precede, semantic encoding operations.

- *Sin 5: Expressive actions have fixed effects.* We presented research suggesting that contrary to widespread assumptions, the meaning and influence of affective expression and action depend on the mental context at the time.

- *Sin 6: Low-route stimulation causes human emotion.* An idea that has captured the imagination of science writers is that emotion is triggered via a fast "low route" (LeDoux, 1996) that does not involve cortical processing. We noted that some evidence indicates that this particular low route may not exist in humans. Further, limitations in its processing capacity make it unable to handle the effects of stimuli known to elicit human emotion.

- *Sin 7: Emotions occur too quickly to require appraisals.* We note that appraisal theories address the underlying structure of emotion variation, not the process of emotion elicitation, as critics often assume. Since they are evaluative reactions, emotions necessarily require appraisals, and these are typically fast, unconscious, and based on simple associations. We suggested that it is helpful to view the relation between appraisal theory and everyday emotion elicitation as similar to the relation between the rules of syntax and everyday speech.

ACKNOWLEDGMENTS

Support is acknowledged from National Institute of Mental Health grants to Gerald L. Clore (No. MH 50074) and Michael D. Robinson (No. MH 068241).

NOTES

1. Thanks to Piotr Winkielman for these words, which succinctly summarize our initial point. In addition, thanks to Piotr for years of friendly debate about the issues addressed in this volume.
2. The point of citing the excellent work by Lodge and associates is not to criticize it but to show that misinterpretations by us psychologists inevitably affect even the best work in other fields that draw on psychology.

REFERENCES

Bargh, J. A. (1997). The automaticity of everyday life. In R. S. Wyer (Ed.), *Advances in social cognition* (Vol. 10, pp. 1–61). Mahwah, NJ: Erlbaum.

Bornstein, R. F. (1989). Exposure and affect: Overview and meta-analysis of research, 1968–1987. *Psychological Bulletin, 106,* 265–289.

Bower, G. H. (1981). Mood and memory. *American Psychologist, 36,* 129–148.

Cacioppo, J. T., Priester, J. R., & Berntson, G. G. (1993). Rudimentary determinants of attitudes. II: Arm flexion and extension have differential effects on attitudes. *Journal of Personality and Social Psychology, 65,* 5–17.

Cahill, L., Haier, R. J., Fallon, J., Alkire, M. T., Tang, C., Keator, D., Wu, J., & Mcgaugh, J. L. (1996). Amygdala activity at encoding correlated with long-term, free recall of emotional information. *Proceedings of the National Academy of Sciences, 93,* 8016–8021.

Cahill, L., & McGaugh, J. L. (1998). Mechanisms of emotional arousal and lasting declarative memory. *Trends in Neuroscience, 21,* 294–299.

Centerbar, D. B. (2003). *Contextual meaning of isometric arm flexion and extension and implications for affective processing.* Unpublished doctoral dissertation, University of Virginia, Charlotterville.

Centerbar, D. B., & Clore, G. L. (2004). *Do approach–avoidance actions create attitudes?* Unpublished manuscript.

Christianson, S. A., & Loftus, E. F. (1991). Remembering emotional events: The fate of detail information. *Cognition and Emotion, 5,* 81–108.

Clore, G. L., & Colcombe, S. (2003). The parallel worlds of affective concepts and feelings. In J. Musch & K. C. Klauer (Eds.), *The psychology of evaluation: Affective processes in cognition and emotion* (pp. 335–369). Mahwah, NJ: Erlbaum.

Clore, G. L., & Ortony, A. (1991). What more is there to emotion concepts than prototypes? *Journal of Personality and Social Psychology, 60,* 48–50.

Clore, G. L., & Ortony, A. (2000). Cognition in emotion: Always, sometimes, or never? In R. D. Lane & L. Nadel (Eds.), *Cognitive neuroscience of emotion* (pp. 24–61). New York: Oxford University Press.

Clore, G. L., Wyer R. S., Dienes, B., Gasper, K., Gohm, C., & Isbell, L. (2001). Affective feelings as feedback: Some cognitive consequences. In L. L. Martin & G. L. Clore (Eds.), *Theories of mood and cognition: A user's handbook* (pp. 27–62). Mahwah, NJ: Erlbaum.

Conrad, C. (1974). Context effects in sentence comprehension: A study of the subjective lexicon. *Memory and Cognition, 2,* 130–138.

Darwin, C. (1965). *The expression of emotion in man and animals.* Chicago: University of Chicago Press. (Original work published 1872)

Dehaene, S., & Naccache, L. (2001). Towards a cognitive neuroscience of consciousness: Basic evidence and a workspace framework. *Cognition, 79,* 1–37.

Dehaene, S., Naccache, L., Cohen, L., Bihan, D. L., Mangin, J. F., Poline, J. B., & Riviere, D. (2001). Cerebral mechanisms of word masking and unconscious repetition priming. *Nature Neuroscience, 4,* 752–758.

De Houwer, J., & Randell, R. (2004). Robust affective priming in a conditional pronunciation task: Evidence for the semantic representation of evaluative information. *Cognition and Emotion, 18,* 251–264.

Dijksterhuis, A., Bargh, J. A., & Miedema, J. (2000). Of men and mackerels: Attention and automatic behavior. In H. Bless & J. P. Forgas (Eds.), *Subjective experience in social cognition and behavior* (pp. 36–51). Philadelphia: Psychology Press.

Dolan, R. (2000). Functional neuroimaging of the amygdala during emotional processing and learning. In J. P. Aggleton (Ed.), *The amygdala: A functional analysis* (pp. 631–654). New York: Oxford University Press.

Edelman, G. M. (1989). *The remembered present: A biological theory of consciousness.* New York: Basic Books.

Fazio, R. H., Sanbonmatsu, D. M., Powell, M. C., & Kardes, F. R. (1986). On the automatic activation of attitudes. *Journal of Personality and Social Psychology, 50,* 229–238.

Freud, S. (1959). Instincts and their vicissitudes. In E. Jones (Ed.), *Sigmund Freud: Collected papers* (Vol. 4). New York: Basic Books. (Original work published 1915)

Frijda, N., Ortony, A., Sonnemans, J., & Clore, G. (1992). The complexity of intensity: Issues concerning the structure of emotion intensity. In M. Clark (Ed.), *Emotion: Review of personality and social psychology* (Vol. 13, pp. 60–89). Newbury Park, CA: Sage.

Fukuda, M., Ono, T., & Nakamura, K. (1987). Functional relations among inferior-temporal cortex, amygdala, and lateral hypothalamus in monkey operant feeding behavior. *Journal of Neurophysiology, 57,* 1060–1077.

Glaser, J., & Banaji, M. R. (1999). When fair is foul and foul is fair: Reverse priming in automatic evaluation. *Journal of Personality and Social Psychology, 77,* 669–687.

Graf, P., & Schacter, D. L. (1985). Implicit and explicit memory for new associations in normal and amnesic subjects. *Journal of Experimental Psychology: Learning, Memory, and Cognition, 11,* 501–518.

Greenwald, A. G., McGhee, D. E., & Schwartz, J. L. K. (1998). Measuring individual differences in implicit cognition: The implicit association test. *Journal of Personality and Social Psychology, 74,* 1464–1480.

James, W. (1955). *Principles of psychology.* New York: Dover. (Original work published 1890)

Kudo, M., Glendenning, K., Frost, S., & Masterson, R. (1986). Origin of mammalian thalamocortical projections: I. Telencephalic projection of the medial geniculate body in the opossum (*Didelphis virginiana*). *Journal of Comparative Neurology, 245,* 176–197.

Laird, J. D. (1974). Self attribution of emotion: The effects of expressive behavior on the quality of emotional experience. *Journal of Personality and Social Psychology, 29,* 475–486.

LeDoux, J. (1996). *The emotional brain: The mysterious underpinnings of emotional life.* New York: Simon & Schuster.

LeDoux, J., Romanski, L., & Xagoraris, A. (1989). Indelibility of subcortical emotional memories. *Journal of Cognitive Neuroscience, 1,* 238–243.

Lodge, M., & Taber, C. S. (in press). Implicit affect for political candidates, parties, and issues: An experimental test of the hot cognition hypothesis. *Political Psychology.*

Lowery, B., Hardin, C., & Sinclair, S. (2001). Social influence effects on automatic racial prejudice. *Journal of Personality and Social Psychology, 81,* 842–855.

McRae, K., & Boisvert, S. (1998). Automatic semantic similarity priming. *Journal of Experimental Psychology: Learning, Memory and Cognition, 24,* 3, 558–572.

Murphy, S. T., & Zajonc, R. B. (1993). Affect, cognition, and awareness: Affective priming with optimal and suboptimal stimulus exposures. *Journal of Personality and Social Psychology, 64,* 723–739.

Nielson, K. (2003, November 17). Paper presented at the annual meeting of the Society for Neuroscience, Orlando, FL.

Pashler, H., Johnston, J., & Ruthruff, E. (2001). Attention and performance. *Annual Review of Psychology, 52,* 629–651.

Pavlov, I. P. (1960). *Conditioned reflexes* (G. V. Anrel, Trans.) New York: Dover. (Original work published 1927)

Pearson, H. (2002). Bloody teeth boost memory. *Nature: Science Update,* Nature News Service. Retrieved December 12, 2004, from www.nature.com/nsv.

Robinson, M. D. (2004). Personality as performance: Categorization tendencies and their correlates. *Current Directions in Psychological Science, 13,* 127–129.

Rolls, E. T. (1999). *The brain and emotion.* Oxford, UK: Oxford University Press.

Roser, M., & Gazzaniga, M. S. (2004). Automatic brains, interpretive minds. *Current Directions in Psychological Science, 13,* 56–59.

Russell, J. A. (2003). Core affect and the psychological construction of emotion. *Psychological Review, 110,* 145–172.

Scherer, K. R. (1984). On the nature and function of emotion: A component process approach. In K. R. Scherer & P. Ekman (Eds.), *Approaches to emotion* (pp. 293–317). Hillsdale, NJ: Erlbaum.

Schwarz, N., & Clore, G. L. (1983). Mood, misattribution, and judgments of well-being: Informative and directive functions of affective states. *Journal of Personality and Social Psychology, 45,* 513–523.

Simon, H. A. (1967). Motivational and emotional controls of cognition. *Psychological Review, 74,* 29–39.

Sloman, S. A. (1996). The empirical case for two systems of reasoning. *Psychological Bulletin, 119,* 3–22.

Squire, L. R., & Zola-Morgan, S. (1991). The medial temporal lobe memory system. *Science, 253,* 1380–1386.

Storbeck, J., Robinson, M. D., & McCourt, M. (in press). Semantic processing precedes affect retrieval: The neurological case for cognitive primacy in visual processing. *Review of General Psychology.*

Storbeck, J., & Robinson, M. D. (2004b). Preferences and inferences in encoding visual objects: A systematic comparison of semantic and affective priming. *Personality and Social Psychology Bulletin, 30,* 81–93.

Strack, F., Martin, L. L., & Stepper, S. (1988). Inhibiting and facilitating conditions of the human smile: A nonobtrusive test of the facial feedback hypothesis. *Journal of Personality and Social Psychology, 54,* 768–777.

Tamir, M., Robinson, M. D., Clore, G. L., Martin, L. L., & Whitaker, D. (2004). Are we puppets on a string?: The contextual meaning of unconscious expressive cues. *Personality and Social Psychology Bulletin, 30,* 237–249.

Wegner, D. M. (2002). *The illusion of conscious will.* Cambridge, MA: MIT Press.

Wells, G., & Petty, R. (1980). The effects of overt head movements on persuasion: Compatibility and incompatibility of responses. *Basic and Applied Social Psychology, 1,* 219–230.

Whalen, P. J. (1998). Fear, vigilance, and ambiguity: Initial neuroimaging studies of the human amygdala. *Current Directions in Psychological Science, 7,* 177–188.

Willingham, D. B., & Preuss, L. (1995). The death of implicit memory. *Psyche, 2*(15). Retrieved October 1995 from psyche.cs.monash.edu.au/v2/psyche-2-15-willingham.html.

Wilson, T. D. (2002). *Strangers to ourselves: Discovering the adaptive unconscious.* Cambridge MA: Belknap/Harvard Press.

Wundt, W. (1897). *Outlines of psychology.* Leipzig, Germany: Englemann.

Zajonc, R. (1980). Feeling and thinking: Preferences need no inferences. *American Psychologist, 35,* 151–175.

Zajonc, R. (2000). Feeling and thinking: Closing the debate over the independence of affect. In J. P. Forgas (Ed.), *Studies in emotion and social interaction: Vol. 2. Feeling and thinking: The role of affect in social cognition* (pp. 31–58). New York: Cambridge University Press.

Index